Body *into* Balance

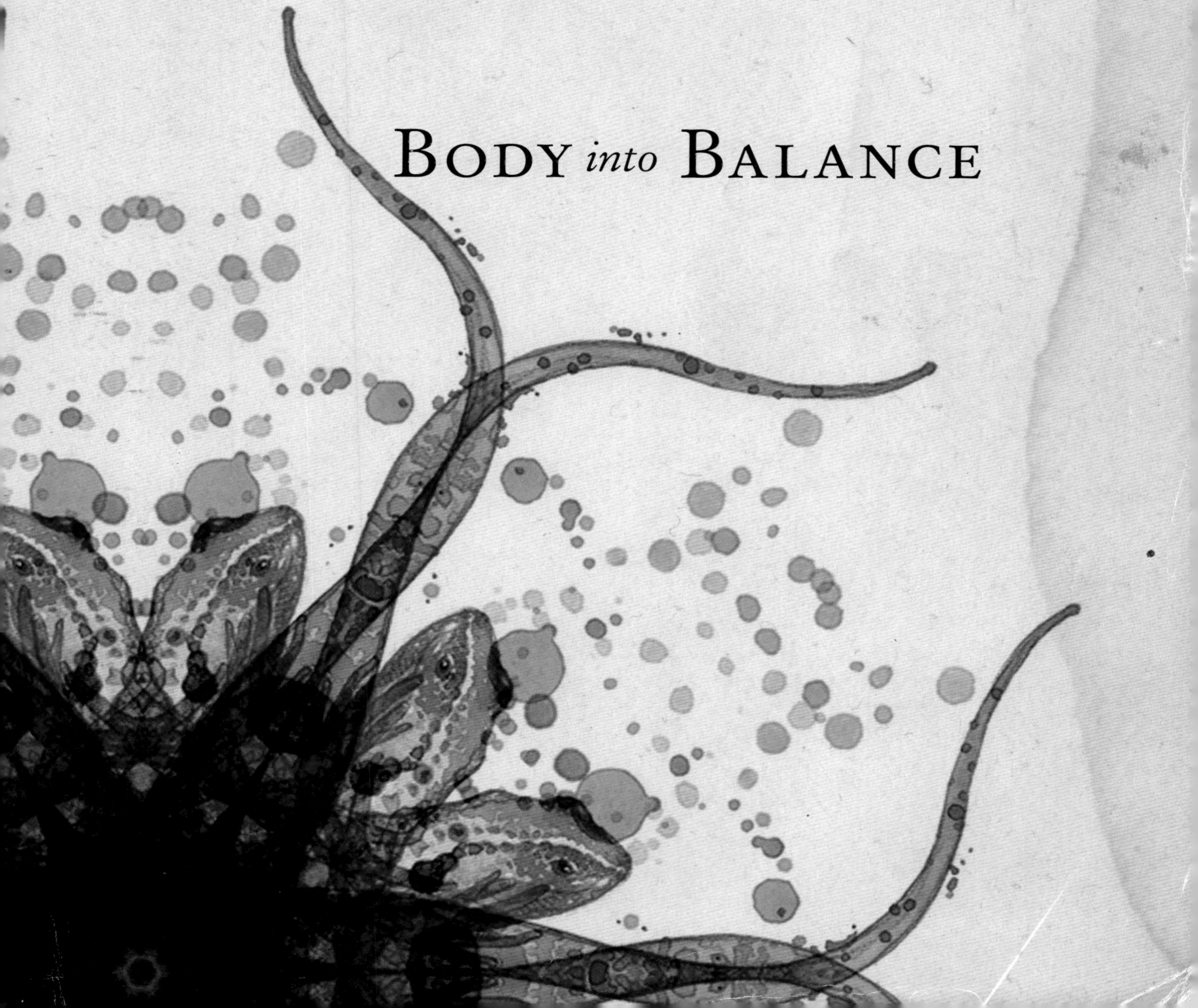

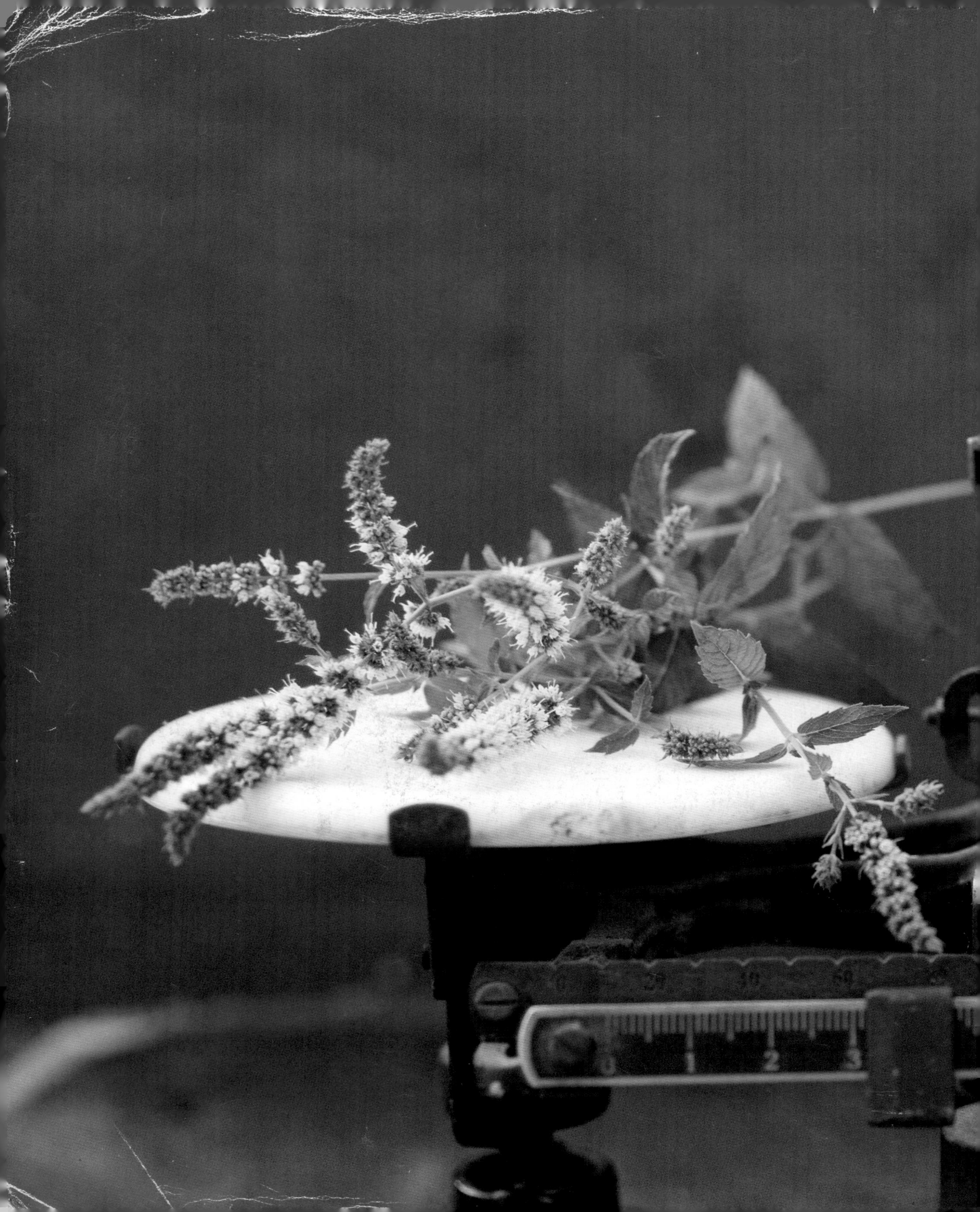

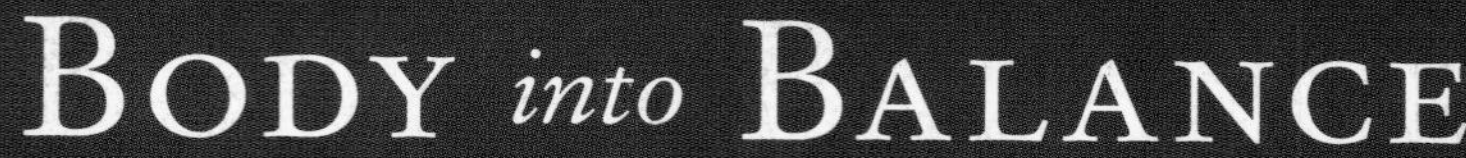

BODY *into* BALANCE

AN HERBAL GUIDE *to* HOLISTIC SELF-CARE

Maria Noël Groves

The mission of Storey Publishing is to serve our customers by publishing practical information that encourages personal independence in harmony with the environment.

EDITED BY Deborah Balmuth and Nancy Ringer
ART DIRECTION AND BOOK DESIGN BY Michaela Jebb
INDEXED BY Christine R. Lindemer, Boston Road Communications

COVER AND INTERIOR ILLUSTRATIONS BY © Narda Lebo
COVER PHOTOGRAPHY BY © Kimberly Sanders Peck (back & author) and Mars Vilaubi (spine)
INTERIOR PHOTOGRAPHY BY © Kimberly Sanders Peck except as noted below

© 4kodiak/iStockphoto.com, 206; © abadonian/iStockphoto.com, 78; © Adam Smigielski/iStockphoto.com, 173 (bottom); © aleks1949/iStockphoto.com, 152; © alexmak72427/iStockphoto.com, 51; Carolyn Eckert, 274; © Dave Alan/iStockphoto.com, 256; © Diana Taliun/iStockphoto.com, 147; © Difydave/iStockphoto.com, 129; © dolnikow/iStockphoto.com, 62; © duckycards/iStockphoto.com, 131; © eurobanks/iStockphoto.com, 299; © Image Source/Alamy, 229; © John Seller/iStockphoto.com, 224; © lenta/iStockphoto.com, 250; © Mantonature/iStockphoto.com, 178; © marilyna/iStockphoto.com, 245; Mars Vilaubi, 117, 134, 161, 225, 243, 288, 313; Michaela Jebb, 25; © Natalia Bulatova/iStockphoto.com, 289; © nbehmans/iStockphoto.com, 73; © Oktay Ortakcioglu/iStockphoto.com, 205; © Pleio/iStockphoto.com, 173 (top); © P_Wei/iStockphoto.com, 212; © princessdlaf/iStockphoto.com, 283; © SchmitzOlaf/iStockphoto.com, 222; © sd619/iStockphoto.com, old index card (throughout); © 2015 Steven Foster, 99, 126, 191, 253; © stocksnapper/iStockphoto.com, 81; © subjug/iStockphoto.com, 220; © tomograf/iStockphoto.com, old paper sheets (throughout); © Vladimir Floyd/iStockphoto.com, 263; © Xifotos/iStockphoto.com, 317

This publication is intended to provide educational information for the reader on the covered subject. It is not intended to take the place of personalized medical counseling, diagnosis, and treatment from a trained health professional.

The information in this book is true and complete to the best of our knowledge. All recommendations are made without guarantee on the part of the author or Storey Publishing. The author and publisher disclaim any liability in connection with the use of this information.

Storey books are available for special premium and promotional uses and for customized editions. For further information, please call 1-800-793-9396.

Storey Publishing
210 MASS MoCA Way
North Adams, MA 01247
www.storey.com

Printed in the United States by Versa Press
10 9 8 7 6 5 4 3 2 1

Library of Congress Cataloging-in-Publication Data on file

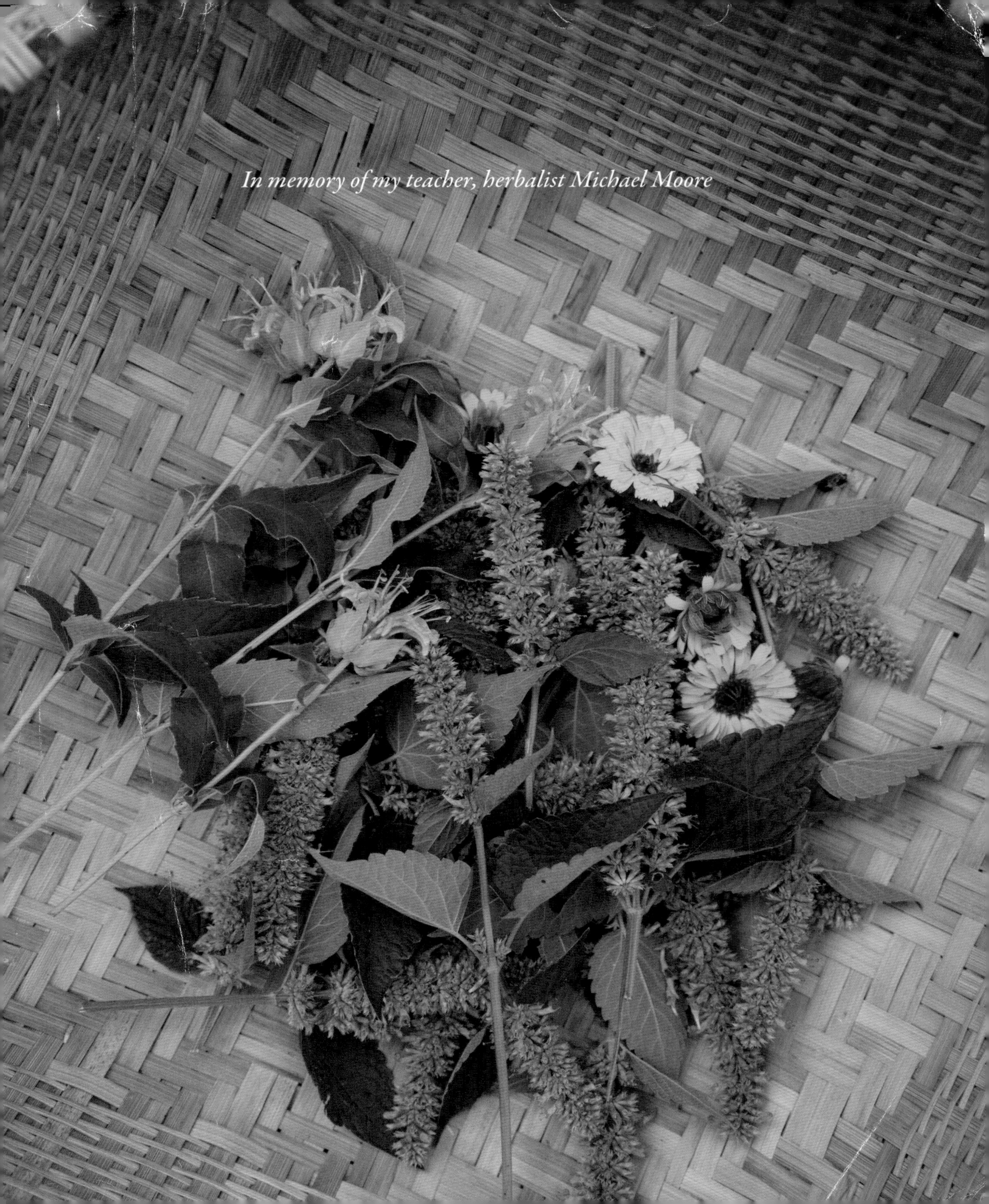

In memory of my teacher, herbalist Michael Moore

Acknowledgments

No herbalist comes into the world knowing everything there is to know about plant medicine. We learn from one another. We learn from experience. We learn from the plants. I'm incredibly grateful to the many people who influenced my study and helped bring this book together.

Herbalist Michael Moore, with whom I studied at the Southwest School of Botanical Medicine, remains my most influential teacher. He opened my eyes to the body systems and made me realize how utterly fascinating the nexus of herbal medicine and the human body can be. Although I have learned remedy-making techniques from many other herbalists, Michael's unique techniques remain my favorite and can be found in this book. Though we lost this herbal icon in 2009, his profound contributions to the herbal community live on through his books, course, wife, and students.

To round out my education, I'm grateful to many other herbal teachers: Rosemary Gladstar is not only a wonderful herbalist but also probably the most inspiring human being I have ever met. Nancy and Michael Phillips introduced me to the way of living herbs. Christine Tolf taught me to look beyond the more chemical aspect of herbs and work with flower essences. Other people who greatly influenced my approach to herbs — through reading their work and interviewing them for articles — include Mary Bove, Rosalee de la Foret, James Duke, Henriette Kress, Greg Marley, Rob McCaleb, Jim McDonald, Joe Pizzorno, Aviva Romm, Kiva Rose, Julie Bruton-Seal, Sharol Tilgner, and Maia Toll. My work at *Natural Health Magazine, Herb Quarterly*, and *Remedies Magazine*, along with teaching classes, seeing clients, and working the supplement aisles of various natural food stores, has provided constant exposure to other people's stories — what has worked for them and what has not. I'm always listening and taking notes, and I thank all those people who have taken the time to share their experiences with me.

In my life, I'm grateful for the loving support of my parents, my grandparents, and my husband. I must admit that Shannon was a little anxious to have his wife quit her "day job" after our honeymoon to be a full-time herbalist, but we made it happen! I also thank everyone who kept asking when I would write a book, especially Susanna Hargreaves, who finally made it "click" and helped ignite my vision and drive for these pages. Thank you, too, to friends and colleagues Mimi Alberu (the animal herbalist), Dr. Cora Rivard (the naturopath), and Tiffany Coroka (my first-pass editor) for their invaluable input on my manuscript.

Lastly, my deepest gratitude to the team at Storey, without whom this book wouldn't be possible: Deborah Balmuth, Nancy Ringer, Michaela Jebb, Kimberly Peck, and Sarah Armour. Thank you for believing in me and bringing the book into being.

Contents

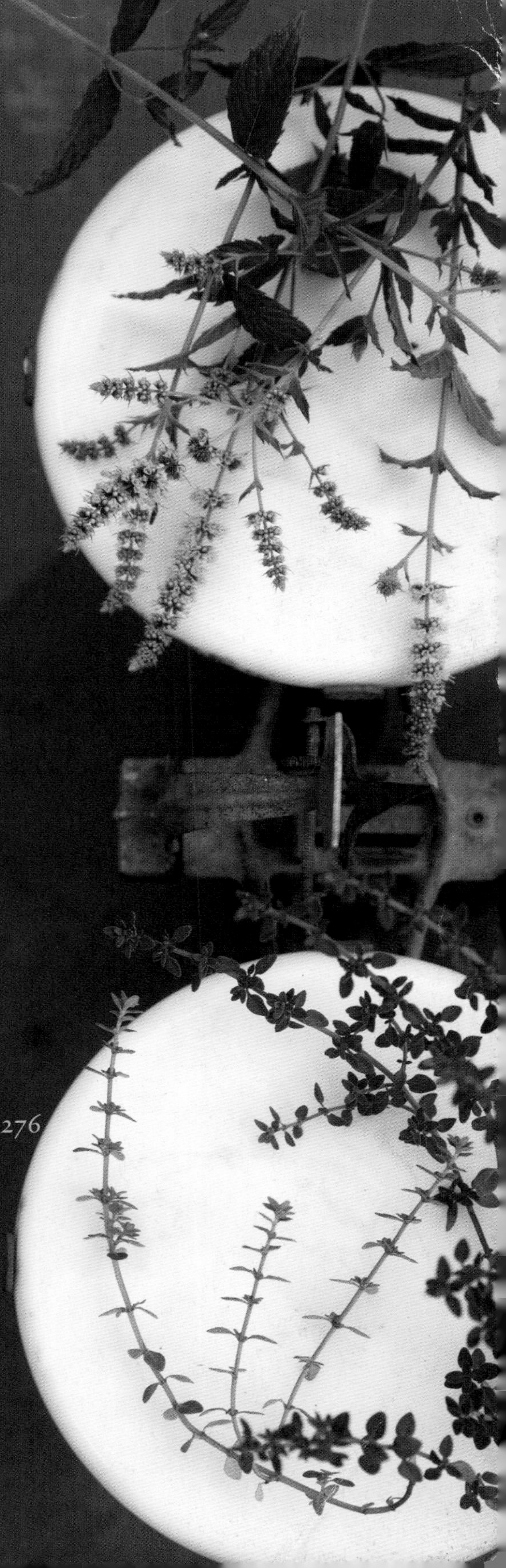

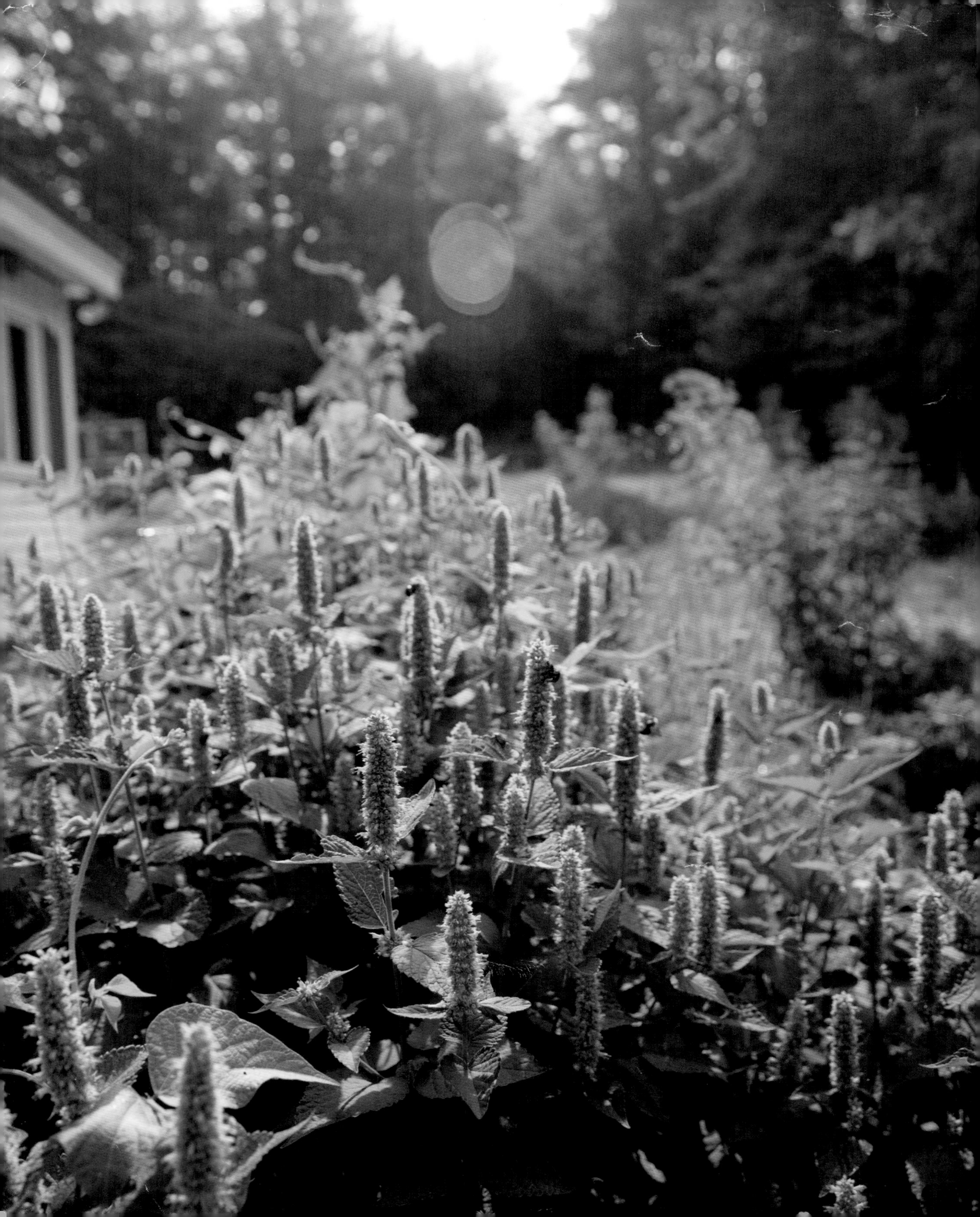

Introduction: Achieving a Natural Balance

Good health grows in nature. It's really that simple.

We thrive in nature. We feel better, we feel healthier, when we rely on real food, spend plenty of time outdoors, bring the elements of nature into our daily life, and use herbs as our primary form of medicine. Many of the common ailments and diseases we see in modern society stem from the fact that we have shifted away from our primal connection to nature. Health and disease in the body interact in fascinating interconnected patterns, and when we make use of our connection to nature — employing herbs and natural therapies — we can shift those patterns to bring the body into greater balance and vitality. Plants heal. Nature heals.

Whether you have a multitude of serious diseases or you're relatively healthy, with just a couple of minor complaints, your symptoms are not something to overcome. Instead, they're your body's way of telling you that something is out of balance. These symptoms are your taskmasters — that is, the alarm system for your body and clues about the underlying imbalance. This book will teach you how to listen to your body. It may take some detective work and a multifaceted healing approach, but it's worth it. The earlier you recognize your body's distress signals, the easier it will be to heal disease naturally. But no matter where you are in your health, you *can* make improvements with herbs and holistic therapies.

Americans are gradually realizing that our current allopathic medical system — its approach *and* its medicines — often makes us sicker (not to mention broke) in the long run. In this profit-driven system, we spend more on health care than any other nation, yet we come in at a dismal number 38 worldwide for our actual health and well-being. Doctors rely heavily on an arsenal of pharmaceuticals, but side effects from these strong drugs kill more than 100,000 Americans annually. Even if you survive the treatment, you'll often experience a slew of serious side effects. With this myopic approach to treating symptoms, the body continues to scream for help, and new issues (backup alarms) sound off. Side effects build. You might be taking a handful of pills each day, but you still don't feel *well.*

Enter herbal and natural medicine.

Natural therapies are generally less expensive, significantly safer, better suited to self-care, and more holistic than allopathic medicine, and they have a host of side *benefits*. In fact, just one herb can contain hundreds of compounds that work together in synergy to address a range of health conditions. So that hawthorn you're taking for blood pressure may ultimately also improve your mental clarity, energy levels, and mood.

What's really fascinating is how they do this. Herbs rarely force the body in a particular direction or supply a single isolated compound with a specific effect on the body. Instead, herbs encourage your body to heal and balance itself. For example, the reproductive herb vitex doesn't *contain* progesterone; instead, it encourages your brain and ovaries to produce healthier levels of this hormone over time. Most immune-system herbs don't act directly as antibiotics or antivirals; they fortify your body's natural immune response so that white blood cells and disease-fighting mechanisms work better. What's more, many herbs have a *modulating* effect on the body, not a one-way action. For example, astragalus and medicinal mushrooms (fungi are honorary "herbs" in this book) balance over- *and* underactive immune systems. Modest doses of eleuthero raise low blood pressure or reduce high blood pressure, depending on what's needed. Holy basil and other adaptogenic herbs amp up or turn down the production of stress hormones, like cortisol, as needed. It's really quite amazing.

Don't think of herbs as mere substitutes for drugs. Herbs act like training wheels to help your body relearn patterns of health, breaking away from patterns of disease and improving day-to-day functioning. For this reason, this book is *not* an A-to-Z list of helpful herbs. I want you to *understand* your body, what it needs to be healthy, and common themes of disease. You'll learn how to listen to your body and understand what it's telling you. You'll grasp *how* the herbs work so that you can put together the best blend of herbs and natural therapies to nudge *your* body back into balance, no matter what your starting point.

How *to* Use This Book

In this book, we'll look at the root causes of disease, patterns of imbalance, and how to sleuth out clues to find the most appropriate herbs and therapies for you.

First, it's important to understand your body's basic needs. When those needs aren't met, it's almost impossible for your body to stay in balance. When they *are* met, many diseases and symptoms simply disappear. A whole-foods diet and good nutrition, adequate sleep, stress management, and regular exercise and movement — how well you attend to the pillars of health makes an enormous impact on how healthy or sick you will be. If you've got a long way to go, never fear. Take baby steps, make slow changes, and address the specific areas that seem to have the most impact for you. Achieving vitality and a healthy lifestyle is a lifelong journey.

Herbs make the journey easier. Plant medicine helps your body shift into healthier patterns. But herbal medicine is more than just taking plant remedies. Any herbal or holistic practitioner will tell you: herbs work *best* when combined with a healthy diet and lifestyle. As we delve into the individual body systems, you'll see Protocol Points sections that clarify approaches for addressing common health concerns. These sections will recap the specific dietary guidelines, lifestyle practices, and herbs that tend to work best for the health condition in question.

The bulk of this book will explore specific body systems and patterns of health and disease. The first body systems it discusses make the biggest impact for the most people: nervous-endocrine (stress, sleep, mood), digestion, and detoxification. These body systems affect *everything* else, and when you bring them into balance, it becomes easier to overcome seemingly disparate health issues.

In herbal medicine, we identify underlying disease patterns and select herbs and other natural therapies that address those patterns. For example, many people suffer from poor digestion (especially poor *fat* digestion), combined with constipation, high cholesterol, cardiovascular inflammation, chronic pain, diabetes, and sometimes also skin issues. These folks tend to run hot, eat poorly, and not get enough exercise. Cooling, digestion-enhancing, detoxifying, anti-inflammatory herbs like artichoke, turmeric, dandelion, and schizandra work wonders as the base of a formula for turning the tide. In another pattern (often relating to food sensitivities), migraines, allergies, digestive upset, rashes, sinusitis, and asthma often run together, and just one thorough treatment approach may eliminate *all* of them.

Even if you have serious health issues, and even if you are taking pharmaceutical drugs, you *can* still use the herbal approaches outlined in this book to improve your situation. These methods are not an either/or option, and herbs often work fantastically alongside conventional medicine, helping you get better results with fewer side effects. If you're taking pharmaceuticals, you *will* want to proceed cautiously when choosing herbs and work closely with your health practitioner; see page 15 for more discussion of herb-drug safety.

You'll get an herbal vocab lesson as you peruse this book, getting to know the specific primary herbal actions, what they mean, how to use them, and which herbs have them. You'll quickly come to understand what nutritives and adaptogens are and why they make a great base for almost any formula, why demulcent and astringent herbs heal damaged tissue, and precisely how antioxidants fend off age-related diseases. Though herbs have many, many synergistic effects on the body, these primary actions are worth reading about in depth, and you'll find them referred to throughout the book because they have tremendous benefit for many different body systems.

The Basic Principles *of* Herbal Medicine

Although it's entirely possible to use herbs in an allopathic way ("plug X herb in for Y disease"), herbal medicine works much better when incorporated into a more thorough, holistic approach. The following basic principles set herbal and natural medicine apart from conventional medicine in a variety of ways.

- Nature heals, in many different ways.
- Start with the safest, most gentle (yet sufficiently effective) approach.
- Try an integrative approach of herbs, diet, and lifestyle to get the best results.
- Address the root cause and patterns of disease.
- Treat the whole person, not just the disease or symptoms.
- Help your body to heal itself.
- Educate and empower yourself.
- Know your limits and when to seek guidance.
- Cultivate a good health-care team (see page 12).

A KEY TO THE HERB PROFILES

Each of the herb profiles in this book includes a brief notation on the herb's availability indicating whether the plant can be grown in the garden, harvested from the wild, or purchased from an herb seller, and how easy (or difficult) it is to do each of those things. The "codes" are as follows:

G garden herb

W wild herb

C common in commerce

\+ easy to grow/find

– more difficult to grow/find

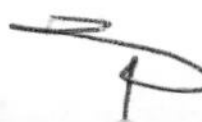

WHO'S ON YOUR HEALTH-CARE TEAM?

HERBAL MEDICINE EMPOWERS you to take a more active role in your well-being, but you'll also want a good health-care team to turn to for guidance, especially when you reach your limits in self-care and knowledge. Sometimes it's hard to step back and see the big picture, or a condition may warrant therapies that you can't provide for yourself. Here are some types of practitioners to consider for your team. At the minimum, I'd recommend a doctor or naturopath. Remember that *you* hire them. If you don't like a particular professional or aren't getting desired results, find a different practitioner. Ask around for recommendations, and schedule a short meet and greet. It's also helpful to understand what different practitioners can and can't do.

Your Doctor

This category includes doctors of medicine (MDs) and doctors of osteopathy (DOs). We may as well also include here nurse practitioners (NPs) and physician's assistants (PAs); though NPs and PAs aren't technically "doctors," they perform similar functions and work within the standard medical system. Unfortunately, the doctor tends to become "the enemy" when we begin to explore alternative medicine. The truth is, although our conventional medical *system* is broken, many great doctors do exist, and the number is growing. Modern medicine can be a powerful ally and may sometimes be the best approach for treating disease. Find a doctor who is willing to listen to you, answer your questions, and respect your decisions. It's important that you trust your doctor so that you can take his or her advice seriously. Doctors can perform useful diagnostic tests, prescribe drugs, and perform or refer you to surgery when needed. Most doctors don't have the training to recommend herbs and natural medicines, though some do, and many more are coming to respect their patients' decisions to use natural remedies. In an insurance-driven system, they may also be your most affordable practitioners.

Your Naturopathic Doctor

Like MDs and DOs, licensed naturopathic doctors (NDs) receive intensive medical training and can run diagnostic tests, prescribe a wide variety of drugs, and perform minor surgeries. However, NDs tend to favor holistic approaches like diet, herbs, dietary supplements, and homeopathics over conventional medical treatments. Depending on your state and insurance carrier, your ND may be covered by your health insurance and be able to act as your primary care practitioner. While NDs can provide many of the same services as conventional medical practitioners and generally spend more time with you than MDs, they may not be covered by insurance, so they can be expensive. Note that not every state licenses naturopathic doctors, and in states that don't license, someone could call him- or herself a "naturopath" with only a correspondence-course education. Find a *licensed* naturopathic doctor near you via the American Association of Naturopathic Physicians (www.naturopathic.org).

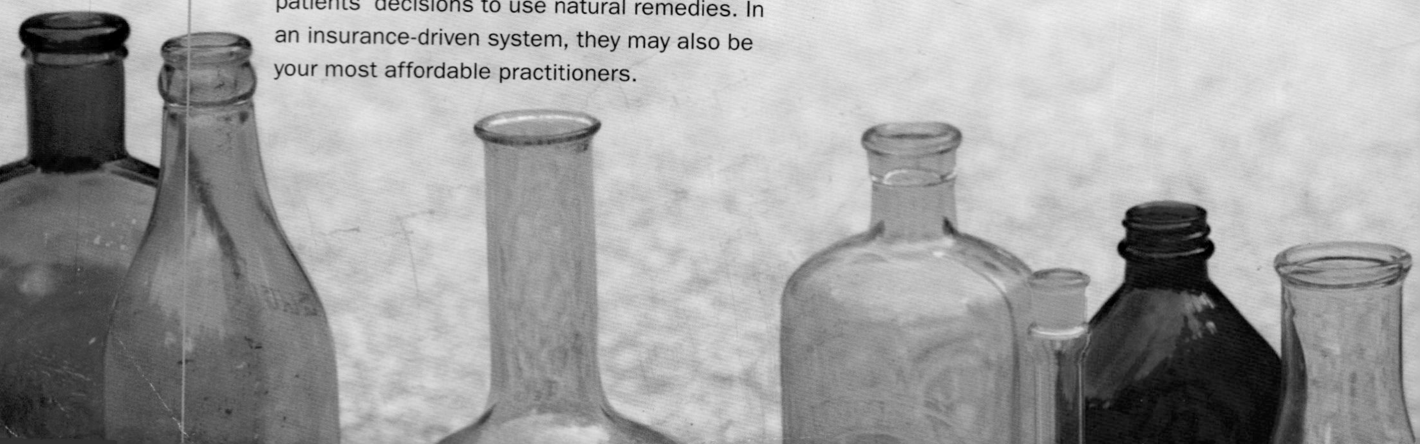

Your Herbalist

Most herbalists are not trained as doctors and can't legally diagnose or prescribe; however, they will generally look at your current diagnosis and health patterns and recommend a protocol specific for you. Typically they can't run diagnostic tests. They usually have more herbal training and a more intimate understanding of the plants compared to other types of practitioners, and they often incorporate diet and lifestyle recommendations into your treatment plan. Herbalism is an unlicensed profession in the United States, and insurance rarely covers your visits, but herbalists' services (and their recommended remedies) often cost less out of pocket than those of doctors and NDs. They may offer economical options like free clinics, sliding-scale rates, or barter payment systems. Herbalists registered with the American Herbalists Guild — identified with "RH (AHG)" after their names — must have a minimum of 400 education hours, 400 clinical hours, and peer review, and you can find one near you via the AHG website (www.americanherbalistsguild.com). However, many other great herbalists are not registered AHG professional members.

Your Nutritionist/Dietitian

These practitioners can give you more detailed advice from a dietary perspective. Training varies widely. Compared to other types of nutritionists, registered dietitians (RDs) and registered dietitian nutritionists (RDNs) generally have more education and are more likely to enjoy mainstream medical status — including insurance coverage; however, their approach may be more conventional.

Your Pharmacist

Though mainly in the business of dispensing drugs per your doctor, most pharmacists can provide extra information about the drugs, their safety, and herb-drug interactions upon request. Some are trained in herb-drug interactions, and most have good databases at their disposal. They may be able to provide more detailed information about interactions than your doctor, but they can't tell you what to take or not take, and you should always keep your doctor in the loop.

And Then Some!

Depending on your specific health needs and philosophies, you may want a chiropractor, massage therapist, physical therapist, acupuncturist, energy worker, yoga instructor, fitness trainer, or other specialist on your team.

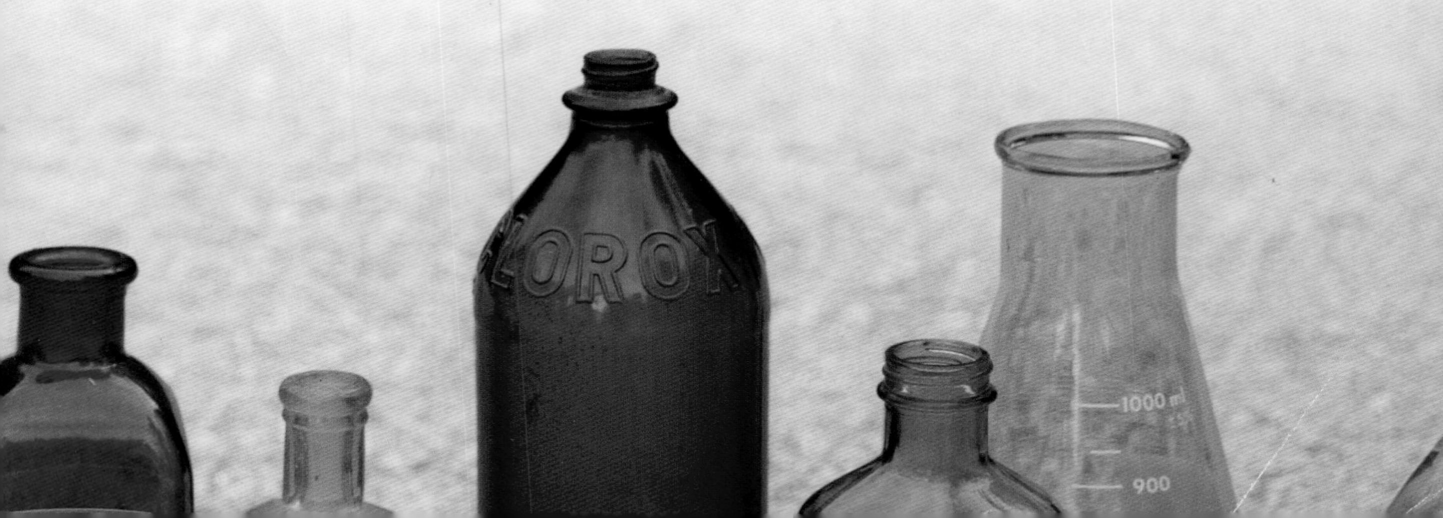

An Ounce *of* Prevention: Herb Safety

As much as mainstream media would like you to believe otherwise, herbal medicine is one of the safest forms of medicine in existence. Evidence suggests that humans have relied on plant medicine since at least the Stone Age, and formal written herbal healing practices date back several millennia. Herbs remain the number one form of medicine worldwide. They're affordable, accessible, effective, and empowering.

So why should you be concerned about herb safety at all? Because different herbs suit different people better, and you want to find the best herb for you and your situation. Herbs *can* have side effects, though fortunately they're usually mild and go away if you stop taking the herb. Many herbs just aren't a good fit for certain individuals. Cinnamon works well to staunch diarrhea, but if you already tend toward constipation, it could make that worse. Hot and spicy ginger gets stagnant digestion going, but it might aggravate acid reflux in certain people. If you're researching your herbs and listening to your body, you'll figure out pretty quickly what does and doesn't work for you.

That said, not *every* herb or natural remedy is safe. Some have high rates of toxicity and can even be deadly, such as foxglove, datura, aconite, and the destroying angel (amanita) mushroom. Though they can have medicinal actions when used properly at low doses, they're not appropriate for self-treatment and are not generally available for purchase. When you're harvesting herbs from the wild, you will want to be aware of these deadly plants and be sure to distinguish them from safer plants, lest your cup of mullein tea turn out to be a deadly dose of foxglove.

Potency vs. Safety

Everything exists along a safety continuum. When possible, start with the gentlest option. As you move across the continuum, the medicine becomes more potent, but the risk of negative side effects increases as well. Keep in mind that some situations warrant a more heavy-hitting approach right from the start. For example, a kidney infection requires immediate medical attention and antibiotics. Pussyfooting around with nettle tea delays appropriate treatment and increases the risk of kidney failure.

Part of taking a holistic approach to medicine is knowing which approach will be the most effective for the situation at hand and when to turn to a trained professional for stronger medicines with a higher likelihood of side effects.

The Four Safety Rules

Most of the sources you can go to for health and herb information — including this book — offer general information rather than specific, personalized advice for *you*. You'll need to do some digging to pick out the best options for self-treatment or see a practitioner whose approach will take into account your particular health issues and constitution, any potential herb-drug interactions that could arise during your treatment, and so on. Before you begin taking high doses of an herb (or anything, really) on a regular basis, I recommend the following.

1. Do Your Research

Information about herbs is constantly evolving and varies across cultures, time, and the herbalist you're learning from. Before you begin taking an herb, research it in at least three good sources, whether online or in print. Look for sources that come from the perspective of herbalists as well as those that are research driven — folk use *and* science. Herbal practitioners generally offer a better understanding of the nuances of herbs and the ways that they can be used. Researchers (who may not actually use herbs themselves) are more likely to list every potential side effect and drug interaction under the sun while discrediting folk uses that haven't been researched. (Do we *need* a double-blind, placebo-controlled study to prove prunes are laxative?) Both perspectives are useful.

Science can help us better understand herbs; however, research on the use of herbs is very limited in scope. Scientists are notorious for using inadequate doses and treatment time frames, active placebos, or uncommon extracts of the plants and for having a vested interest in antiherb outcomes. Well-designed studies also rarely test the crude, whole-plant medicine that most of us use, partly because such studies are harder to fund — there's no profit in finding out whether a whole plant that anyone can grow themselves is medicinally useful.

Relying on a mix of quality sources for your research gives you a broader understanding of a plant's actions and potential pitfalls. See appendix II for a list of some of my favorite resources to get you started.

2. Listen to Your Body

While you *should* do your research, also listen to your body to see if the herbs agree with you. A tea that makes some people feel absolutely vibrant may not resonate with others or may even subject them to a mild side effect like stomach upset. If an herb's side effect is mild, you may want to try taking it a couple of times (perhaps with a meal?) to see if the symptoms pass or if perhaps they were unrelated to the herb. No matter how much science or folk use is out there for a particular plant, ultimately only *your body* can tell you whether or not the herb is working for you.

3. Confirm the Plant's Identity

If you're harvesting your herbs from the wild or garden to make medicine, be sure you've correctly identified the plant. Don't take *anything* for granted. Even if you grew the plant from seed or someone identified it for you, mistakes happen. Keep some comprehensive plant identification guides on hand. Field guides focused specifically on edible or medicinal plants aren't sufficient; their exclusion of plants not deemed edible or medicinal makes it difficult to guarantee the identity of the plant in front of you. The most effective identification guides are organized with botanical keys such as flower color and shape as well as leaf structure and include a range of plants.

Plants are best identified while they're in flower, and secondarily when in fruit or seed, so you may need to watch a plant for a full cycle before going back to harvest the following year.

It's important to develop good identification skills before you start harvesting plants from the wild. Though most plant misidentifications are benign (e.g., dead nettles for stinging nettle), some plants are mildly toxic and others are downright deadly (e.g., foxglove instead of mullein). Don't get overwhelmed, though — you don't need to know the identity of every plant in the universe, but you should know the one you're harvesting, as well as the deadly plants common to your area. And watch out for hitchhikers — errant leaves, stray bugs — in your harvesting basket.

4. Ensure Herb-Drug Safety

If you use pharmaceutical medications, be aware of the potential for herb-drug interactions. While we have used herbs for millennia, and pharmaceuticals for about a century, we have been combining the two for only a few decades, and the potential for combinations are endless. It's difficult to be 100 percent sure that an herb and a drug won't interact, but the truth is that actual cases of herb-drug interactions are relatively few and far between.

Most of the drug interactions we know about are theoretical, but I still err on the side of caution. When there's the potential for a negative interaction, you can usually find an alternative herb with a lesser chance of interaction.

The most common herb-drug interactions include the following:

- St. John's wort interacts with about half the pharmaceuticals on the market, usually by clearing them from the body too quickly.
- A long list of herbs, foods, and dietary supplements can interact with the blood-thinning drug warfarin (brand name Coumadin) and aggravate bleeding.

- Sedative herbs (valerian, hops, kava, et cetera) may interact with most sedative, psychiatric, and pain medications.
- Combining herbs and drugs with similar effects may cause them to have a synergistically greater action and increase the risk of side effects. You should be cautious, for example, when combining diuretic herbs (dandelion, parsley) with diuretic medications, seaweed with thyroid medications, caffeine with stimulant-based asthma medications, cinnamon with insulin, or sedative herbs with sedative medications.
- Combining herbs and drugs with opposing effects — for example, vitex with birth-control pills — may make each less effective.

Be cautious when using herbs that affect digestion or detoxification, especially if the drugs you are taking are metabolized by that particular pathway. For example, fiber supplements and mucilaginous herbs may slow drug absorption if taken in the same gulp, and liver or kidney detox herbs may clear drugs from the system too quickly. Diet, lifestyle, and dilute remedies like homeopathics and flower essences are the least apt to interact with medications.

You aren't expected to know every possible side effect. Talk with your doctor and ask your pharmacist before adding a new herb to your regimen. Pharmacists are now equipped with extensive databases to look for herb-drug interactions. You may also want to seek the assistance of a qualified herbalist or naturopath who can recommend herbs with the least likelihood for interaction. My go-to reference guide is *Mosby's Nursing Drug Reference,* which is updated regularly and includes detailed information about each herb-drug interaction as well as drug side effects and how each drug is cleared from the body. The *Botanical Safety Handbook* offers more measured, realistic guidance, whereas the online database WebMD tends to list every possible interaction, even if it's not likely.

Don't reduce or stop taking your pharmaceutical drugs without talking with your doctor. If you find that your medical team is unwilling to work with your holistic interests or that they don't seem to listen to and respect you, find a new doctor and pharmacy.

The good news is that serious safety issues rarely occur when people take herbs. However, the more informed and proactive you are, the healthier you'll be and the more you'll feel confident and comfortable with the herbs you choose.

COMMON VS. LATIN NAMES

WE OFTEN REFER TO HERBS by their common names because they are easy to remember. But sometimes multiple plants have the same common name — for example, the names "brahmi," "betony," "hemlock," and even "oregano" and "rose" can each refer to different plants, some with very different uses. Also, a single plant often has multiple common names, especially if it's used in different countries. In contrast, in the scientific nomenclature, each plant is assigned a unique Latin name.

Though the nomenclature may evolve over time, you can generally assume that each plant has just one botanical Latin name and shares it with no other plant. (Botanists sometimes update and change Latin names, most recently as a result of genetic research. While this renaming confuses things for the humble herbalist and herb student, it's important to note that whether or not you're using an outdated Latin name, it still refers to the *one* plant. Wikipedia comes in handy for providing both the up-to-date and the old name to clear up any

THE SAFETY CONTINUUM

	Safe and gentle	Usually safe and gentle	Stronger	Even stronger	Highly potent and potentially dangerous
Treatment Modalities	Diet, lifestyle, energy work, massage, etc.	Functional food and focused diets, rigorous exercise, herbal and naturopathic medicine	Conventional medicine	Pharmaceuticals with a low risk of side effects, most over-the-counter drugs	Pharmaceuticals, surgery
Remedies	Dilute remedies (e.g., homeopathics, flower essences, hydrosols)	Foodlike remedies (tea, broth, herbs as food, herb-infused honey), topical remedies	Kitchen medicine (e.g., tinctures, vinegar extracts, crude capsules), low/modest-dose dietary supplements	Lab-made remedies (e.g., standardized extracts, carbon dioxide extracts, high-dose dietary supplements, essential oils for topical use)	Essential oils for internal use, potentially toxic herbs
Specific Herbs	Herbs that are almost always safe for everyone, especially nutritives and tonics (e.g., nettle, rose hips, marshmallow)	Herbs that generally are safe but may not be appropriate for everyone (e.g., chamomile, holy basil, ginger)	Herbs with specific actions, like stimulating adaptogens or hypoglycemic herbs (e.g., rhodiola, licorice, gymnema)	Herbs likely to have serious side effects if used inappropriately or in high doses (e.g., comfrey, laxative herbs)	Herbs that are potentially toxic in standard doses (e.g., pulsatilla, thuja)

As your options become more potent, your risks also tend to increase.

mysteries.) The Latin names provided in the herb profiles and in appendix I (page 322) will help ensure that you know exactly which plant the text is referring to.

Most Latin names have two parts: the genus (capitalized) followed by the species (lowercase). The genus refers to a group of closely related plants, and the species describes exactly which plant in the genus we're talking about. For example, roses are in the genus *Rosa*. The Latin name for dog rose is *Rosa canina*, whereas the Latin name for apothecary rose is *Rosa gallica*.

If you really want to tend to your inner herb geek, look up the meanings of the different Latin names. They may refer to where the plant grows, who identified it first, what it looks like, or even its medicinal uses. For example, *angustifolia* means narrow leafed, and *officinalis* means that the plant was once considered the official medicinal species. As you get to know the names, your understanding of plants and herbal medicine will deepen.

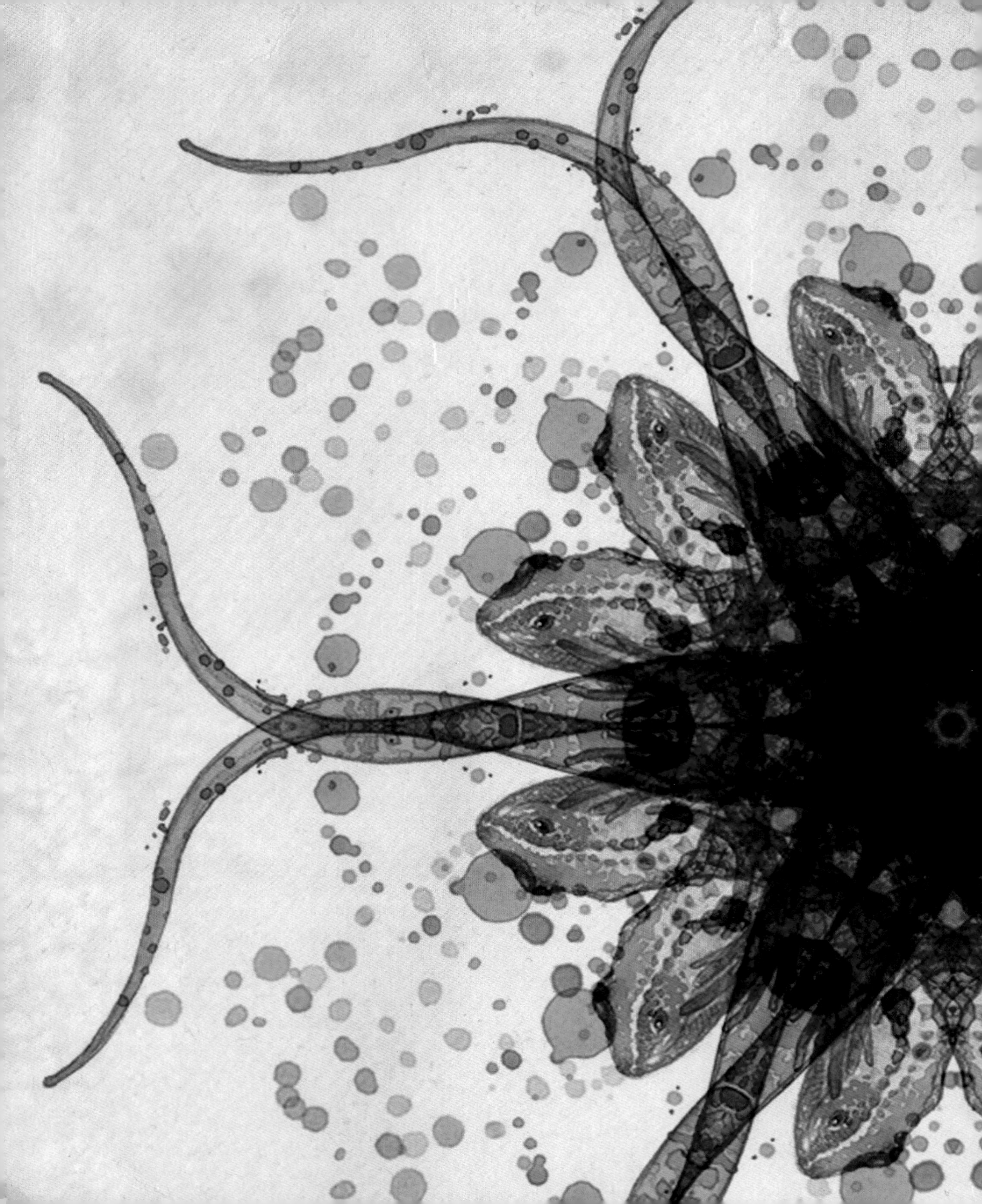

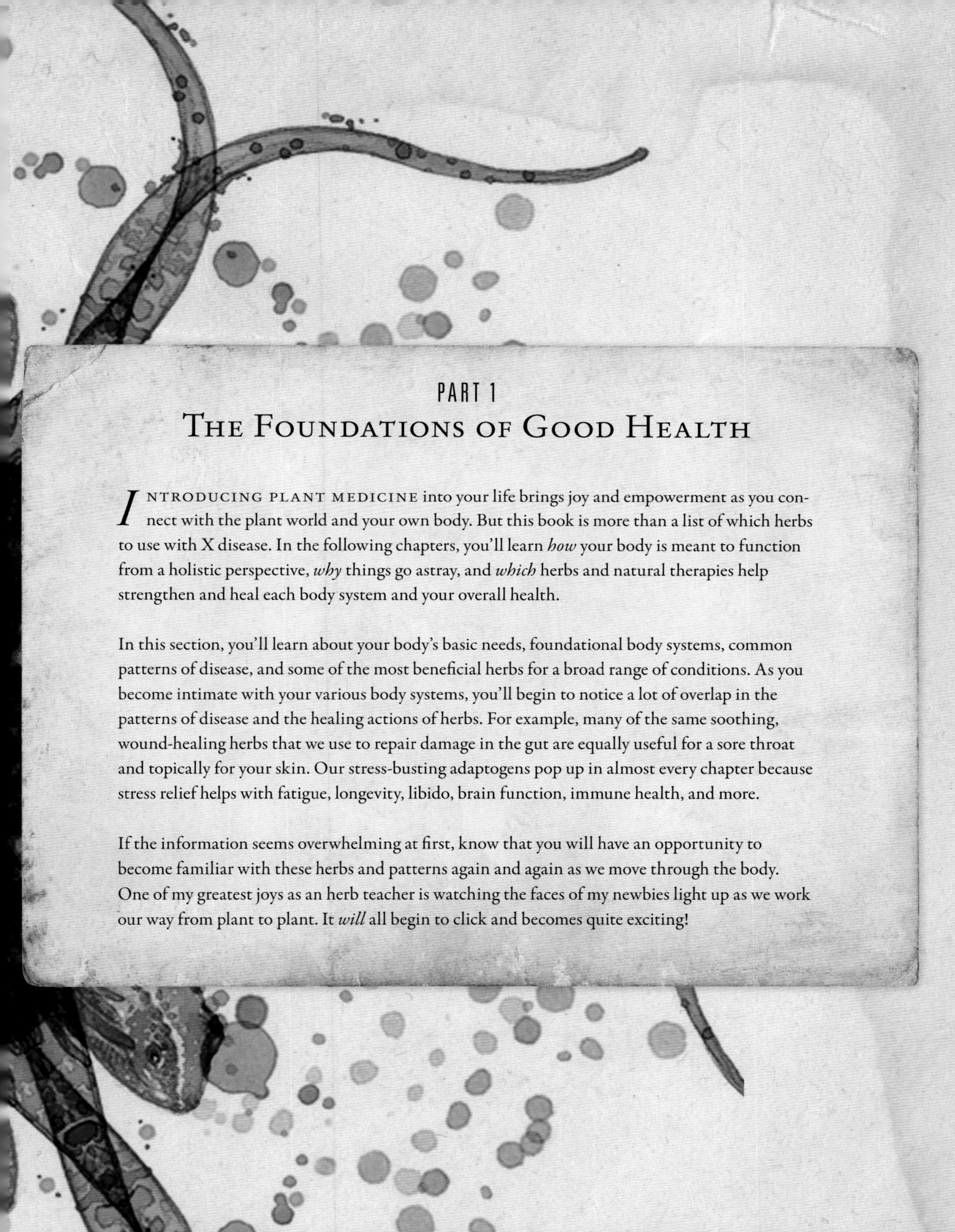

PART 1
The Foundations of Good Health

INTRODUCING PLANT MEDICINE into your life brings joy and empowerment as you connect with the plant world and your own body. But this book is more than a list of which herbs to use with X disease. In the following chapters, you'll learn *how* your body is meant to function from a holistic perspective, *why* things go astray, and *which* herbs and natural therapies help strengthen and heal each body system and your overall health.

In this section, you'll learn about your body's basic needs, foundational body systems, common patterns of disease, and some of the most beneficial herbs for a broad range of conditions. As you become intimate with your various body systems, you'll begin to notice a lot of overlap in the patterns of disease and the healing actions of herbs. For example, many of the same soothing, wound-healing herbs that we use to repair damage in the gut are equally useful for a sore throat and topically for your skin. Our stress-busting adaptogens pop up in almost every chapter because stress relief helps with fatigue, longevity, libido, brain function, immune health, and more.

If the information seems overwhelming at first, know that you will have an opportunity to become familiar with these herbs and patterns again and again as we move through the body. One of my greatest joys as an herb teacher is watching the faces of my newbies light up as we work our way from plant to plant. It *will* all begin to click and becomes quite exciting!

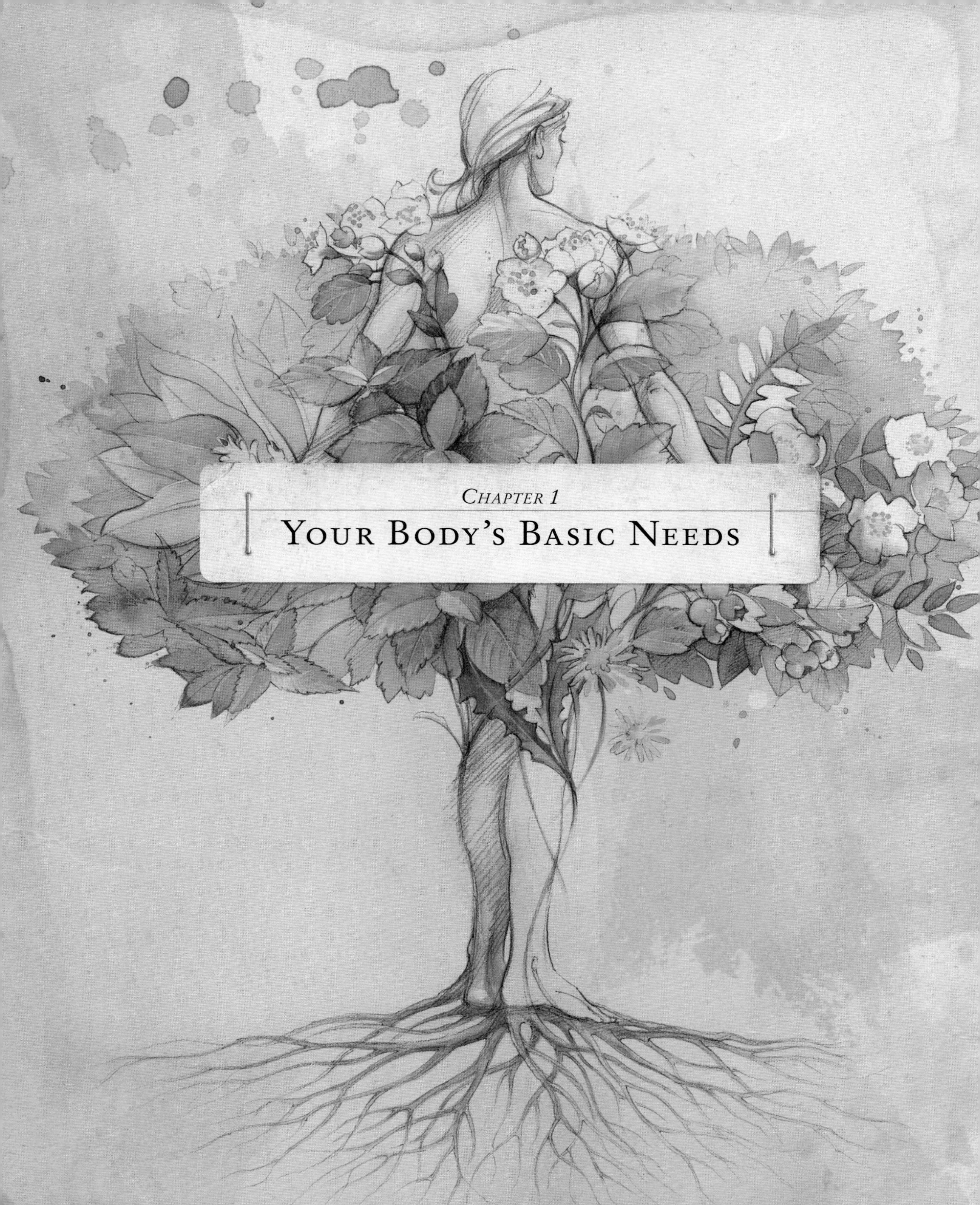

Chapter 1

Your Body's Basic Needs

To really make vital changes to your well-being, look beyond a simple "take some herbs" approach. While herbs alone *can* dramatically improve health and alleviate disease and discomfort, they work much better as part of a multifaceted, holistic approach. Diet, lifestyle, and mind-body balance are the pillars of health, and no amount of tinctures or capsules can take their place. Attending to these key areas will resolve or improve almost any health concern.

You Are What You Eat: Diet *and* Nutrition

Everything you eat or drink influences your body. Your digestive system breaks food and drink down into tiny bits and absorbs or eliminates them. The bits that enter your bloodstream serve as the building blocks for skin, bones, organs, blood, hormones, neurotransmitters, enzymes, glucose your body uses for fuel, and so on. Specifically *what* you consume — and how it's balanced in the context of your overall diet — in large part determines your overall health, good or bad. Sometimes the effects are immediately noticeable, and sometimes they accumulate gradually and don't become apparent until years or decades later.

Aiming for dietary perfection may be futile, and fortunately the human body can handle a surprising amount of junk. But strive for good habits, and listen to your body to figure out what your body likes best. No one rigid diet works for everyone. Your constitution, taste buds, food sensitivities, cultural training, budget, and food availability will all play a role in which diet makes you feel most vital. That said, let's talk about some general "good diet" principles to keep in mind.

Balance Your Plate

Enjoy good-quality produce, protein, carbohydrates, and fat at every meal and ideally at snack time, too. Avoid dietary ruts — which get boring and can cause you to miss out on essential nutrients over time — by eating a rainbow of (natural) colors and mixing things up regularly. In general, your plate should comprise the following:

- **One-half produce.** Plants provide an abundance of micronutrients (like vitamins and minerals), fiber, antioxidants, and protective phytochemicals that fight disease, improve digestion and detoxification, and help you feel great. Aim for five to nine servings (heavy on the veggies) daily. Salads, stir-fries, beds of greens, and fruit for snack and dessert make it easy. Go organic and/or local if you can; it's generally more nutritious, better tasting, and free of herbicides and pesticides.

- **One-quarter protein.** Protein helps you feel satisfied, reduces the glycemic effect of your meal, and ultimately serves as building blocks for the structure and chemicals of your body. Focus on fish, seafood, nuts and nut butters, seeds and seed butters, beans, poultry, hard cheeses, yogurt, eggs, mushrooms, and seed "grains" (quinoa, buckwheat, millet, amaranth). In moderation: dairy products, meat (preferably from pasture-raised or wild sources), and whole or fermented soy. Vegetables and whole grains provide some protein as well.

- **One-quarter carbohydrates.** Carbs primarily serve as fuel. Complex whole-food carbs eaten as part of a balanced diet provide a steady energy source without a blood sugar roller coaster. Focus on root vegetables, winter squash, beans, fruit, whole grains (wheat, corn, oats, rice, barley, rye, teff), and seed "grains." Most forms of dairy also provide carbohydrates, and vegetables provide some as well. In moderation: whole-grain flour, white potatoes, honey, and maple syrup. Avoid or limit sugar, refined and white flours, and fried potatoes.

- **A little bit of fat.** Fats are a key component of cell membranes, and they have a profound effect on your entire body, particularly your nerves, brain, heart, hair, skin, and nails. Fats help your body absorb fat-soluble nutrients (vitamins A, D, E, K, carotenoids, and more) and are building blocks for various essential compounds, including hormones and cholesterol. Focus on fatty fish, nuts and nut butters, seeds and seed butters, extra-virgin olive oil, unrefined coconut oil, tea seed oil (a.k.a. camellia seed oil), avocados, olives, and eggs. In moderation: whole-fat dairy, meat, and butter from pasture-raised sources.

Add Herbs for Nutritional Punch

Adding tea, herbs, and spices to your daily cuisine amps up your antioxidants, vitamins, minerals, and other key compounds that help keep you healthy. Everyday seasonings and tea blends can improve digestion, fight inflammation, fend off cancer, enhance the benefits of other foods you eat, and even counteract some of the detriment of certain foods like sweets and grilled meat. So enjoy herbs liberally, fresh or dry, in teas, in salads, in smoothies, as seasonings for your meals, as flavorings for your beverages.

Keep It Real

As much as possible, work with foods in their whole, unprocessed form. Limit or avoid flour, sugar, artificial sweeteners, artificial flavors, anticaking agents, preservatives, monosodium glutamate (key words that reveal its presence include "hydrolyzed," "glutamate," and "natural flavors"), and ingredients you can't pronounce. Purchase seasonal, fresh, local ingredients when you can.

Select Better Animal Products

If you eat animal products like meat, dairy, and eggs, opt for pasture-raised, wild, or organic sources that have been treated humanely. This improves the nutrient profile dramatically while minimizing the problematic fats and chemicals associated with "factory farm" production. Limit grilled meats (grilling causes cancer-causing compounds to form), and marinate them when you can. A homemade watery marinade based on tea, wine, beer, honey, or vinegar can reduce carcinogen formation in grilled meats by up to a whopping 90 percent. Why watery? Watery marinades do a more thorough job (compared to thick marinades) of penetrating the meat to deliver antioxidant compounds throughout. An antioxidant-rich marinade — with plenty of herbs and spices — is even better.

Take a Hint from Healthy Traditions

The diets most closely linked with disease prevention and longevity include the Mediterranean diet, Indian and Asian cuisine, and the vegetarian or (especially) vegan diet. But we're not talking chain restaurant fare here. Instead, opt for the traditional cuisine consumed by long-lived common folk. There are a lot of great cookbooks and blogs focusing on healthy cuisines. (One of my favorite sites for recipes is www.eatingwell.com.)

Hydrate Wisely

Adequate water intake keeps everything running smoothly. Aim for half your body weight in ounces daily — so a 130-pound person should drink 65 ounces of liquid, or about eight 8-ounce glasses. Focus on water, unsweetened all-natural seltzer, tea, herbal tea, soup, broth, and juicy fruits and veggies. Drink juices (especially high-sugar fruit juice), alcohol, and coffee in moderation. Avoid or limit drinking from plastic containers, which can leach toxins, in favor of glass, stainless steel, and ceramic containers.

Listen to Your Body

As mentioned, no one diet fits all people, and no one food is friend or foe to everyone. You might do better with more or less protein, vegan or flexitarian, gluten-free, dairy-free, egg-free, raw or cooked veggies, and so on. The perfect diet for *you* will depend on your health issues, your constitution, and even your genetics. Don't get too stuck on diet dogma

WHY HYDRATE?

WE KNOW WE SHOULD DRINK plenty of water, yet 75 percent of Americans are chronically dehydrated. Water — mixed with sodium, electrolytes, and other compounds — constitutes 60 percent of your body, including 75 percent of your muscles and 85 percent of your brain. As my teacher Michael Moore would say, "There is an ocean inside of you," and you need to regularly replenish it with plenty of clean water.

The color and scent of your urine will give you a hint to your level of dehydration. It should be light and straw colored (if you take a multivitamin or B vitamins, it might be bright yellow in the hours afterward). Here are some symptoms of mild to moderate dehydration. Severe dehydration can be dangerous and may require medical attention.

- Dark, scant, stinky urine
- Dry, sticky mouth
- Chapped lips
- Thirst (but not always!)
- Headache
- Fatigue
- Joint pain
- Brain fog
- Skin that is dry or lacks vitality
- Constipation
- Dizziness or lightheadedness
- Weight gain
- Ulcers

and trends. Simply eat a balanced healthy diet based on whole foods; then listen to your body to determine what specifically works best for you. Keep a food diary to help you sleuth things out. Pay attention to how you feel after you eat a particular food, or a food prepared in a particular way. Do you feel more or less vibrant? Do you have digestive distress? Mood, inflammation, energy levels, and specific disease markers can all serve as clues. Some effects are immediate, while others take time to build. And of course, your needs and food sensitivities may change with your health status and as you age. (See page 84 for more discussion of food sensitivities.)

You Are How You Live

Lifestyle is more than an important piece of the health puzzle; it is the table you piece the puzzle together on, the foundation upon which all aspects of well-being are built. You can take all the herbs in the world, and you can work with the finest doctors in the land, but if, for example, you never get outside and are chronically stressed out, you still won't feel *well.*

Basically, lifestyle is what you do, day in and day out. Fitness, sleep, work, relationships, activities, point of view, your connection with nature, and the environment you live in all play a role in determining your overall lifestyle. Even your spiritual practices play a role because they affect how you spend your time, think, feel, connect to others, and find spiritual solace.

Improving your lifestyle habits can yield significant improvements to your health and energy levels. Some people plunge right in, letting the momentum of big life changes carry them forward. Other people find lifestyle changes overwhelming, and they may prefer to start slowly or to tackle different aspects of their life one by one. Small changes can lead to more small changes that, over time, build up to new perspectives on life and living and well-being. But whether you're making big leaps or taking baby steps, focus on the following biggies.

Daily Movement

Exercise — or lack thereof — has an enormous effect on your overall well-being, equal to or surpassing diet. Human beings were meant to move, yet modern culture has made it tricky. Most of us don't have to physically harvest our food, wash clothes by hand, walk around the village to do our daily errands, or make our living from manual labor anymore. Unfortunately, our bodies weren't meant to sit in front of a screen and push papers around a desk all day. Enter exercise. Setting aside specific times to move and working activity into your daily routine help compensate for a more sedentary lifestyle.

The advantages of regular movement go beyond a slim physique and increased muscle mass. If you need motivation to take that midday walk around the block or plan a more physically active weekend, consider the following perks of regular activity:

- Improved cognition and brain volume
- Resistance to the effects of aging
- Longer life span
- Better energy levels
- Improved mood (exercise is equal to or better than antidepressants in this regard!)
- Better sleep
- Decreased stress levels
- Improved metabolism and weight management
- Decreased pain
- Balanced blood sugar
- Improved markers of cardiovascular health, including circulation, cholesterol levels, and blood pressure
- Reduced risk of heart disease, diabetes, stroke, and cancer
- Improved reproductive health and sexual vitality
- Stronger bones
- Better balance and a reduced risk of falls

Exactly how much time should you spend moving around? The Centers for Disease Control and Prevention (CDC) recommends 2½ hours of moderate physical activity (e.g., walking) each week — for example, 30 minutes 5 days a week — *plus* muscle-strengthening activities (e.g., weight lifting, lunges, sit-ups) twice a week. That's about as much time as it takes to watch a movie, once a week. For more vigorous activity like jogging and running, you can cut that time in half. Doubling your fitness time beyond the recommendations provides even more benefits. You still reap the rewards if you break it up into 10- or 15-minute blocks.

Also remember that *some exercise is always better than none*. Use the recommendations as a guide, not a guilt trip.

Sleep

Sleep is the ultimate panacea. During a good night's sleep, your body has the chance to relax muscles, repair damage, detoxify, fortify your immune system, balance out hormones and neurotransmitters, and restore itself. If you're coming down with a cold, dealing with a stressful period in your life, or trying to diet and lose weight, your day will go *much* more smoothly if you slept well the night before. Unfortunately, the reverse is also true, and at least one-third of Americans live in a bleary-eyed state of sleep deprivation.

We deteriorate with chronic sleep deprivation: heart health, blood sugar metabolism, libido and reproductive health, psychological health, and skin appearance all go to pieces. Just one or two nights of sleep deprivation diminish your cognition, mood, and immune function. Sleeping less than 7 hours a night *triples* your risk of viral infection. On the other hand, if you get extra rest when you're sick, you'll recuperate more quickly. Sleeping for just 5 hours per night can cause you to up your calorie intake, make it harder to stick to a healthy diet and make good self-care decisions, and cause you to gain a whopping 2 pounds in a mere 5 days compared to sleeping 8 hours a night. Worse, British researchers found that workers who slept 5 or fewer hours per

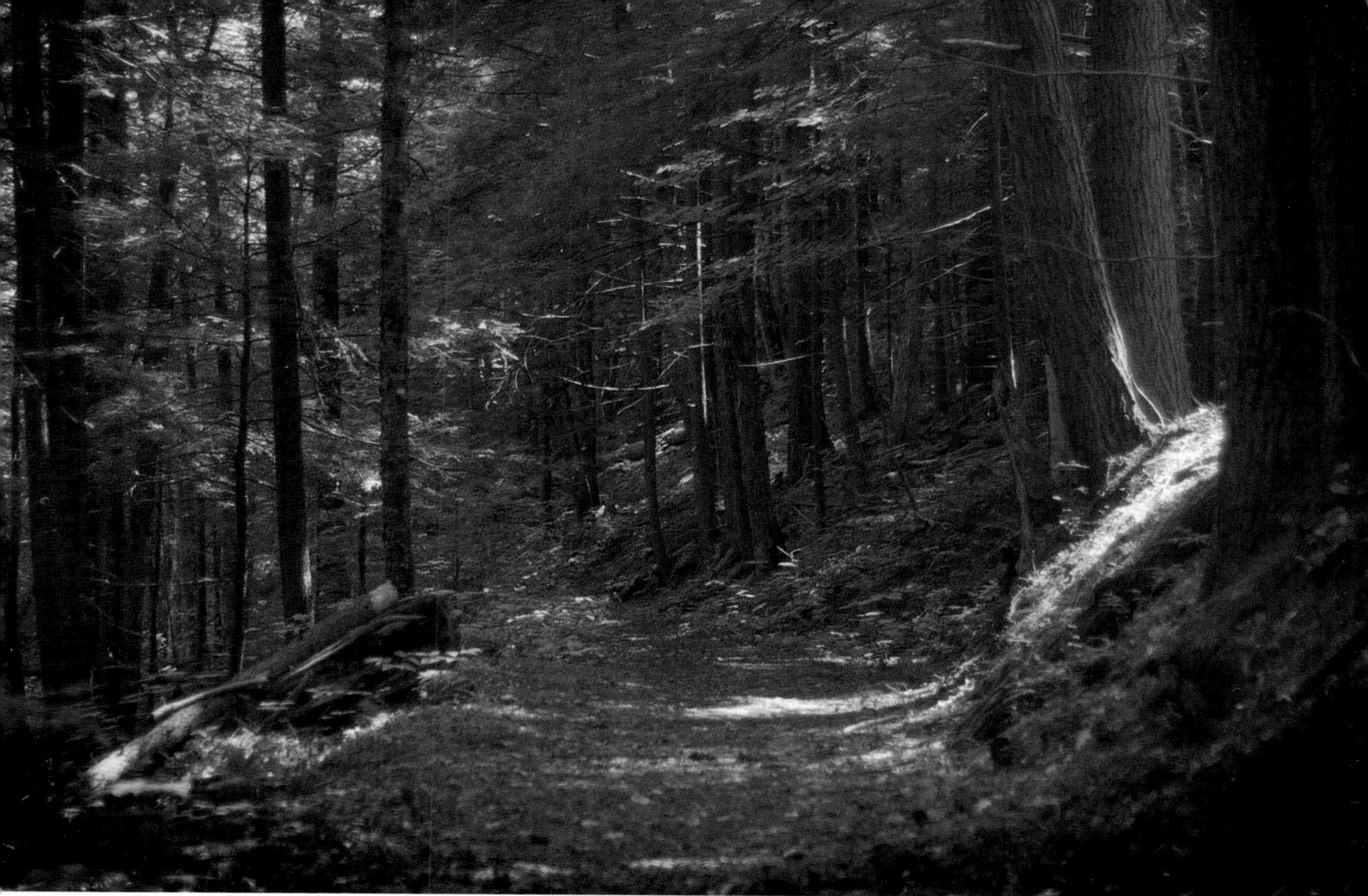

FOREST BATHING

WE CAN LEARN A LOT FROM JAPAN, a country so obsessed with work productivity and long hours that *karoshi*, or death by overwork (both work-related suicide and stress-related diseases like heart disease and stroke), has become a major problem. The solution? Forest bathing. The Forest Agency of Japan introduced the concept in 1982 and, with dedicated research, has shown that walking, meditating, exercising, and playing among trees in a forest-like environment has physical and emotional benefits that surpass those of the activities alone. Even sitting in a chair gazing at forest scenery has merit: in one Japanese study, just 20 minutes spent staring at a natural vista decreased stress hormones by 13 percent compared to those in a city environment. A view of water — such as a lake, pond, river, or other water feature — improves the effect. Other benefits of forest bathing include the following:

- Improved cardiovascular health, including blood oxygenation and heart rate variability (which also relates to nervous system health), along with decreased pulse rate and blood pressure
- Reduced levels of cortisol, a stress-triggered hormone related to blood sugar balance and metabolism
- Improved mood, improved self-esteem, and decreased stress, resulting in fewer symptoms of depression, less hostility, and increased liveliness
- Decreased brain fatigue and attention deficit; improved cognition, focus, and creativity

night had double the risk of death from all causes versus those who averaged 7 or more hours.

The flip side of this dismal scenario is that getting adequate sleep (which is really quite enjoyable and free!) improves almost every aspect of health. Aim for 7 to 9 hours of sleep per night. You'll begin to reap the rewards almost immediately. Having a hard time getting to sleep and staying there? In chapter 4 we'll discuss sleep remedies and good sleep hygiene tips.

The Healing Power of Nature

One of the remarkable aspects of nature is its ability to nurture and heal the human body. Herbs and good food are elements of nature, but so are sunlight, clean air, and beautiful restorative vistas. Forget taking herbs — sometimes all you need to do to feel better is sit under a tree for 15 minutes, walk by the river, or dig your hands in the garden.

Studies now suggest that many of the ills of our youth trace back to "nature deficit disorder" and lack of unstructured playtime in natural environments. Stress, depression, anxiety, and attention issues creep up when kids go from school to screen or an endless stream of lessons. I'd argue the same is true for adults.

The natural world calms, intrigues, and challenges us. Temperature fluctuations in your environment give your thyroid (which regulates your body temp) a mini workout. Sunlight helps your body make vitamin D and keeps your endocrine system in sync with the day's cycle. Exposure to minute amounts of bacteria and soil organisms refocuses a wayward immune system, reducing the tendency for autoimmune disease and allergies.

Children and adults alike benefit from *daily* time outdoors, if only a 15-minute walk in the woods or through a park. While actually getting outside is ideal, you can also reap rewards by infusing nature into your indoor space at work and home. Improve window access to natural or garden views, decorate with houseplants (even artificial ones), and hang pictures of beautiful views like mountains, trees, or water, which studies show improve work performance and well-being. As someone who spends a lot of time in front of my laptop, I can personally attest to the advantages of incorporating houseplants, pretty pictures, and beautiful window views. It helps that my chickens come by periodically to knock on my office window, reminding me to take a break and, on good days, get out for a quick midday walk in the sun . . . oh, and toss my sweetie pies some treats! No chickens? Set a reminder on your computer or phone to take a break, even if it's just to sip tea and look out the window for a few minutes.

Clean and Green Living

The truth is, you are constantly bombarded by low-level toxins that can increase your risk of cancer, mess with reproductive and metabolic hormones, and damage your nervous system. They may also cause skin rashes and respiratory issues like asthma. The individual toxins may not pose a big threat on their own at low exposure, but they can accumulate and work in synergy with one another. Common sources of problematic toxins include processed and factory-farmed food, plastic (especially in food and drink packaging), pesticides and herbicides, personal-care products, home renovation products, flame retardants in furniture, and cleaning products.

The good news is that you can drastically limit your exposure to these chemicals by choosing products with more natural ingredients. We have more options than ever before. Even if you can't change everything, here are some easy places to start.

- **Eat more whole foods and less "factory" food.** A diet based on whole foods (heavy on plants and rich in fiber) encourages your body's natural detoxification systems. Highly processed foods — chips and crackers, packaged snacks, mass-marketed prepared meals — are convenient, but they also tend to have preservatives and artificial ingredients that are potential toxins and can dampen your detox response.

- **Limit your use of plastic containers, plastic-packed food, and canned food.** Choosing fresh foods over foods that come packed in plastic quickly and significantly drops your levels of plastic-based toxins like bisphenol A (BPA) and di(2-ethylhexyl) phthalate (DEHP). Store food and drink in glass, stainless steel, wood, or ceramic. Don't heat food in plastic.

- **Use all-natural personal-care and cleaning products or make your own.** Specific ingredients to avoid include synthetic fragrances, parabens, and phthalates. Companies design labels to make products appear better than they are; read the ingredients list or use a database to decipher the best store-bought options. Natural food stores generally carry greener options, and some of the best things can be made easily and cheaply at home with simple ingredients like vegetable oils, beeswax, baking soda, vinegar, and lemons. My favorite "make-your-own" authors include Annie B. Bond (for green cleaning) and Donna Maria, Stephanie Tourles, and Rosemary Gladstar (for body care).

- **Minimize your exposure to chemical toxins and mold.** Look for no- or low-VOC options when buying paint and home renovation materials. Flame retardants, mold inhibitors, and stain guard on fabrics, furniture, and new cars can be a source of toxins. Generally, the stronger the smell, the more toxic the product is. Opt for natural materials and ingredients when possible. Be sure to wear proper protective gear like masks and gloves when you work. Avoid mold by keeping areas dry, installing fans when needed, and fixing leaks promptly. And when you're hiring contractors, look for LEED or Green Building certified professionals.

- **Check out the Environmental Working Group.** The EWG website (www.ewg.org) offers handy consumer-guide databases for personal-care products, pesticides in produce, cleaning products, mercury in seafood, and more. They've done the sleuthing for you!

You Are How You Think *and* Feel: Mind-Body Balance

A less tangible, but equally important, pillar of health is mind-body balance, or mind-body-spirit balance. How you think and feel has a direct effect on your overall health and vice versa. While taking care of your body via diet, exercise, and reduced toxin exposure will also benefit your mind and spirit, consider giving mind-body wellness some direct TLC. This will specifically help your nervous and endocrine systems and stress response and augment your resistance to a range of diseases, from mood disorders and heart disease to cancer.

Of course, just telling yourself to be calm, think positive, and stay centered won't always do the trick. Changing your perspective and thinking habits can seem daunting. Fortunately, certain activities directly nourish your mind and spirit to make this transition easier. Bringing some of these tasks into your daily life will slowly and profoundly shift your reality toward one of health and balance.

- **Meditate:** Just 8 weeks of mindfulness meditation approximately 30 minutes a day can help you feel calmer and make positive changes in various areas of your brain, including improved memory, empathy, sense of self, and stress regulation. Studies also support meditation's ability to decrease blood pressure, heart disease risk, anxiety, depression, insomnia, and addictive behaviors. Some of the most profound research on meditation is focused on mindfulness-based stress reduction techniques and programs. Classes and books will help you get started. Once you have the basics, you can meditate anywhere, even in short bursts.

- **Breathe:** Sure, you're always breathing. But specific breathwork can help pull you out of the fight-or-flight stress response and shift your focus inward. Most forms of meditation and yoga incorporate breathwork, but you can also try specific short breathing exercises. One of my favorites is the 4-7-8 breath touted by integrative healing expert Dr. Andrew Weil. In a sitting position, place your tongue gently on the roof of your mouth, by your teeth. Breathe out through your mouth with a "whoosh" sound. Inhale through your nose to the count of four. Hold your breath for the count of seven. Then exhale through your mouth to the count of eight. Practice this breath at least four times in a row, and up to eight times (but no more than that in one sitting). You can do this as often as you'd like throughout the day, but doing it at least once or twice is ideal. Dr. Weil describes it as "water cutting the Grand Canyon." It can single-handedly make profound changes, but it doesn't happen overnight. I once led a multifaceted course on happiness for 50 people through my local co-op, and this breathing exercise ranked number one among students for helping them feel calmer, happier, and more at peace. To learn more, check out Dr. Weil's book *Spontaneous Happiness*.

- **Try yoga, tai chi, or qigong:** These ancient practices from India and China were developed by masters of mind-body-spirit balance to help guide their students to a better state of being. They incorporate gentle movement and breathwork to increase your vital force. They also improve strength, flexibility, and balance.

- **Be grateful and cultivate optimism:** As you will see, little tasks done regularly can accumulate for really phenomenal positive changes in your well-being. Gratitude and optimism are key traits that improve your mental and physical health, and they're surprisingly easy to develop. Consider keeping a gratitude journal where you write down three good things that happen to you each day. Research suggests that daily gratitude alone can improve your overall happiness by as much as 25 percent.

You Are Your Own Healer: How *to* Use Herbs *for* Health

Herbal medicine offers infinite possibilities for ways to create a personalized protocol for the individual. Your own particular health concerns, personal preferences (including convenience and cost), herb availability, and other factors all come into play. That said, here are some ways in which I approach herbal medicine that you can use to get started.

Double- (or Triple-) Dip

For any health concern, you have a wide range of options to choose from, including lifestyle approaches, various conventional and alternative therapies, and a myriad of herbs. A multifaceted approach that includes lifestyle *and* herbal remedies often works best, but don't feel like you need to incorporate anything and everything into your new daily routine.

For herbs, choose one or two forms of remedies that suit your needs well: perhaps a pleasant-tasting daily tea that happens to address some of your health goals plus a more focused tincture blend, or a capsule formula, or an herb-infused broth.

Also try to incorporate at least one lifestyle therapy that seems particularly well suited for your needs, such as improved diet, increased exercise, meditation, breathwork, or something that incorporates several aspects of this, like tai chi or yoga. Think about what might best address your concerns — weight-bearing exercise for stronger bones, meditation for stress relief, a more plant-based diet for heart health — as well as what feels most manageable and sustainable for the long term.

General Well-Being vs. Specific Health Concerns

The basic concepts behind building a personalized protocol don't differ too much whether you're addressing a significant health concern or simply want better overall health and disease prevention. What changes are the specific herbs involved and often also the dose.

- **General well-being:** If you simply want to support overall health, you're likely to stick primarily with supportive tonic herbs — plants that are generally very safe and improve various aspects of health. These include nutritive herbs, stress-relieving adaptogens, antioxidant culinary herbs and spices, and perhaps some digestion-enhancing bitters. You might just drink a cup of tea daily, throw a teaspoon of mixed powders into your smoothie, or take a few squirts of tincture.
- **Chronic disease:** Addressing chronic disease often involves a more thorough approach, perhaps two or more herbal remedies taken a few times daily. Tonics still form the backbone of your formulas, but you'll also want more targeted herbs and formulas such as anti-inflammatories, immune modulators, and pain relievers.
- **Acute conditions:** These conditions usually call for very specific herbs used in frequent doses throughout the day until the condition passes. For example, you might take echinacea tincture, elderberry syrup, or fresh ginger tea every hour at the onset of a cold or flu; two squirts of cramp bark tincture every 15 minutes as needed for menstrual cramps; a cup or two of "herbal aspirin" tea for a few days for pain associated with an injury; antimicrobials (topically) for a skin infection; or elderflower and peppermint tea to break a fever. Just taking the herbs once or twice a day or taking a tonic formula probably won't suffice for an acute condition. On the flip side, once the acute condition has passed, it's usually not necessary or appropriate to continue taking the herbs or the dosages you used to address it. (Of course, if the acute condition occurs commonly, a different approach may be needed for day-to-day care in between flare-ups, which will look more like a chronic disease or general well-being protocol.)

By combining an herbal protocol with diet and lifestyle therapies, you can profoundly affect your health for the better. Be patient; although you may notice improvements within the day or week, they often take several weeks or months to fully build. Consider writing down all your health issues before you make changes, then revisit the list a month or two later. You might be surprised by how much you've improved!

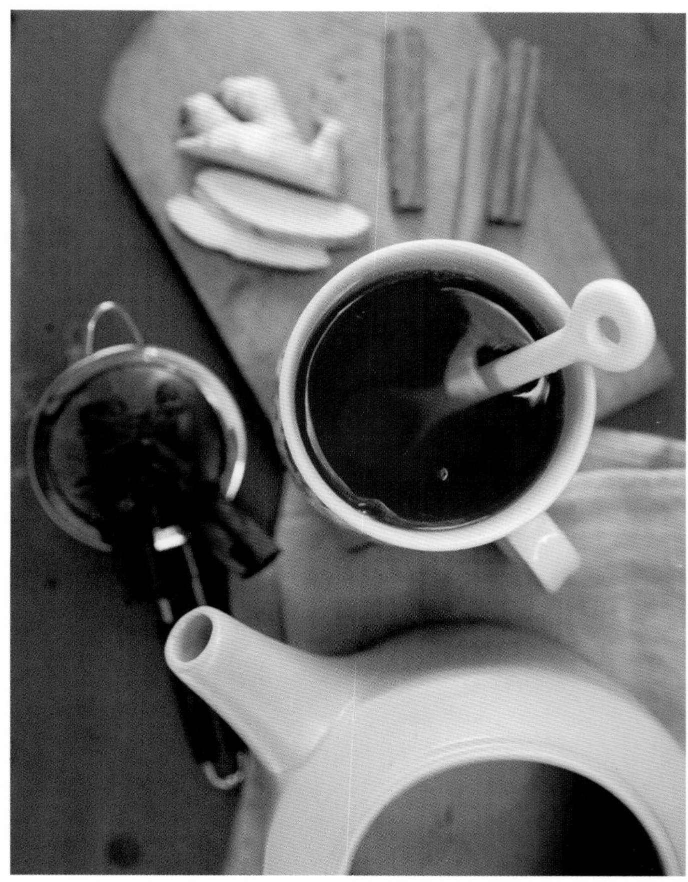

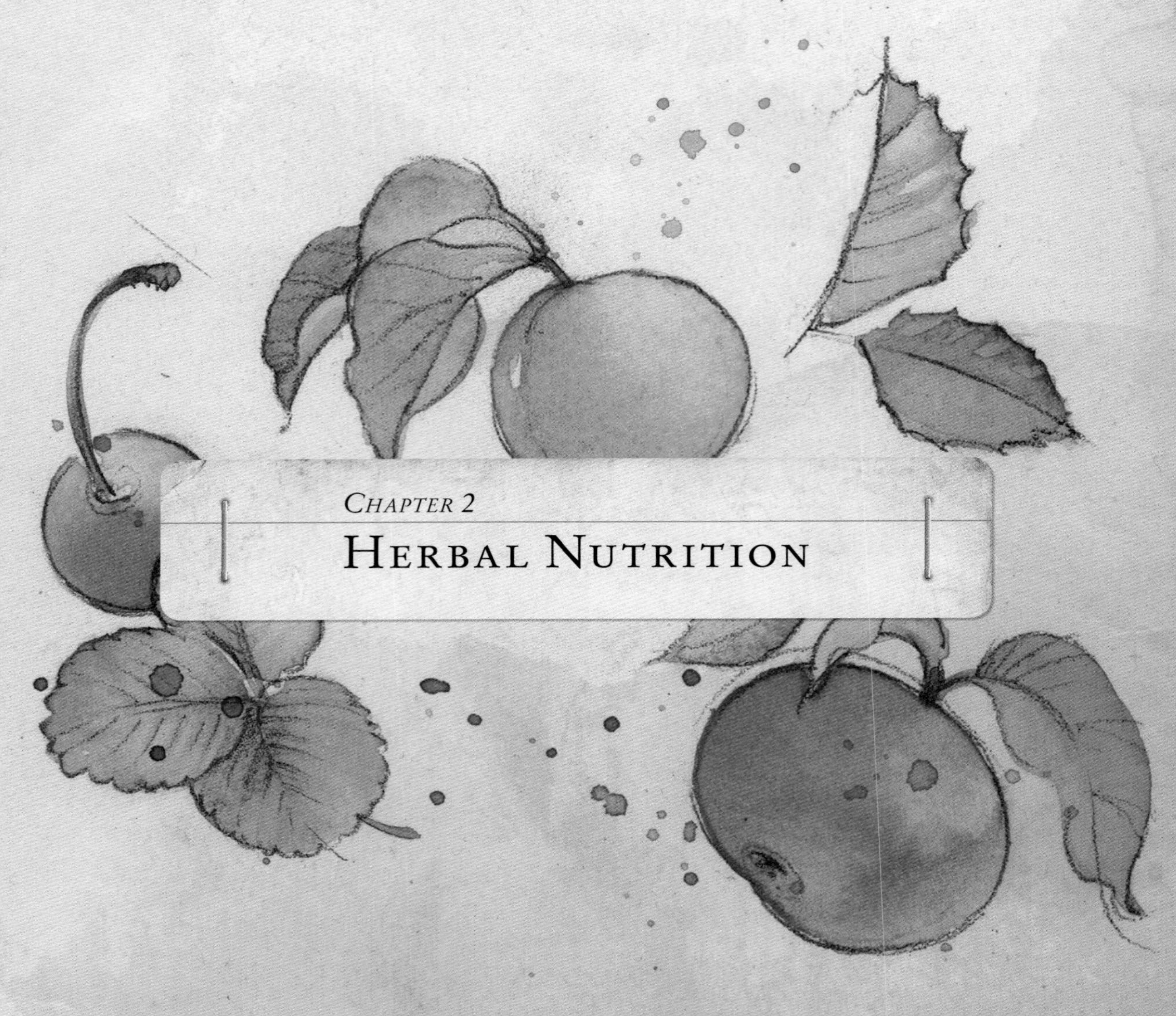

Chapter 2

Herbal Nutrition

CERTAINLY YOUR DIET should serve as the basis of your nutritive needs, and we discussed some basic dietary goals in chapter 1. But nutrient deficiencies are incredibly common, particularly with specific nutrients like vitamin D, iron, vitamin B_{12}, folic acid, calcium, and so on. These deficiencies can add up to diseases and also lost vitality for your body. Dietary supplements can be helpful — not as a replacement for a good diet but as insurance. Herbalists tend to take this a step further by turning to nutrient-dense herbs and tonics.

Nutritive herbs bridge the gap between diet and dietary supplements, providing concentrated nutrition in a whole-foods package. A nutritive is a kind of tonic — that is, an herb that supports your overall health by improving the function of one or more systems in your body. Like most tonics, nutritive herbs are generally quite safe, with few or no negative side effects, and they are often gentle enough to use even with children. And they are multifaceted — one herb can provide several different nutrients, as well as other health benefits, and can serve as a tonic for more than one system. Incorporating nutritive herbs into your daily diet will result in many improvements for your overall health, including better mood and energy, more vibrant skin, stronger bones, shinier hair and harder nails, more efficient detoxification, and a better-functioning immune system.

Get the Most *from* Nutritive Herbs

How you take nutritive herbs will make a huge difference in the level of vitamins and minerals they actually deliver to your body. For example, you'll get almost no calcium from nettle tincture, a little bit from nettle-infused vinegar, maybe 40 to 80 mg from a cup of regular tea, or a whopping 500 mg from a nettle super infusion, decoction, broth, or soup.

Generally, the nutrients will be most potent and absorbable if you simply *eat* the herbs, incorporating them — fresh, dry, or powdered — into everything from broth, soups, and stews to casseroles, smoothies, and stir-fries. Teas do a pretty good job of extracting the nutrients, and nutritive herbs can be added as supportive ingredients to almost any tea blend. Super-infused teas (steeped for at least 4 hours and up to overnight; see page 302 for instructions) concentrate those nutrients.

Minerals are simultaneously difficult to extract from herbs *and* may not be adequately absorbed by your body (especially if you have poor digestion), and you may need a substantial dose to get the effect. Super infusions, decoctions, and food forms (broths, smoothies, pesto) give you the best mineral bang. Standard infusions and herbal vinegars provide a light fizz of minerals, while capsules are at the mercy of dose and digestion and tincturing won't extract minerals at all.

WHAT IS A TONIC?

"Tonic" is a general term referring to herbs that are known for their high degree of safety as well as for their many different positive effects on your overall health.

General Uses: Tonics form the backbone of herbal medicine. We turn to them for daily use, overall well-being, disease prevention, and supportive treatment for serious health conditions. They can generally be taken in large or regular doses without safety concerns.

Examples: This is a really broad class of herbs with a range of actions. Tonic herbs include herbs that are nutritious (nutritives like nettle), improve your resistance to stress (adaptogens like holy basil), nourish the nervous system (nervines like milky oat seed), decrease inflammation (anti-inflammatories like turmeric), squelch free radicals (antioxidants like hawthorn), support your immune system (immunomodulators like medicinal mushrooms and astragalus), and so on.

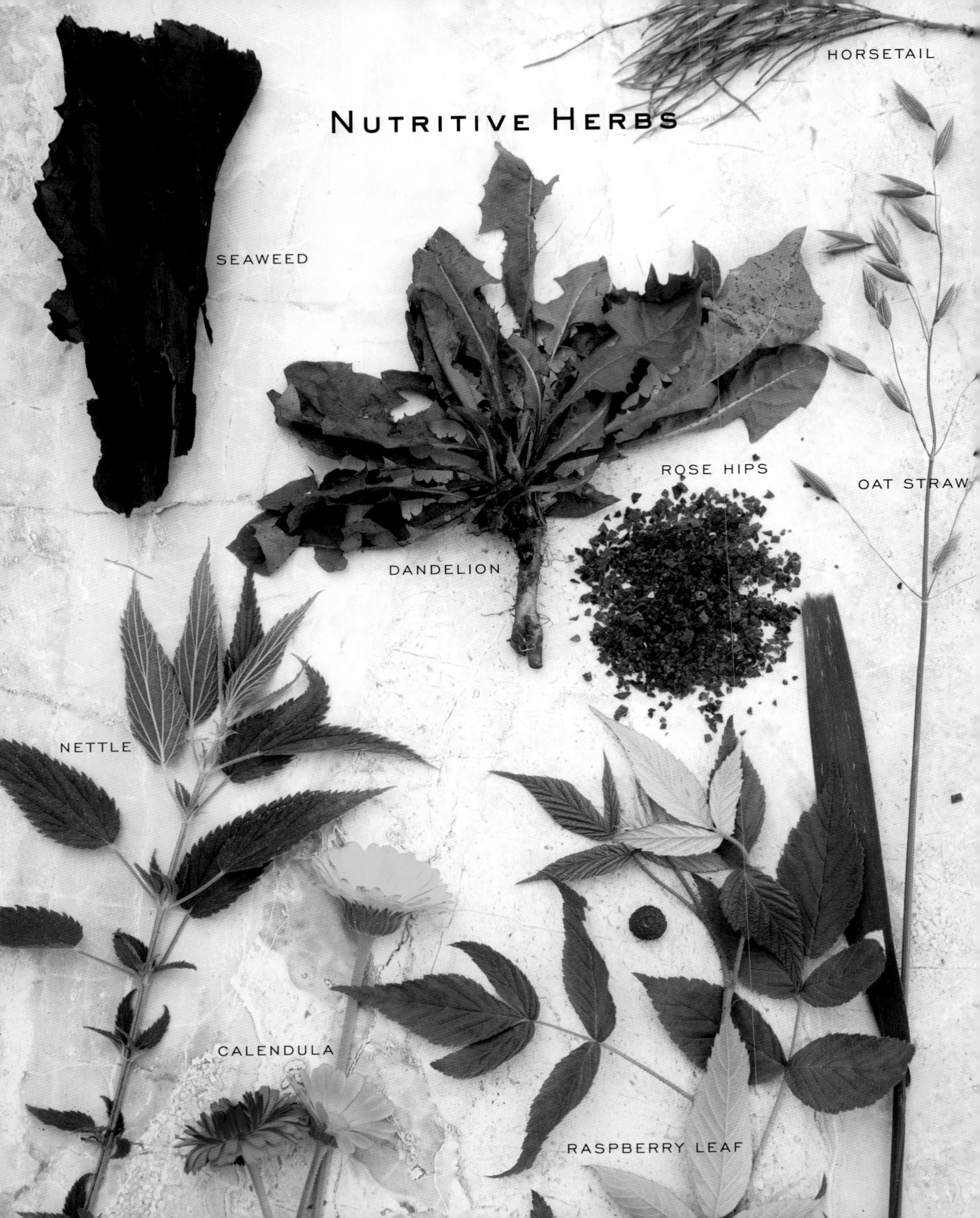

Nutritive Herbs
HORSETAIL
SEAWEED
ROSE HIPS
OAT STRAW
DANDELION
NETTLE
CALENDULA
RASPBERRY LEAF

Nutritive Herbs *to* Know

While many herbs provide nutrition, the following herbs are the most potent, safe, and common options available. They offer a superlative nutritional boost to your daily diet, providing large doses of the vitamins, minerals, and other compounds your body needs for optimal function. They make great additions to tea and broth, and some can be eaten on their own.

▸ Nettle

Urtica dioica, U. spp.

Availability: G W C+ (see A Key to the Herb Profiles, page 11)

Key Properties: These spring greens get the spotlight as one of the most nutritious and safe herbal remedies on land. One cup of super-infused nettle leaf tea offers approximately 500 mg of bone-building calcium in a highly bioavailable form. (Bioavailability refers to how easy it is for the body to absorb a nutrient and put it to use.) In contrast, the calcium from most of the foods that are touted as good sources (dairy products, oxalate-rich leafy greens, beans, seeds, and grains that contain phytic acid) is poorly absorbed because other compounds in those foods block the absorption or increase the excretion of calcium. Nettles also provide significant doses of magnesium, potassium, and silica. As a superb green food, they're also rich in chlorophyll and support the alkalinity of the body.

Additional Benefits: Nettle leaves act as a diuretic (they make you pee), gentle kidney cleanser, and mild antihistamine. They help you eliminate uric acid, which may relieve gout. Stinging yourself by whacking your skin with fresh nettles causes hives, but some people use that for health-promoting purposes. The body releases anti-inflammatory compounds to bring down the inflammation, and in the process, chronic inflammation like joint pain may also disappear temporarily.

Preparation: Harvest happy green nettle leaves and tops in the spring. Cook, dry, or juice the nettles to remove the sting. You can also knock the sting back (or out) by puréeing, like when you're making smoothies and pesto, depending on the strength of your blender and the bite of your nettles. This is a true food herb — enjoy nettles in broths, soups, and stir-fries or as a steamed vegetable. Use the powder in capsules, smoothies, or other treats. Oftentimes we simply use nettle to make tea. This herb does well as an infusion, super infusion, or decoction, though you'll get more nutrition from the latter two preparations. Anywhere from 1 teaspoon to a full ounce of nettles can be taken daily.

Cautions and Considerations: Nettles are very safe, although their diuretic effect can be annoying and dehydrating or drying for some, and they can sometimes cause atypical negative reactions. Of course, the sting of a fresh plant can

WHAT IS A NUTRITIVE?

Nutritive herbs contain high levels of a particular vitamin or mineral or contain modest levels of several nutrients.

General Uses: Without adequate nutrition, your body can't function properly. Nutritive herbs nourish your body, correct deficiencies, and bring you to optimal health. Use them for diseases related to specific nutrient deficiencies — including osteoporosis, poor hair/skin/nails, and anemia — as well as general health and well-being.

Examples: Common nutritive herbs include nettle, horsetail, oats and oat straw, raspberry leaf, seaweed, rose hips, dandelion leaf and root, alfalfa, red clover blossoms, and calendula flowers, as well as edible weeds and culinary herbs like chickweed, lamb's-quarter, pigweed, parsley, and sorrel and more exotic superfoods like amla, acerola, maca, and cacao.

be unpleasant; harvest cautiously and wear thick gloves. If you get stung, there are many antidotes: apply fresh mashed jewelweed, chickweed, or yellow dock leaves or even nettle juice. You may want to watch your nettle plants for a full year to see them in flower and ensure their identity. Several unrelated mint-family "nettles," including *Lamium* species, are sometimes mistaken for the real deal because they look so similar before flowering. Spring nettles are preferred; nettles harvested after the plants have flowered can cause mild kidney irritation.

▸ Horsetail

Equisetum arvense

Availability: W+ C

Key Properties: Horsetail is a pernicious and ancient weed of damp places. Its green growth is 35 percent silica, and though no recommended daily amount has been set for this mineral, it helps build healthy connective tissue and collagen, including bones, hair, skin, and nails. Horsetail also provides significant amounts of calcium and iron as well as some potassium and magnesium. Its combination of nutrients makes it useful for broken bone, sprains, and osteoporosis, especially in combination with like-minded herbs, including oat straw, nettle, and alfalfa.

Additional Benefits: Horsetail is diuretic, so it's sometimes used to cleanse the kidneys. Interestingly, even though horsetail's silica is not well extracted by alcohol, the tincture appears to be useful for breaks and sprains (often combined with Solomon's seal and mullein roots, per the wisdom of herbalist Jim McDonald). Horsetail extracts are sometimes added to topical formulas as well for collagen and connective tissue support.

Preparation: Harvest horsetail in early summer while it is still bright green and tender, with tight bunches pointing up. To get the silica from the plant, super-infused or long-decocted teas and capsules work best. The plant is too tough to eat; its relative scouring rush was used by early pioneers to scour pots and pans. Standard herb doses (see page 298) apply.

Cautions and Considerations: Horsetail is generally safe, but you do need to be careful of some things. First, ensure that you don't have other species of horsetail; *E. palustre* looks similar and is toxic to horses and possibly people. Second, ensure that you're harvesting from a clean source because horsetail will bioaccumulate kidney-toxic nitrogenous compounds from farms (fertilizer, manure waste), agribusiness, and chemical plants upstream. (Because of horsetail's potential to irritate the kidneys, herbalists do not generally recommend taking

Nutri-Tea

This is a classic herbal tonic tea with many variations. The theme: a base of nutritive herbs, some herbs for flavor, and a few flowers for color. Feel free to play around with this recipe and incorporate other herbs specific to your needs.

- 1 teaspoon nettles
- ½ teaspoon horsetail
- ½ teaspoon oat straw
- ½ teaspoon red clover
- 1 teaspoon mints of choice
- ¼ teaspoon calendula
- Honey or stevia (optional)

Combine all the herbs. Pour 2 cups boiling water over the herbs and let steep, covered, for 5 to 15 minutes. Sweeten with honey or a pinch of stevia, if desired.

Nettle-Oat Chai

Not warming up to nettle tea? Turning it into chai really perks up the flavor. For even more nutrition, you can prepare a super-infused nettle–oat straw tea, and then simmer it with the chai spices for 20 minutes. For extra energy and immune support, add 1 slice astragalus root, ½ teaspoon ashwagandha root, and ½ teaspoon codonopsis root. Chaga (a medicinal mushroom) also blends well with simmered chai. Play around with these recipes to make them your own!

- 1 heaping teaspoon nettles
- 1 teaspoon oat straw
- 1 teaspoon rolled or quick oats
- ½–1 teaspoon yerba maté, rooibos, or black tea* (optional)
- 1 pinch powdered or cut/sifted licorice root
- 1 pinch freshly grated nutmeg
- 5 whole cloves
- 1–3 thin slices fresh ginger
- 2–3 cardamom pods, cracked
- 1–2 cinnamon sticks
- 1 whole star anise
- Maple syrup (optional)
- Cream or milk (optional)

Combine all the herbs with 2 cups water over high heat. Bring to a boil, then reduce the heat and let simmer, covered, for 20 minutes. (Alternatively, pour 2 cups boiling water over the herbs and let steep, covered, for 30 to 60 minutes.) Strain. Add maple syrup and cream to taste, if desired, and enjoy.

***If you're using black tea, add it in the last few minutes of steeping or simmering to avoid an overly bitter brew. Note that both black tea and yerba maté contain caffeine.**

it every day long term.) Fresh horsetail can block vitamin B_1 absorption; however, it shouldn't be an issue once it is dried or tinctured. Horsetail may interact with some medications, such as diuretics, heart medications, lithium, and nicotine.

▸ Oat Straw

Avena sativa

Availability: G C

Key Properties: Oat straw is just one of the many forms of oats you can enjoy as food and medicine. The straw represents the grassy bulk of the herb harvested while it is still green, with or without the tops. Ounce for ounce, it offers approximately four times more vitamins and minerals than oatmeal, and the mild hay flavor works well in tea formulas. Oat straw is almost equally rich in calcium, magnesium, and iron as stinging nettle, with supportive silica and B vitamins. Because of this, oat straw not only blends well with nettle but can also be used as a substitute if you don't like nettle's "green" flavor or its strong diuretic effect.

Additional Benefits: The mild flavor of oat straw makes a nice base for light, flavorful herbs like lemongrass, rose petals, lemon verbena, and Korean licorice mint in tea. The immature oat grain, which exudes a milky sap when squished, is referred to as "milky oats" or "milky oat seed." Alkaloids in this fresh latex relax and nourish the nervous-adrenal system and may also help quell withdrawal symptoms for addicts. Unfortunately, this alkaloid is lost upon drying and is not present in the other forms of oats. (But see page 57 for more on milky oat seed.) Dry oat tops still make a nice nutritive tea akin to the straw.

Preparation: Make oat straw as a standard tea, super infusion, or decoction. You can add oat straw to broth, but you'll want to strain it out — the human digestive system can't break down grass. That said, it can be used in capsule form, usually in combination with other nutritive herbs. Standard herb doses (see page 298) apply, or up to a full ounce per day.

Cautions and Considerations: Oat straw is extremely safe (unless, of course, you're allergic to oats). For those who are sensitive to gluten, note that oat straw itself doesn't contain gluten; however, it might be contaminated with gluten on shared processing equipment (though cross-contamination is more likely for oatmeal than for oat straw). Look for oat straw in a happy shade of light green; brown oat straw is either too old or was not properly processed, though it might still offer some nutrition.

▸ Raspberry Leaf

Rubus idaeus and related species

Availability: G+ W+ C+

Key Properties: Although raspberry leaf is best known as a women's herb, as a nutritive it's beneficial for anyone. When prepared as a super infusion, the freshly dried leaves provide a surprising amount of vitamin C (important for healthy collagen and tissue) as well as significant doses of calcium and iron. They taste pleasant and a bit puckery (thanks to their astringency) and make a nice tea ingredient.

Additional Benefits: In addition to providing a wealth of nutrients, raspberry leaf has important yet gentle astringent effects, which is common among rose-family herbs. As an astringent, raspberry leaf tightens and tones tissue, improving its function, and has a particular affinity for the uterus, digestive tract, and mouth (gums). It even strengthens the muscles of the uterus; standard raspberry leaf tea is often drunk during the last trimester of pregnancy to facilitate a swift, easy birth. In the gut, it can help counter chronic diarrhea as well as leaky gut, though blackberry root provides more potent antidiarrheal support.

Preparation: Leaves from wild raspberry plants are preferred. Harvest the vibrant green first-year leaves in spring or early summer. (Second-year canes have woody stems, less vibrant leaves, and — ultimately — flowers and berries.) Nibble a leaf and harvest from stands that have a slight tang, like raspberry fruits; they'll make a more flavorful and medicinally potent tea. Though raspberry's thorns aren't as vicious as those of its

Red Tea

Using hibiscus and rose hips as your base, play around with whatever other red and fruity herbs you have on hand for an antioxidant-rich brew. If the tea is too tart for your taste, sweeten with your favorite natural sweetener.

- 1 teaspoon hibiscus
- ½ teaspoon rose hips
- ½ teaspoon dried elderberries, hawthorn berries, blueberries, and/or bilberries
- ½ teaspoon lycii (goji) berries
- ½ teaspoon rooibos

Combine the herbs. Pour 2 cups boiling water over them and let steep, covered, for 20 minutes. Strain and reheat if necessary.

relatives, you may want to wear gloves. We use raspberry leaf almost exclusively as tea, whether as a regular or super infusion; standard herb doses (see page 298) apply. Super infusions will provide more nutrients but may be too astringent and bitter for some.

Cautions and Considerations: Raspberry leaf is very safe, even in pregnancy. Although studies suggest that up to 6 cups of raspberry tea daily is safe during pregnancy, I'd recommend just 1 or 2 cups daily of a standard (not super) infusion during the second and third trimesters. Raspberry's astringent action may aggravate constipation, and strong tea on an empty stomach may cause nausea and low blood sugar in sensitive folks.

▸ Rose Hips

Rosa spp.

Availability: G+ W+ C+

Key Properties: The rose family provides many delicious and nutritious fruits, including hawthorn, raspberry, apple, cherry, and peach. The matriarch of this family is no exception. Rose hips, the fruit that develops on rosebushes, contain more vitamin C per ounce than almost any other natural source. They also contain antioxidant, anti-inflammatory, and antihistamine bioflavonoids that work in synergy with vitamin C. Bioflavonoids improve vitamin C's ability to strengthen connective tissue, bolster immune health, promote healing, and boost cellular energy. Rose hips have a pleasant flavor reminiscent of slightly tart raisins or tomatoes. They combine well with hibiscus and other red or fruity herbs.

Additional Benefits: New research suggests that rose hip flesh and seeds decrease inflammation and arthritis pain. Rose petals (and rose flower water and rose essential oil) have very different benefits; they are astringent, like raspberry leaf, and can gladden the heart and calm the nerves. See page 158 for more about rose petals.

Preparation: Gather rose hips from any rose that makes a nice-looking hip and hasn't been sprayed with chemicals, preferably heirloom or wild species. Popular species include seaside or rugosa (*R. rugosa*) and dog (*R. canina*). The invasive *R. multiflora* can also be used, but take care not to compost or otherwise spread the seeds. Choose hips that are deep red and taste sweet, typically after the first frost (note that peak flavor and quality vary by locale and species and may occur earlier or later than the first frost). Slice them open to check for worms (especially in large hips like those of *R. rugosa*). The tiny hairs found within the hips can irritate the throat, so either remove the hairs with a small spoon, dry hips whole (and risk a few worms), or thoroughly strain your tea/preparation using a tightly woven cloth or coffee filter before serving. Truth be told, sometimes hips are easier to just buy, but it's nice to have some plants on hand in the garden to play with.

Rose hips are most often used as tea but can also be taken in capsules, powder, jam, cordials, and oxymels. Standard herb doses (see page 298) apply. Rose hips lose potency quickly in storage and are best used within 6 to 12 months.

Cautions and Considerations: Rose hips are extremely safe. Just be careful to strain out the irritating hairs (if you're processing your own), and know that the vitamin C and other benefits dissipate with long storage or with excess heat during processing.

▸ Dandelion

Taraxacum officinale

Availability: G W+ C+

Key Properties: This weedy ally grows almost anywhere and is edible from petal to root. The nutrient-dense plant offers a range of vitamins and minerals in both the root and leaf. The bitter leaves contain more iron and calcium (though the roots are still considered good sources of these nutrients), whereas the sweeter yellow flowers contain carotenoids like lutein. The dried raw or roasted roots have a woody, bitter chocolaty, coffeelike flavor that blends well with burdock

GETTING NUTRIENTS FROM HERBS

Nutrient	Benefits	RDA	Good Herbal Sources (per 1 ounce)*
Vitamin A/ beta-carotene	Supports vision and eye health, immune function, red blood cell production, healthy lubrication/mucous membranes; functions as antioxidant. Severe deficiency causes blindness.	5,000 IU vitamin A or 600 mg beta-carotene	Violet leaf (3,400 mg), alaria (2,406 mg beta-carotene), calendula (850 mg mixed carotenoids), lycii/goji berry (rich in zeaxanthin)
Vitamin C	Strengthens immune function (increases resistance to infections and cancer, reduces histamine in allergies and colds); serves as antioxidant; supports eye health, cardiovascular health, energy production, connective tissue integrity. Deficiency can cause scurvy, which causes connective tissue to disintegrate.	60 mg	Rose hip (710 mg), alfalfa (265 mg), raspberry leaf (75 mg), violet leaf (75 mg), lycii/goji berry (42 mg), hibiscus flower (33 mg)
Calcium	Promotes bone formation (with vitamin D and weight-bearing exercise); maintains electrolyte balance alkaline-acid balance, and blood pressure balance; helps regulate muscle contractions; helps prevent kidney stones and colorectal cancer. Deficiency can cause osteoporosis (bone loss) and dental problems.	1,000 mg	Nettle leaf (935 mg), kelp (860 mg), horsetail (680 mg), alfalfa (490 mg), oat straw (405 mg), dandelion leaf (370 mg), red clover flower (370 mg), raspberry leaf (345 mg), alaria (310 mg)
Iron	Enriches red blood cells with hemoglobin, improving oxygen transport and energy levels. Deficiency results in anemia, characterized by pale skin, fatigue, depression, anxiety, and heart and breathing issues.	18 mg	Dandelion leaf (140 mg), chickweed (70 mg), burdock root (40 mg), horsetail (35 mg), marshmallow root (33 mg), raspberry leaf (29 mg), oat straw (28 mg), dandelion root (27 mg), yellow dock root (20 mg)
Magnesium	Supports energy metabolism, cardiovascular health; helps regulate muscle relaxation, nerve function, and blood pressure; promotes bone formation; helps prevent migraines. Mild deficiency aggravates muscle cramps/tension.	400 mg	Oat straw (420 mg), kelp (245 mg), nettle leaf (245 mg), burdock root (150 mg), alfalfa (125 mg), horsetail (125 mg), cacao/cocoa (100 mg), red clover flower (100 mg)
Potassium	Works with sodium to maintain fluid balance, acts as enzyme cofactor, supports cardiovascular system, prevents kidney stones, promotes bone formation, regulates blood pressure. Deficiency can cause electrolyte imbalance, fatigue, muscle cramps, intestinal issues, and cardiovascular issues and can be fatal in extreme cases.	4,700 mg	Oat straw (2,235 mg), dulse, alaria (2,187 mg), dandelion root (2,125 mg), nettle leaf (1,050 mg), dandelion leaf (780 mg), alfalfa (576 mg), red clover flower (565 mg), horsetail (510 mg), lycii/goji berry (473 mg)
Iodine	Supports thyroid function primarily, but also immune function. Deficiency results in hypothyroid disease, with symptoms of fatigue, weight gain, goiter, depression, and sensitivity to cold.	150 mcg	Kelp (153,000 mg), dulse (56,400 mg), alaria (56,100 mg)
Silica	Contributes to healthy hair, skin, nails, bones and helps maintain the elasticity and strength of connective tissue. Deficiency can cause brittle, ridged nails and poor skin and hair health.	N/A	Unrefined rice (2,970 mg), horsetail (2,750 mg), oat straw (210 mg), nettle leaf (185 mg)

*These numbers give the nutrient content in the whole plant. They don't take into account how much will actually become soluble/bioavailable when the plant is prepared as a tea, tincture, or other remedy. And some herbs may not be well tolerated or may have side effects at a dose of 1 ounce (dry). For example, seaweeds (kelp, dulse, alaria) would provide an overdose of iodine, which may cause a hyperthyroid storm.

and chicory root in tea. You might find the leaves unpleasantly bitter in tea, but they pair well with strong flavors like garlic and lemon alongside milder greens in recipes.

Additional Benefits: Dandelion is an herbal pharmacopoeia! The leaves and roots offer similar benefits. Alongside their nutrient density, they offer digestive bitters that stimulate all aspects of digestive function as well as detoxification via the liver (increasing bile production and excretion) and kidneys (the diuretic action makes you pee). But each part has its affinities. The leaves have a greater affinity for the kidneys as a diuretic, whereas the roots focus more on the liver. Their diuretic effects vary, too; the leaves act as a volume diuretic (making you pee, lots), whereas the roots are more sodium leaching (encouraging the body to eliminate more sodium in the urine, and then the water follows by osmosis). Diuretics generally also eliminate potassium, but dandelion is rich in potassium, helping to replace what is lost. These diuretic effects can help with edema, water retention, and, in some cases, hypertension. The bitter, liver-supportive properties of dandelion make it useful for aiding digestion, relieving constipation, improving fat digestion and absorption, improving skin issues, and lowering cholesterol and blood sugar levels. The fresh roots may also relieve allergies, acting as a natural antihistamine.

Preparation: The leaves taste best (less bitter) before dandelion blooms in early spring, and the roots are most potent after a hard frost. But you can harvest any part of dandelion at any time to use it fresh or dry. Dandelion makes a great tincture, tea (especially if made with the root, roasted or not), capsule, infused vinegar, or digestive cordial. Standard herb doses (see page 298) apply. As mentioned, the leaves can be eaten and make a fabulous pesto when combined with pumpkin seeds, garlic, lemon, olive oil, and Parmesan (see the recipe on page 274). Don't be alarmed by a cloudy white substance at the bottom of dandelion root tincture; it's just the inulin.

Cautions and Considerations: Dandelion is generally safe. The French name, *pissenlit*, which means "piss the bed," reminds us that bedtime is not the best time to take diuretics. Though it has a much weaker action than pharmaceuticals, be cautious when using therapeutic doses of dandelion with medications that interact with pharmaceutical diuretics. Dandelion may aggravate acute gut inflammation and some (but not all) cases of reflux. If you've got an intestinal, bowel, or bile duct blockage, don't try to fix it with dandelion — call your doctor. And be sure to properly identify dandelion using a field guide, because many plants look similar.

Weed Pesto

This isn't a formal recipe so much as an idea and inspiration. Walk through your garden and grab a couple of handfuls of nutritious and flavorful weeds and herbs. Toss them in the blender. Experiment with nettles (if you have a good blender — otherwise they might give a mild sting), basil, parsley, oregano, chives, arugula, kale, dandelion, bee balm, lemon balm, purslane, lamb's-quarter, sorrel, pigweed, chickweed . . . Add to the blender some pumpkin seeds, pine nuts or tree nuts, grated Parmesan, a few cloves of garlic, a healthy dose of olive oil, a squeeze of lemon, salt, or whatever strikes your fancy. Process the ingredients until they form a paste.

Spread the pesto on toast and sandwiches, use it as a dip for crackers or vegetables, dollop into soup, smear on homemade pizza, use to marinate meats or tofu, and so on.

▸ Seaweed

Availability: W C+

Key Properties: "Seaweed" represents a broad class of sea vegetables that are rich in minerals like calcium as well as trace minerals like iodine and selenium. Depending on the species, seaweed can also be a good source of beta-carotene, iron, B vitamins, and fiber. Popular and common seaweeds include various species of kelp, alaria, wakame, dulse, nori, bladderwrack, kombu, and hijiki.

Additional Benefits: Brown seaweeds like kelp and bladderwrack contain therapeutic doses of iodine, which help prevent hypothyroid disease and other iodine deficiency disorders and may protect against radiation exposure. Bladderwrack also contains fucoxanthin, a carotenoid that may promote fat burning and aid weight loss. Brown seaweeds also contain sodium alginate, which binds to heavy metals and other compounds, making them potentially beneficial for detoxification. Furthermore, kombu and kelp contain special enzymes and compounds that break down complex starches, so adding a strip of either type of seaweed to a pot of simmering beans will reduce their "toot factor."

Preparation: You can make capsules and decoction-style tinctures with seaweed; under a practitioner's supervision, standard herb doses (see page 298) apply, but otherwise use smaller quantities. More often we eat small quantities of seaweed as part of a regular diet, particularly in soup or as a seasoning blend. The iodine content can dissipate with poor storage, high heat, and powdering, but toasted seaweed tastes great and will still offer other minerals. Sesame seeds and sesame oil improve the flavor of seaweed dramatically.

Cautions and Considerations: Purchase seaweed from a reputable supplier who harvests it from clean waters because seaweed can be contaminated with heavy metals and other unpleasantries from polluted oceans. Maine Coast Sea Vegetables tests its seaweed for purity. If you have hypertension or salt sensitivity, you may want to limit seaweed since it is high in sodium. However, it may still be useful as a salt substitute because it contains much less sodium than salt, with a better balance of other minerals. Unless you're working with your health-care practitioner, stick to low doses. Excessive amounts iodine from seaweed can cause hyperthyroid toxicity. Limit brown seaweed intake in cases of hyperthyroid disease, where any added iodine intake may be dangerous, unless under the supervision of a practitioner.

Salt Plus Seaweed Seasoning

This blend is inspired by In Joy Organics' Sea Shakes. Combining seaweed and salt helps you trim down on sodium while boosting the calcium, iodine, and potassium content in your food. It's surprisingly tasty, particularly on popcorn.

- ½ ounce dried dulse
- ½ ounce dried kelp
- ½–1 ounce sea salt (iodized or regular)

Grind your dulse and kelp to a powder using a blender or grinder. Mix with the salt. Pour into a saltshaker, and keep it by the stove or on the table.

▸ CALENDULA

Calendula officinalis

Availability: G+ C

Key Properties: These bright blossoms bring cheer to any garden with their vibrant yellow, orange, and sometimes red-tinged petals, and they just won't quit putting out new blooms from late spring through autumn frosts. The fresh petals and dried flower heads provide 100 times more carotenoids (including lutein and beta-carotene) than a sweet potato by weight. These antioxidant carotenoids support the eyes, immune health, and mucous membranes. Enjoy a sprinkle of petals in everything from eggs to salad. The fat-soluble nutrients will color soup broths golden, hence the common name pot marigold. Fed to livestock, the beta-carotene transfers to egg yolks and butter, enhancing their yellow hue and boosting their vitamin A content.

Additional Benefits: Calendula is healing, soothing, anti-inflammatory, detoxifying via the lymph, and slightly antimicrobial. Its soothing, vulnerary properties help heal the gut when taken in tea, broth, or food, and the herb-infused oil makes fabulous all-purpose skin salves and baby-care formulas for dry skin, rashes, and minor wounds.

Preparation: Pinch off the flower tops every few days (your fingers will get sticky with the healing resin), and use them fresh or dry them for later use. You'll get more blooms and, consequently, more medicine this way. Let some flowers go to seed in autumn, and this annual might continue to self-seed for future years. Use calendula in tea, tincture, broth, and food and infused in oil for topical use. Calendula gets bitter if you overdo it in tea or broth, but it's mild and nearly flavorless if you stick to the petals and combine it with other flavors. Standard herb doses (see page 298) apply.

Cautions and Considerations: Though the flower is generally safe, the central florets can irritate the throat of sensitive people. If you're allergic to other flowers in the daisy-ragweed family, approach calendula with caution. If you're purchasing calendula, be willing to pay more for recently harvested plants from small-scale producers, and use color as a cue to how potent it is. Carotenoids lose potency during storage. You'll notice a dramatic loss of color within 6 to 12 months of harvest, but you can still use older calendula (with varying effects).

Super-Infused Nutri-Tea

You'll get 15 to 30 times the nutrients in your cup of tea if you super-infuse it. Use this technique for the gentle nutritive and tonic herbs, like nettle and oat straw, which are safe to use even in large quantities, and not for really potent medicinal herbs (stimulants, laxatives, et cetera). You'll need a quart-size container, like a mason jar or French press, for brewing the tea.

1 ounce nutritive herbs

Put the herbs in a quart jar. Pour enough boiling water over the herbs to fill the jar. Stir, cover, and let steep for 4 hours or overnight. Strain, squeezing as much liquid as you possibly can from the herbs. (This is where a French press comes in handy! Otherwise, strain the tea through a tightly woven cloth or jelly bag and squeeze the spent herbs with your hands.)

Drink as desired, warming the tea first if you like. Store leftover tea in the refrigerator, where it will keep for up to 2 days.

Nutritive Bone Broth

Simmering leftover bones in water makes a nutrient-dense broth rich in minerals like iron and calcium, as well as beneficial gelatin. Adding a splash of apple cider vinegar increases the breakdown of minerals from the bones. But you don't have to stop there. Add nutritive, adaptogenic, and tonic herbs and immune-enhancing mushrooms to give yourself a boost whenever you use the broth in recipes. For a vegetarian version, simmer everything but the bones, and add 1 tablespoon of miso paste per cup of hot water before serving. Feel free to adapt the recipe to your taste buds and the ingredients you have on hand.

BROTH BASE

- About 1 gallon water
- 1–2 poultry carcasses, or 12 cut beef bones, or 1–3 fish carcasses
- Splash of apple cider vinegar
- Basic stock vegetables (onions, garlic, carrots, celery, or whatever you prefer)

NUTRITIVE HERBS

Add any of the following:

- 1–2 tablespoons nettles, oat straw, and/or horsetail
- 1 tablespoon seaweed flakes or 1–3 large strips seaweed
- 1 tablespoon calendula

SEASONINGS

- ¼–1 teaspoon turmeric
- Pinch of cayenne
- Salt and freshly ground black pepper

IMMUNE, ADAPTOGENIC & TONIC HERBS

Add any of the following:

- 3 slices astragalus root
- 1 tablespoon codonopsis root
- 1 tablespoon ashwagandha root
- 1 fresh burdock root, sliced, or 1 tablespoon dried
- 6 ounces fresh shiitakes and/or maitakes, or 1 tablespoon powdered
- 1 slice reishi

Combine all the ingredients in a large pot or slow cooker. Bring to a slow simmer, and let simmer over low heat for 3 hours or longer (up to 3 days in a slow cooker). Strain and use as desired in recipes calling for broth. To concentrate the broth, after you strain it, simmer the broth uncovered until it is reduced to one-quarter to one-half the original volume. You can freeze it for later use (in ice-cube trays if you like, for preportioned servings). For therapeutic uses, aim to consume 1 cup of broth or 1 ounce of concentrated broth (that's one ice cube) once or twice daily.

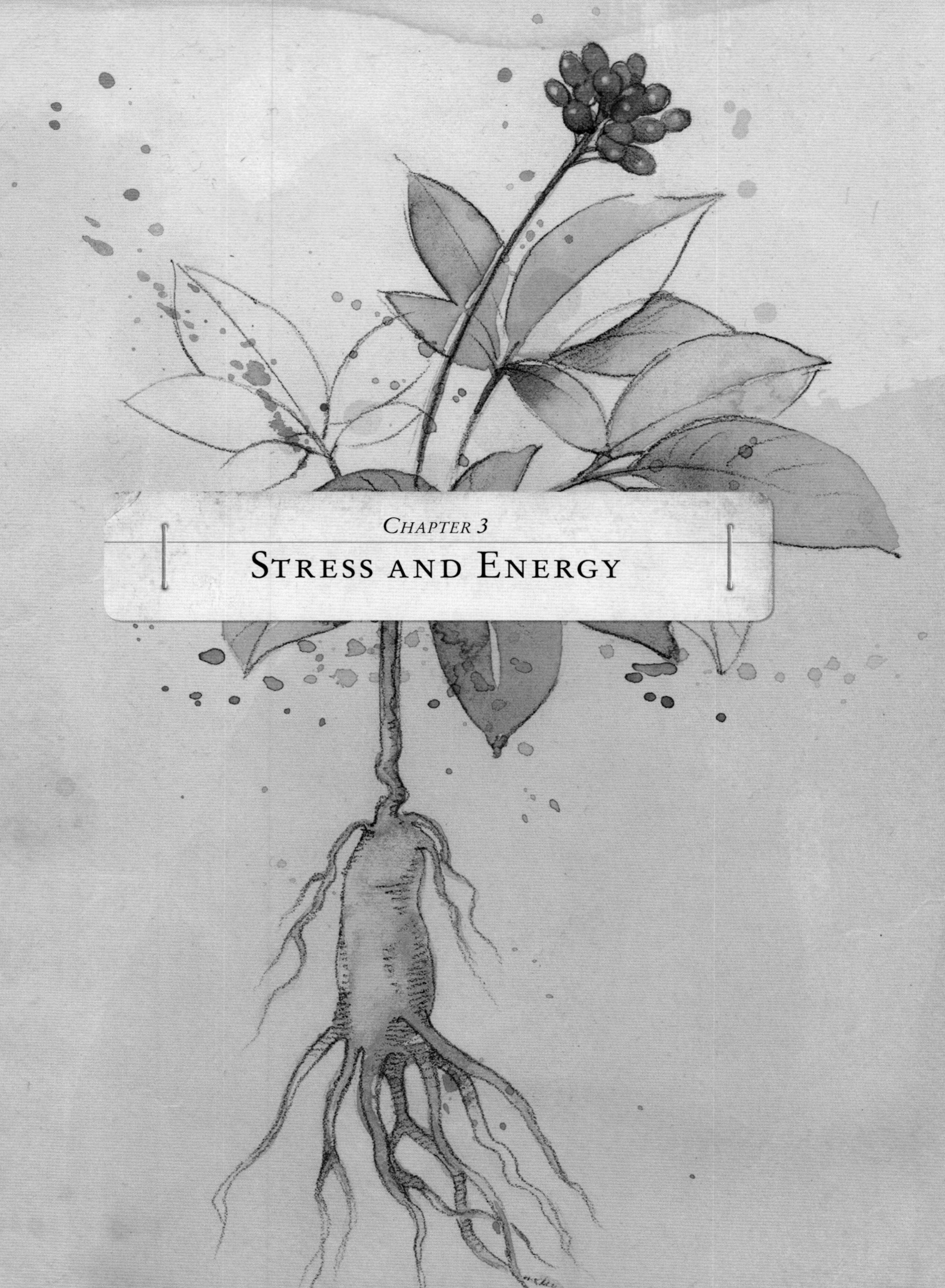

Chapter 3

Stress and Energy

If you feel like stress interferes with your quality of life, you're not alone. More than 75 percent of Americans stress out regularly. Common culprits include work, money, relationships and family, health, sleep deprivation, poor nutrition, and media overload. These and other stressors can put your nervous-system stress response into overdrive, which sets off a chain of bad reactions throughout your body. The good news? Healthy habits and herbs can help flip the switch in your favor.

Why Is Stress So Bad?

The term "stress" can mean many things. Most often, it refers to the sympathetic nervous system response known as "fight or flight." An interconnected surge of neurotransmitters (nervous system) and stress hormones (endocrine system) triggers widespread effects throughout your body to help you meet the demands of the perceived threat. The foremost result is a burst of energy, which would have been crucial for helping our ancestors fight or flee from imminent threats like large wild beasts. Today some of us actually enjoy and rely on those quick bursts of stress-induced energy. Other positive effects of short-term stress include the following:

- Increased brain activity
- Expanded airways
- Increased heart strength, blood viscosity, and clotting
- Increased blood flow to the organs involved in fighting and fleeing
- Decreased blood flow to the periphery and the "rest and repair" organs

But your body isn't meant to sustain the stress response over the long term, and doing so causes wear and tear on many body systems. Some of the negative effects of long-term stress include the following:

- Cognition and memory issues
- Insomnia
- Fatigue and/or feeling "wired"
- Depression and/or anxiety
- Increased inflammation
- Poor metabolism, including elevated cortisol and blood sugar, which can lead to diabetes and abdominal weight gain
- Slow digestion, indigestion, gas, pain, bloating, irritable bowel syndrome, and/or constipation
- Reduced cardiovascular health, including increased risk of stroke, high blood pressure, and high cholesterol levels
- Decreased libido and impaired reproductive health and function
- Decreased detoxification
- Slower, less adequate digestion and elimination
- Decreased immune function
- Slower, less effective wound healing and reduced connective tissue integrity

So you can see how just one little thing — stress — can affect your entire well-being and factor into a range of diseases. In my clinical practice, chronic stress is a *major* player in most of my clients' health concerns and general state of vitality. Just addressing stress levels and helping the body balance stress hormones can correct or reduce the severity of conditions that may not otherwise seem related.

Because stress played an integral role in humans' early survival, the compounds that elicit the stress response are incredibly potent. Adrenaline (a.k.a. epinephrine) functions as both a neurotransmitter and a hormone. Why is this important? Neurotransmitters travel through your nervous system quickly, jumping from synapse to synapse, which triggers a lightning-fast response. Enzymes break neurotransmitters down very quickly, too, which means the effects are short lived. In contrast, hormones travel through your blood, acting on cell receptor sites. Hormones move more slowly than neurotransmitters but take longer to be broken down and eliminated (via liver detoxification). Eventually, the stress hormone cortisol gets in on the action, releasing a steady stream of sugar from storage into your bloodstream to fuel the perceived stress demands and shifting your levels of energy and fatigue, wakefulness and sleepiness, and metabolism.

These stress-related compounds are an essential part of health, but chronic stress throws them out of whack and pulls your body out of balance quickly. If you really were responding to a primal source of stress, such as a saber-toothed tiger, the physical acts of fighting or fleeing would help clear these stress hormones from your system more quickly. However, modern sources of stress don't generally give you a physical outlet. This is one reason chronic stress causes so much damage across your body systems — and it explains why regular exercise does such a nice job decreasing the effects of stress.

Addressing stress culprits should be your main goal. You can do a number of things in your routine — from quitting a terrible job and saying no more often to taking up a regular meditation practice and exercising regularly — to reduce your stress levels. But you can also take action with herbs that help the body adapt to stress, and you can encourage your body to return to the parasympathetic rest and repair state. Enter the wonderful world of adaptogens.

Managing Stress *with* Adaptogens

Adaptogens help your body adapt to stress. Soviet researcher Nikolai Vasilyevich Lazarev coined the term in the mid-1940s, and the concept was researched heavily in the region during that time. Adaptogens are not bound to a particular plant family or categorized by a specific group of plant chemicals but are defined by their actions:

- They're relatively nontoxic and safe.
- They have beneficial effects on a range of body systems.
- They often have a modulating effect. For example, depending on whether levels of a particular hormone are low or high, an adaptogen may increase or decrease the body's production of that hormone.
- They seem to work by affecting the stress response and the hypothalamic-pituitary-adrenal axis of the nervous-endocrine system.

WHAT IS AN ADAPTOGEN?

Adaptogenic herbs help your body adapt to stress, mainly by supporting the production of stress-related neurotransmitters and hormones. They're sometimes called "trophorestorative" or "modulating," in reference to the fact that adaptogens can increase or decrease the function of any particular system based on what the body needs most. Generally speaking, adaptogens help you feel less stressed while increasing energy levels; some are zippy, while others are more balancing or calming.

General Uses: We use adaptogens for a range of conditions whenever stress is a primary or underlying factor — which it often is! They are especially helpful when stress has left you feeling fatigued and sluggish (physically and/or mentally). Most support fertility, libido, reproductive function, longevity, overall vitality, mood, and immune strength and modulation. Depending on the herb, some also calm, invigorate, protect the body from toxins, decrease inflammation, balance blood sugar, improve circulation, and/or improve digestion. Most are warming, to varying degrees, which makes them more or less suitable for a person's individual constitution.

Examples: Zippy adaptogens include the ginseng species, eleuthero, rhodiola, codonopsis, jiaogulan, and cordyceps. Balancing and calming adaptogens include reishi, schizandra, ashwagandha, gotu kola, holy basil, bacopa, shatavari, and possibly chaga.

Though the term "adaptogen" isn't even a hundred years old, the herbs that fall into this category have been revered in herbal medicine for millennia. They're mainstays in traditional Chinese medicine as qi tonics and in the Indian medicine system of Ayurveda as rasayana herbs — herbs that improve the vital force or energy within a person. Both of these ancient systems of medicine place a high value on maintaining optimal health — not just treating disease when it occurs — and adaptogens help us do just that. These herbs have long been known to improve vitality, longevity, and energy. Side benefits can include improved brain function, better thyroid health, increased fertility and libido, improved immune system function, decreased inflammation and pain, and enhanced liver detoxification, although the properties vary depending on the herb. Adaptogens can be the core of an herbal formula, but they also play a supporting role in almost any blend because of their antistress effects and side benefits. These adaptogens fall on a continuum: some are more stimulating while others are more calming, even though they all improve energy levels. (See the chart on page 68 for a big-picture breakdown.)

WHAT ABOUT CAFFEINE?

WHEN IT COMES TO ENERGY, most of the world relies on caffeine-containing stimulants, not adaptogens. Caffeine plants like coffee, tea, maté, and cacao are *not* adaptogens — and none of our adaptogens contain caffeine. Caffeine plants do not modulate stress hormones or have the same set of benefits. However, they are quite stimulating. Instead of helping your body adapt to the stress response, however, they *elicit* the stress response. Caffeine acts on a variety of stress- and mood-related hormones and neurotransmitters, increasing the effects of some (like adrenaline and cortisol) while outcompeting and decreasing the effects of others (like gamma-aminobutyric acid, or GABA). Caffeine-rich plants have many benefits and certainly boost energy, but long-term reliance on caffeine for energy will deplete your overall vitality.

Green and white tea and chocolate may still be worthy additions to your herbal routine because they contain less caffeine while offering antioxidant, anti-inflammatory, blood-sugar-balancing, and mood-boosting benefits. Coffee and yerba maté (preferably "green" or unsmoked) contain more caffeine and semi-impressive benefits. Beware of the high-caffeine kola nut and guarana, as well as "caffeine stacking" (multiple caffeine sources) found in mass-market energy, libido, and weight-loss products. Excessive caffeine can have serious effects on your heart, nerves, brain function, mood, and muscles and may even become life threatening. High-caffeine plants are among the most druglike herbs in common use. One large coffee from Starbucks or a store-bought energy drink can have 300 mg or more of caffeine. That's 10 times more caffeine than what you get from a cup of green tea. And it's highly addictive. Reducing or kicking your caffeine habit can cause unpleasant withdrawal symptoms including headaches, irritability, brain fog, chronic pain, and fatigue. In contrast, adaptogens don't provide the quick hit of energy, but they are completely nonaddictive and offer a greater range of benefits, supporting the body in maintaining balance.

Stimulating Adaptogens

Stimulating adaptogens represent the most potent source of physical and mental energy. Think of them when the body is depleted, deficient, dragging, and depressed. One of the fascinating things about this particular group of plants is that most of them grow in harsh climates, like Siberia or mountain ranges — these plants seem to know what real stress is like!

General Preparations: Stimulating adaptogens can be taken in standard herb doses (see page 298) in any form: tea (preferably decocted), pill, tincture. Some are more palatable than others. You can bring their stimulating properties down a notch by combining them with more balancing and calming adaptogens (ashwagandha, holy basil) and nervine herbs (milky oat seed, lemon balm) or make them more energizing (for better or worse) in combination with caffeine plants (green tea, yerba maté, cacao). Chai spices (cinnamon, ginger, cardamom, nutmeg) tend to improve their flavor and synergize their effects.

General Cautions: Stimulating adaptogens are better taken in the morning; evening doses might interfere with sleep. More is not better. Use caution in a body system that's already overstimulated. These adaptogens can aggravate anxiety, insomnia, mania, hypertension, and heart palpitations in some people. Do not use them during pregnancy without professional supervision. They may interact with some medications.

▸ Ginseng

Panax spp.

Availability: G- W- C

Key Properties: Ginseng has been revered in traditional Chinese medicine (TCM) for more than 2,000 years. According to the herbal theory of the Doctrine of Signatures, a plant looks like the body system or ailment it heals. In the case of Asian ginseng, the freshly dug root looks like the human body, and indeed, it benefits the whole body. Consider ginseng if you feel sluggish, lack vitality, are having fertility or libido issues, suffer from immune deficiency — basically, when you're old or feel old. True ginseng comes in three primary forms: Asian ginseng (*Panax ginseng*) can be found as "white ginseng" (the crude root) or "red ginseng" (the specially cured root, which has a reddish hue and a more warming, stimulating action). American ginseng (*P. quinquefolius*) is used similarly, as a crude root, but it's more popular for women and has a slightly gentler action.

Additional Benefits: Ginseng has many benefits, which is why it is so overused. It protects the liver from toxins, may balance blood sugar in diabetes, corrects erectile dysfunction, improves libido and the vitality and function of sexual organs in men and women, may aid in depression, and much more.

Preparation: See the general preparations, above. Standard herb doses (see page 298) apply.

Cautions and Considerations: See the general cautions, above.

GINSENG, BY ANY OTHER NAME . . .

DURING THE 1980S AND '90S, ginseng's fame as an energy herb — alongside its expense — had created a huge market demand for anything named "ginseng." Companies worked "ginseng" into the name of as many plants as they could: Siberian ginseng for eleuthero (which is at least a ginseng cousin), Indian ginseng for ashwagandha, Brazilian ginseng for suma, and so forth. Ultimately, the American Herbal Products Association put the kibosh on calling anything "ginseng" that isn't in the *Panax* genus.

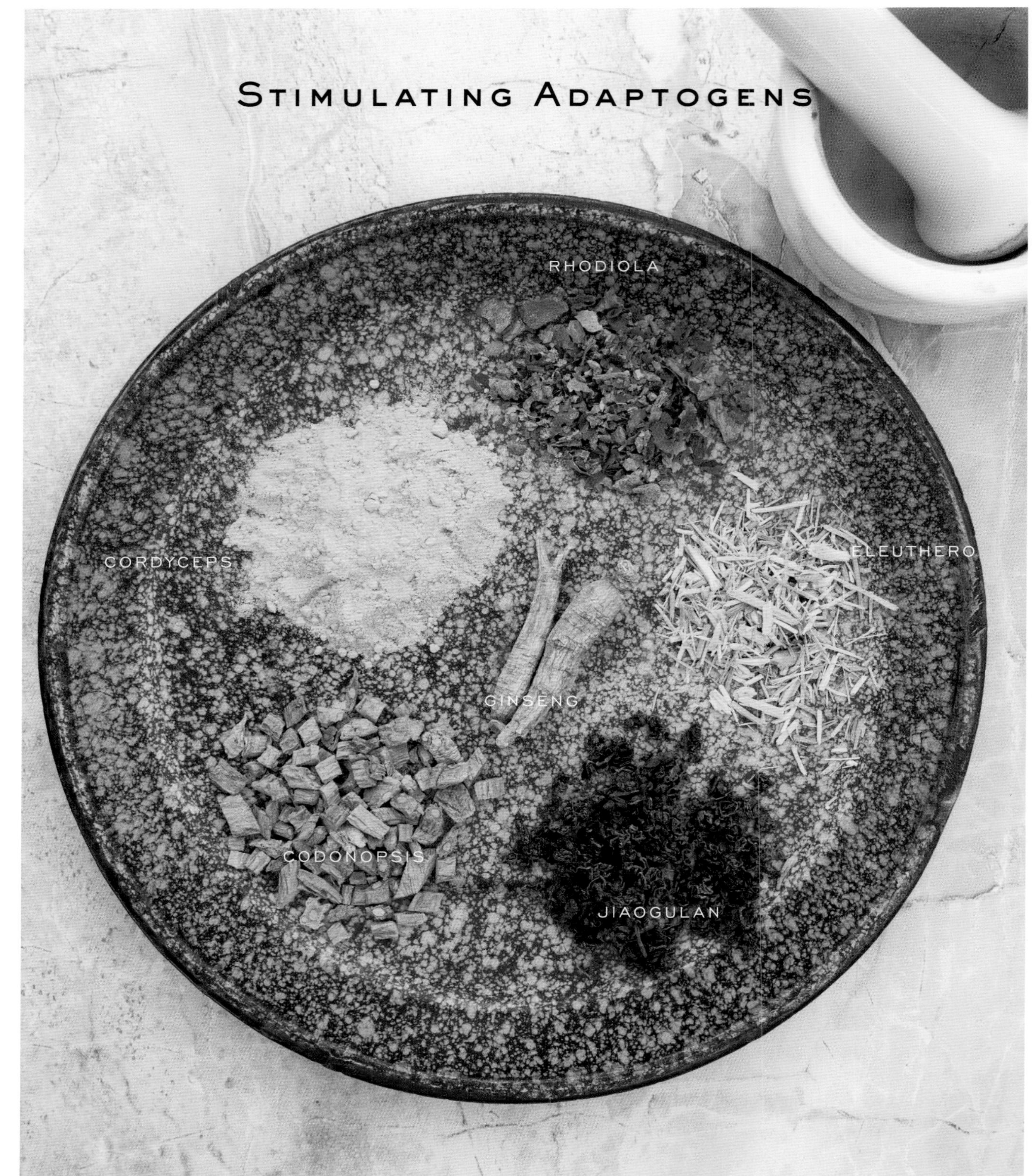
STIMULATING ADAPTOGENS
RHODIOLA
CORDYCEPS
ELEUTHERO
GINSENG
CODONOPSIS
JIAOGULAN

History and Ethical Considerations: China placed such a high demand on the longevity, vitality, libido, and fertility benefits of ginseng that it was nearly dug out of existence. It is notoriously difficult to cultivate because critters and microbes love it as much as people. New World explorers were asked to keep an eye out for similar plants. In 1718 a Jesuit priest "discovered" American ginseng, which grows wild in the Appalachian Mountains. These slow-growing roots — some more than 50 years old — were quickly shipped off to China, and American ginseng trade offered our fledgling country some of its first post-Revolution international trade opportunities. An average of 140,000 tons (and up to a record 600,000 tons in 1824) were exported annually. Even Daniel Boone was in on the action; his family fortune is credited to the ginseng harvest, not animal skin trades. Three centuries later, we are left in a similar state as China. Though both ginseng species can be incredibly useful herbs, the wild stands have been overharvested and the ginseng demand still exceeds the supply. In spite of the law, a lot of ginseng on the market is illegally poached, of poor quality, or adulterated. If you buy ginseng, purchase certified organic plants from a reputable supplier (even though it's expensive) and be wary of imported and too-good-to-be-true cheap products. If you'd like to grow your own, look to herb-growing guru Richo Cech's books and the website of his company, Horizon Herbs, for tips. I keep only a little organic *Panax* tincture on hand and generally favor more sustainable and affordable alternatives.

▸ Eleuthero

Eleutherococcus senticosus

Availability: G- C

Key Properties: This is among our best-researched adaptogens and a favorite for relieving stress and building energy. Soviet researchers tested the effects of eleuthero root — formerly called Siberian ginseng — on approximately 5,000 people during the late 1900s, including factory workers and athletes. They found that eleuthero significantly improved the response to physical and mental stressors, including loud noises, temperature fluctuations, and increased workload. People taking eleuthero were shown to have better performance, health, and vitality under stressful conditions.

Additional Benefits: Eleuthero also improves immune function, lifts depression, protects the liver from toxins, and improves overall health. Even people with serious diseases (including heart disease, diabetes, and cancer) usually tolerate it well. In holistic cancer protocols, eleuthero may be combined with medicinal mushrooms and other tonic herbs as a complement to conventional care to improve vitality and decrease the side effects of treatment.

Preparation: See the general preparations, page 47. Standard herb doses (see page 298) apply.

Cautions and Considerations: See the general cautions, page 47. High doses (4.5 to 6 mL of liquid extract, one to two times per day) of eleuthero tend to raise blood pressure. In low to moderate doses, it has a more beneficial modulating effect, reducing blood pressure in people with hypertension, raising it in people with hypotension.

▸ Rhodiola

Rhodiola rosea

Availability: W- C

Key Properties: Siberians macerate this rose-scented root in vodka to make a tonic that they say improves overall vitality and longevity; some claim it will help them live to be more than 100 years old. Rhodiola is a relative newcomer to Western herbalism but has quickly climbed the ranks of much-loved energy herbs. Studies support its traditional use as a tonic for improving energy, focus, and vitality, and it has been shown to help the body make adenosine triphospate (ATP), which provides energy on a cellular level. It works quickly, and it has proved helpful for night shift workers, students, and athletes alike.

My college students can attest to its ability to improve focus, memory, mental energy, and test scores while reducing exam stress, and menopausal clients love it for relieving brain fog and stress-related memory lapse.

Additional Benefits: Rhodiola has neuroprotective and restorative effects, which can be helpful in conditions and infections that affect the brain and nervous system, such as Lyme disease or after an injury.

Preparation: Rhodiola's ability to improve your level of alertness increases as the dosage goes up, and high doses (500+ mg) can be used short term for increased physical or mental demands. Just 100 mg will suffice for gentle, daily support. Because it's unpleasant tasting, most people take rhodiola as a tincture or capsule.

Cautions and Considerations: Beyond the usual "zippy adaptogen" cautions (see page 47), rhodiola sometimes causes upset stomachs due to its aromatic and astringent properties. Taking it with food usually fixes the issue.

▸ Codonopsis

Codonopsis pilosula and related species

Availability: G C-

Key Properties: Codonopsis is also called dang shen or poor man's ginseng — even though it is completely unrelated to the *Panax* ginsengs — because it has a similar, albeit gentler, action. This fast-growing bellflower vine produces roots much more easily and abundantly, and in a wider range of climates. The long, thin, wrinkly roots are somewhat soft once dried and pleasant tasting, slightly sweet, and nourishing. Use it like ginseng for energy, stress management, overall vitality, recuperation, and immune system strength.

Additional Benefits: Codonopsis has the reputation of being particularly restorative in nature. It is often used in convalescence for debilitated states associated with fatigue and immune dysfunction, as well as in holistic cancer protocols.

Preparation: Codonopsis's affordability and pleasant, sweet flavor make it one of my favorite ingredients for chai tea, broths, and other daily recipes. Some of my fellow herbalists even add it to porridge and rice dishes. It blends well with mushrooms, astragalus, ginger, lycii, and ashwagandha. You can take it in standard herb doses (see page 298).

Cautions and Considerations: See the general cautions, page 47.

▸ Other Energizing Adaptogens

Another energizing adaptogen is **jiaogulan** leaf, also called poor man's ginseng, which can be brewed much like green tea. For more on jiaogulan, see page 266.

From the world of fungi, **cordyceps** also offers stimulating yet tonic effects for physical and mental stamina as well as increasing energy, libido, and respiratory function. Its actions suggest that it may increase oxygen utilization and levels of oxytocin (a "releasing" reproductive neurotransmitter-hormone associated with a good mood and climax). It's most often taken in capsule form; standard herb doses (see page 298) apply.

Balancing Adaptogens

These midrange adaptogens provide stress support for a broad spectrum of people and conditions. They simultaneously energize and calm. Both herbs also have some very useful side benefits, and they are well tolerated, which makes them extremely useful in formulas.

▸ Ashwagandha

Withania somnifera

Availability: G C

Key Properties: The nutty-aromatic root of ashwagandha reportedly gives you the strength and vitality of a horse; however, it also nourishes and strengthens nervous, adrenal, thyroid, and immune function and decreases inflammation. Classic uses include boosting libido, relieving chronic pain, and promoting vigor, while the herb has also become popular for relieving anxiety and post-traumatic stress disorder (PTSD).

Additional Benefits: In spite of ashwagandha's energy effects, it's also a popular sleep aid. The species name *somnifera* means "sleep inducing."

Preparation: Cultivate ashwagandha as you would tomatoes, and dry ashwagandha root before using it, preferably by itself, as its strong scent can infiltrate other herbs. You can use it in any format, in standard herb doses (see page 298). The powder or cut/sifted root can be simmered in milk, and this fatty delivery system may increase benefits for the fat-lined nervous system. Any fatty "milk" will do; if you avoid conventional dairy, try almond, hemp, or coconut milk. Ashwagandha tastes pleasant enough — earthy, woodsy with a hint of malted milk ball — and you can add some honey or maple syrup and sweet spices to make it even tastier. Ashwagandha blends well in decocted teas, including chai, and with cocoa powder.

Cautions and Considerations: Ashwagandha is generally safe. Watch for rare herb-drug interactions, and don't use it during pregnancy without a professional's supervision. If you react negatively to nightshade plants like potatoes and tomatoes, approach ashwagandha (a relative) cautiously.

▸ Schizandra

Schisandra chinensis

Availability: G- C

Key Properties: Known as wu wei zi or "five flavor fruit," schizandra berry tastes simultaneously sweet, salty, bitter, sour, and pungent. (You either love it or hate it, but adding a sweetener makes it much more pleasant.) In traditional Chinese medicine, the flavor of an herb indicates the constitution for which it is most beneficial, and schizandra's multifaceted flavor means it's a balancing, tonic herb for almost any person. Like ashwagandha, schizandra is as likely to be used for sleep and pleasant dreams as it is for energy, vitality, cognition, mood, and libido.

Additional Benefits: What makes this adaptogen stand out to me is its benefits for the liver. Sour and bitter flavors stimulate digestion and liver detoxification, and research suggests that schizandra is one of our best herbs to increase liver detoxification via the bile as well as to protect and heal the liver itself. Schizandra also benefits immune function and can be used in formulas when the immune system is particularly run down (including cases of mononucleosis and cancer). Schizandra blends well with reproductive tonic herbs by supporting balanced hormone levels.

Preparation: Schizandra can be used in any form, in standard herb doses (see page 298). I often use schizandra in tincture form; however, a tea that blends the berries with hibiscus and honey has a sweet-tart tang that makes schizandra's other flavors less noticeable.

Cautions and Considerations: Schizandra stimulates digestion, which may be inappropriate in cases of acute ulcer, reflux, or gastritis. Its liver detoxification actions could theoretically affect drug metabolism.

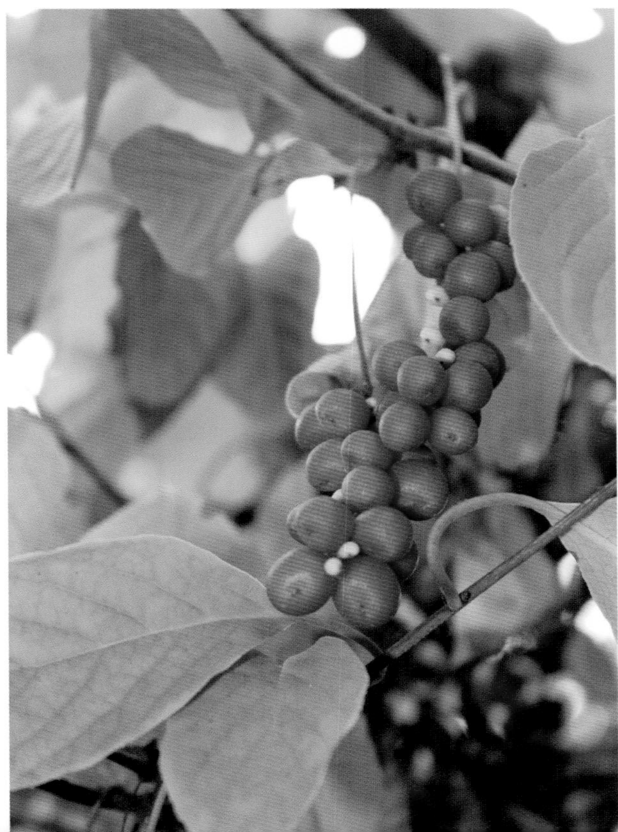

Balancing & Calming Adaptogens

SCHIZANDRA

GOTU KOLA

HOLY BASIL

ASHWAGANDHA

Calming Adaptogens

These are my go-to herbs for calm energy and anxiety relief. Herbal sedatives also quell anxiety, but I often prefer adaptogens — or blend the two — to avoid daytime sleepiness. Both of the following adaptogens come from the healing system of Ayurveda. Someone who needs a kick in the pants may find these herbs ho-hum, but they are well tolerated by almost anyone and can even be given to children.

▸ Holy Basil

Ocimum sanctum, syn. *O. tenuiflorum*

Availability: G+ C+

Key Properties: Holy basil, or tulsi, sprouts from pots dotting the temples of India. The potent aroma wafts through the air when you brush past the plant and elicits a Zen-like state of being. In the past few decades, holy basil has gained popularity in the United States for its ability to calm and energize, relieve anxiety and grief, and balance cortisol and blood sugar levels.

Additional Benefits: Ayurvedic practitioners use tulsi for much more. Think of it as a great protector. It improves immune health to fend off colds and other infections, strengthens digestion, decreases the inflammation response to quell chronic pain, and can even protect against radiation to some degree. On an emotional level, holy basil helps us feel less hopeless and more in tune with the world around us. It's like yoga or meditation in a cup of tea, and it blends well with green tea to amplify the energy and anti-inflammatory effects.

Preparation: This herb is amenable to any kind of remedy, fresh or dry, but it's particularly divine as tea. Holy basil is probably the easiest adaptogen to grow and harvest in abundance. Treat it like culinary basil in the garden; it prefers warm weather and sun with rich, regularly watered soil. Harvest the leaves and flowers regularly. Standard herb doses (see page 298) apply.

Cautions and Considerations: It's generally quite safe, but don't use it during pregnancy without professional supervision. Rarely, it aggravates reflux.

▸ Gotu Kola

Centella asiatica

Availability: G C

Key Properties: The leaves and aerial parts of this creeping ivylike vine are considered a favorite food and the supposed cause of the elephant's great memory. Whether or not this is true, gotu kola's brain-boosting benefits are the best known of its abilities, and it's often used as a purposeful filler in ginkgo pills. The peppery greens are reportedly fed to Indian children before they go back to school. Preliminary research suggests that gotu kola increases mental function while quelling anxiety and also improves circulation throughout the body, including the brain. Of all the adaptogens, I find gotu kola the most subtle. You can blend it with holy basil and other adaptogens for swifter, more obvious effects.

Additional Benefits: In addition to providing these amazing benefits, gotu kola serves as a supreme, smart remedy for healing and strengthening connective tissue, collagen, and the lining of the vascular system. You're as apt to see it in a scar or wound ointment as you are in remedies for varicose veins. It seems to work internally and topically. It's not as fast as comfrey, but it's more sophisticated in its healing action, producing better long-term results.

Preparation: Gotu kola works well in any form, fresh or dry, and is palatable enough to eat and toss into smoothies and tea. Standard herb doses (see page 298) apply. Though difficult to grow from seed and sensitive to cold, gotu kola propagates well from cuttings if you can find a local grower or online source of the starter plants.

Cautions and Considerations: This herb thrives in sludgy conditions with rich, wet soil, which can make it a tad challenging to cultivate (water daily!) but also indicates the need to seek out organically cultivated sources or grow it yourself. It will gladly grow in feces and can be contaminated with *Escherichia coli* (*E. coli*) and other nasties. Don't use it during pregnancy without a practitioner's supervision.

PROTOCOL POINTS

Fatigue

Fatigue can be a temporary or chronic health issue in and of itself, and it also coincides with many chronic and serious health conditions, including chronic pain, depression, and Lyme disease. If you suffer from extreme or long-standing fatigue, work with your doctor to sleuth out underlying causes that should be more directly addressed. However, these holistic recommendations work well for general fatigue and can be incorporated into a broader protocol for more serious conditions that result in fatigue. The herbs and therapies discussed here help lift sluggish fatigue and tend to have a stimulating nature.

Diet: Eat a whole-foods, nutrient-dense diet that promotes balanced blood sugar with plenty of produce, protein, and good fats. Avoid foods that you're sensitive to, as well as sugar and highly processed foods.

Lifestyle: Fit in daily movement and exercise, especially outdoors in the morning and midday. Aim to get a solid night's sleep. Get connected with others in your community, and engage in activities (work, volunteer, a hobby) that you're passionate about. Listen to upbeat music and inhale invigorating scents like peppermint and rosemary.

Herbs: Look to stimulating adaptogens like rhodiola, eleuthero, or codonopsis combined with more balancing adaptogens and nervines such as gotu kola, holy basil, ashwagandha, schizandra, milky oat seed, lemon balm, or damiana. Use nutritives like nettle and oat straw for support and spices to synergize your blend.

Stress and Jitters

At first glance, this might look like "fatigue stress," but really it's a different side of the stress coin that calls for herbs with different properties. Stimulating adaptogens tend to aggravate stress that is accompanied by "jitters," including anxiety, agitation, mania, and insomnia. Gentle adaptogens that help you feel more energized while also calming the nervous system are more appropriate.

Diet: Eat a whole-foods, nutrient-dense diet that promotes balanced blood sugar with plenty of produce, protein, and good fats. Be mindful of your caffeine intake, and consider avoiding it or swapping to green tea.

Lifestyle: Fit in daily movement and exercise, especially in the morning and midday. Aim to get a solid night's sleep, and work in at least one activity that supports mind-body balance, such as meditation or breathwork. Spend time outdoors (for exercise or downtime) most days, and bring elements of peace and nature into your indoor space. Address the stressors that you can.

Herbs: Look to balancing adaptogens like gotu kola, holy basil, ashwagandha, and schizandra. Combine them with nervines and gently calming herbs like milky oat seed, lemon balm, mimosa, motherwort, blue vervain, wood betony, or damiana. Spices, particularly nutmeg, will complement and synergize. Nutritives will support.

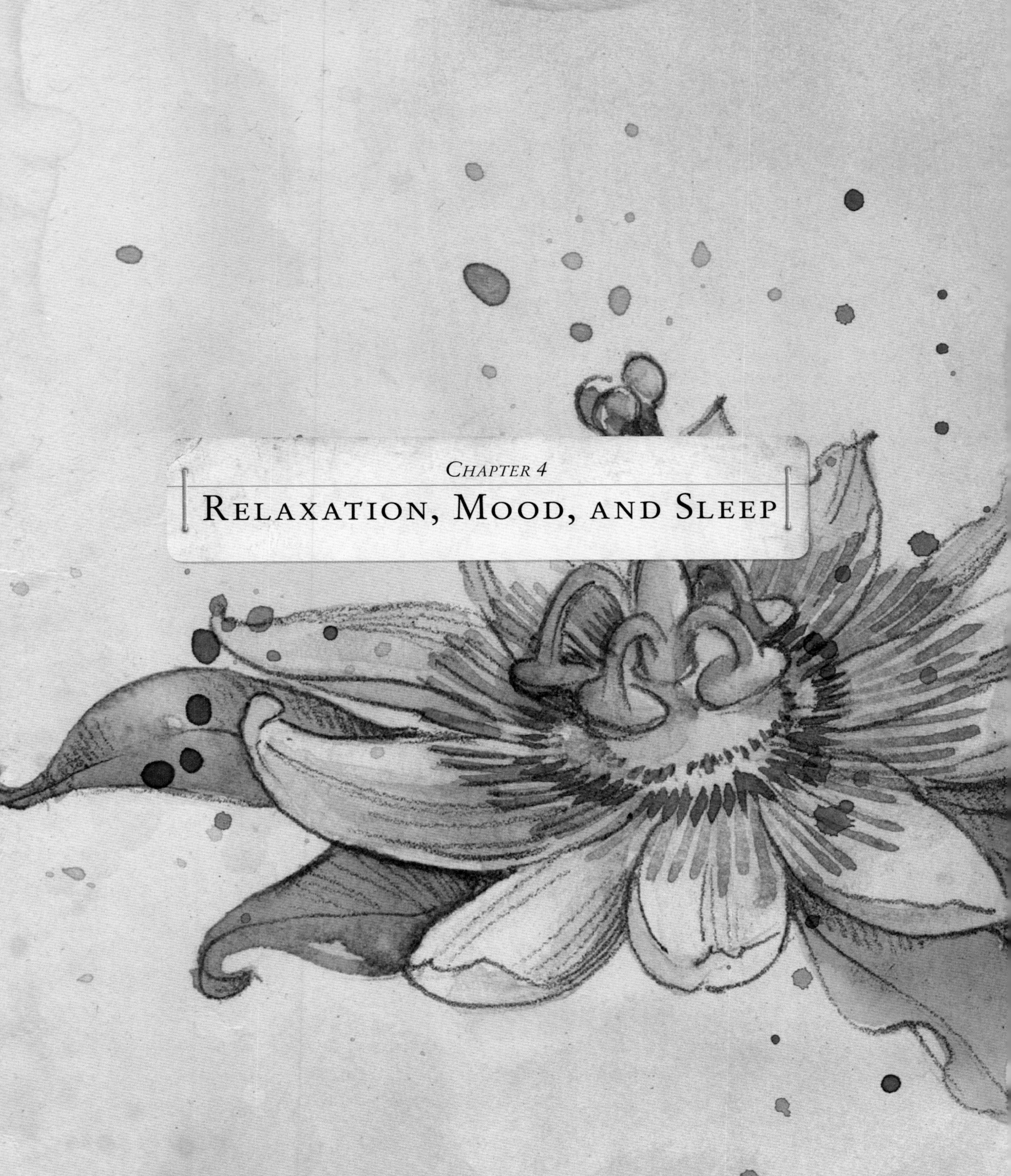

Chapter 4

Relaxation, Mood, and Sleep

Many of our everyday health complaints stem from spending too much time in "fight or flight" mode, and not enough in "relaxation and repair" mode. When you give your body the opportunity to relax, it finally has the opportunity to tend to its maintenance duties, with the following results:

- Improved digestion, absorption of nutrients, and elimination
- Improved immune function
- Increased detoxification via the liver, kidneys, et cetera
- Calmer and stronger cardiovascular system, and decreased blood pressure
- Reduced inflammation
- Better mood and sleep
- Steady metabolism

Eliciting the relaxation response and bringing the central nervous system down a notch can aid a range of common mood and stress issues, including anxiety, panic attacks, hyperactivity, and insomnia. It also plays an important role in alleviating depression. Of course, you don't *need* to take herbs to elicit your relaxation response. Meditation, breathing exercises, yoga, tai chi, spending time in nature, and aromatherapy can all help calm the nervous system. Yet herbs do offer fabulous assistance in soothing the nervous-endocrine system, flipping the switch so that you feel less stressed and enjoy a better mood, more energy, and better overall health and vitality.

The Power *of* Daily Tea

Regardless of plant chemistry, just sipping a cup of tea can have therapeutic effects: studies show that holding a warm cup in your hands encourages warmth and kindness to others and helps you perceive others in a better light. (It's really true — a warm drink makes you a nicer person!) It's also interesting to note that many of the herbs that benefit our nervous system — particularly the relaxing ones — are highly aromatic, so that a cup of tea provides not only the healing constituents you swallow but also the vapors you inhale. For these reasons, a daily tea ritual is one of the best ways to allow herbs to multitask and help you feel better. The simple act of making and drinking tea is an affirmation that you are taking care of yourself and that plants have the power to heal.

That said, tinctures and capsules may be more convenient. You can also try more creative options such as mixing herbal powders into smoothies, ghee, warm milk, or honey or infusing a calming cordial to be sipped after dinner.

RELAXING WITH FLOWER ESSENCES

THESE HIGHLY DILUTE VIBRATIONAL ESSENCES can be used in drop doses for emotional and psychological well-being (as well as spiritual and physical). They are very safe and are unlikely to interact with medications. Blend them with herbal formulas or use them solo. Just a few drops on the tongue or in your drink will do. Bach and FES brands are most commonly found in stores, but you can also make your own. Learn more at www.bachflower.com and www.lichenwood.com, and from Patricia Kaminski's *Flower Essence Repertory*. Some of my favorites include the following:

- **Rescue Remedy**, a blend of five essences, aids trauma, anxiety, and panic attack. The Sleep version adds **white chestnut** for swirling thoughts.
- **Lavender** brings spiritual and emotional calm.
- **Aspen** quells deep fear.
- **Valerian** brings a state of deep peace and calm.
- **St. John's wort** brings light-filled protection for nightmares, dark thoughts, and hypersensitivity to others.
- **Dandelion** helps you relax and feel joy.

Gently Calming *and* Uplifting Nervines

These herbs encourage healthy nervous system function and calm without being overly sedating. Though you could drink them before bedtime to help you sleep, drinking them for frayed nerves during the day won't put you to sleep — an important benefit for those of us who have things to get done during the day! These herbs are also more appropriate for people with a tendency toward depression, as they calm and balance rather than sedate you. (Regular use of stronger sedatives may overly depress the nervous system and bring on feelings of gloom.)

▸ Milky Oat Seed

Avena sativa

Availability: G C

Key Properties: All parts of the oat plant, a member of the grain/grass family, are nutritious and gently calm the nervous system. However, the fresh milky oat offers unique benefits from special alkaloids that relax and nourish your nerves while quelling agitation. Milky oat is neither adaptogen nor sedative (though it blends well with both) — it's food for your nerves and adrenals. Consider it during times of depletion and overstimulation: stress, anxiety, overwork, adrenal fatigue, attention deficit/hyperactivity, all-nighters, coffee-slugging cubicle work, and harried road trips. It quells that obnoxious buzzing feeling.

Additional Benefits: Milky oat seed also eases the side effects of drug withdrawal, including morphine, opium, alcohol, nicotine, and coffee.

Preparation: Harvest immature whole grain tops after squeezing a few to ensure they exude the "milk." Milky oats need to be fresh; once dry, the tops resemble glorified oat straw — nice, but lacking. If you're making a liquid formula (tincture, glycerite, vinegar), whir the fresh tops in a blender with your solvent to improve potency. Milky oats marry well with motherwort, lemon balm, gotu kola, and holy basil but work in many formulas as a supportive herb. Use standard herb doses (see page 298), or more in times of acute need. It can take substantial, regular doses for the effects to build.

Cautions and Considerations: Extremely safe for almost anyone, including kids. Gluten contamination (though unlikely) is possible due to sharing processing equipment with other grains.

▸ St. John's Wort

Hypericum perforatum

Availability: G W+ C+

Key Properties: St. John's wort most famously alleviates mild to moderate depression and seasonal affective disorder (SAD) with an action akin to selective serotonin reuptake inhibitors (SSRIs) like Prozac, without the side effects. However, this is a limited view of an amazing herb. St. John's wort thrives in intense sunlight and brings sun energy to blends. According to folklore, it protects against evil spirits and hexes — in modern terms, dark thoughts, nightmares, and oversensitivity to the negative energy of others.

Additional Benefits: It's an astounding nerve tonic inside and out, not just for stress but also for nerve damage, pain, healing, and mood-related neurotransmitter function. The infused oil applied topically heals wounds, rashes, nerve issues, burns, herpes, and pain. St. John's wort also improves your liver's ability to clear toxins.

Preparation: Look for preparations made with only fresh buds and flowers (best harvested in a dry, sunny spot after a hot-as-Hades week). Red color indicates potency. Poor-quality products (unfortunately common) have minimal impact — read the labels to make sure the product was made from fresh plant material, and look at the color. In terms of dosage, most of the research using St. John's wort for depression with success has used 300 mg standardized capsules three times daily, though the fresh-plant tincture or carbon dioxide extract soft gels can also be used, following label directions or standard herb doses (see

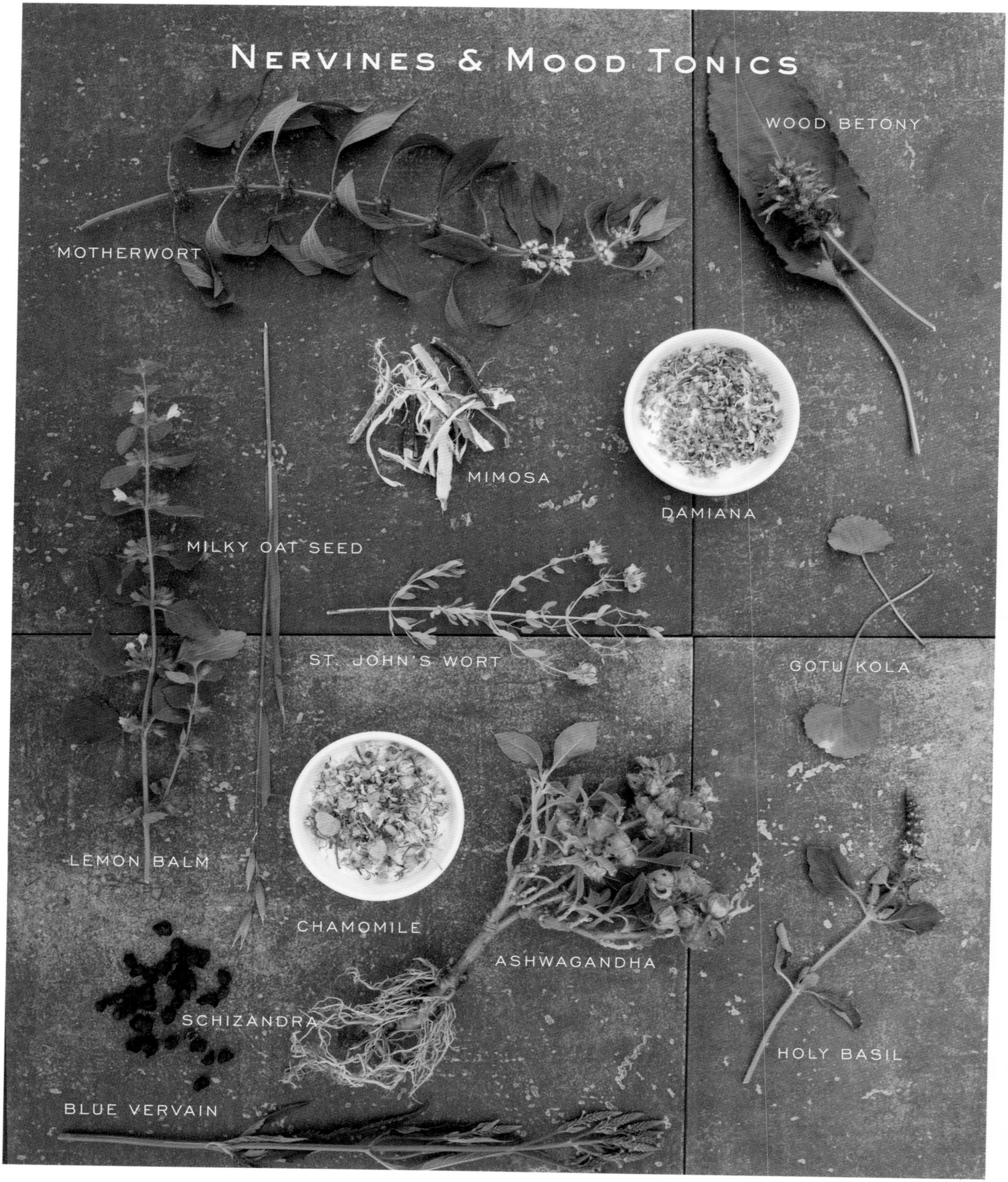

Nervines & Mood Tonics

WOOD BETONY

MOTHERWORT

MIMOSA

DAMIANA

MILKY OAT SEED

ST. JOHN'S WORT

GOTU KOLA

LEMON BALM

CHAMOMILE

ASHWAGANDHA

SCHIZANDRA

HOLY BASIL

BLUE VERVAIN

page 298). Some people notice immediate effects, but, much like SSRIs, it usually takes 4 to 6 weeks of steady use to see results.
Cautions and Considerations: St. John's wort is incredibly safe; however, internal use can interact with many medications. Though rare, it may cause photosensitivity. Don't use it during pregnancy without supervision. St. John's wort alone is not likely to lift major depression — but neither are SSRI drugs.

▸ Lemon Balm

Melissa officinalis
Availability: G+ C
Key Properties: This delightful lemon-scented garden nervine calms without sedating and can improve cognition and mood with as little as one dose in 1 hour! Children and adults alike will find it useful for mild mood funks, anxiety, insomnia, nervous indigestion, restlessness, inattention, mental decline, and hyperactivity.
Additional Benefits: As a mildly bitter mint-family herb, lemon balm improves digestion. Its lemony oils offer antiviral effects against herpes (apply topically and take internally) and possibly the flu. Lemon balm also inhibits an overdrive of thyroid hormone in hyperthyroid disease and offers antioxidant and wound-healing properties.
Preparation: Lemon balm loses potency quickly. You'll get the best results with fresh tincture, tea made from the fresh or freshly dried plant, fresh/frozen juice, and oil infused with wilted or freshly dried herb. Even the tincture loses something after a few years. Standard herb doses (page 298) apply.
Cautions and Considerations: Generally quite safe, but it should be used during pregnancy only with supervision and may (rarely) aggravate hypothyroid disease.

▸ Mimosa

Albizia julibrissin
Availability: G+ W+ C-
Key Properties: This graceful "tree of collective happiness" with its powder-puff pink blooms hails from traditional Chinese medicine (TCM) but grows like a (gorgeous) weed throughout the southeastern United States. Mimosa almost instantly lifts and calms mood. It's appropriate for anxiety, depression, insomnia, grief, and emotional tension.
Additional Benefits: Mimosa stimulates digestive and liver function.
Preparation: Use the bark and twigs (most potent) or flowers, fresh or freshly dried, as a tincture or tea. Standard herb doses (see page 298) apply.
Cautions and Considerations: Mimosa upsets sensitive stomachs if taken without food and shouldn't be taken during pregnancy without supervision. TCM mimosa preparations may be adulterated with magnolia, and the flowers lose potency easily.

▸ Other Nervines to Consider

Other lovely nervines that calm while uplifting the spirits and are appropriate day or night include **damiana, wood betony, blue vervain, motherwort, linden, rose,** and **chamomile.** Many of the adaptogens we discussed in chapter 3 have very good balancing and calming properties, positioning them as a bridge between adaptogenic and sedative herbs. **Ashwagandha, schizandra, holy basil,** and **gotu kola** serve well in this capacity. I really can't overemphasize how valuable these tonic herbs can be for a range of ills. You can amplify their calming qualities by blending them with other relaxing herbs.

Relaxing Sedatives

These herbs help you get a grip and relax. Consider them when your nerves feel fried and you're on edge and overly sensitive. This includes moments of anxiety, panic attacks, agitation, and insomnia. The level of sedation depends on the dose and your individual response. You might find them perfectly calming during the day, or they may make you want to curl into a ball and go to sleep. You can make them a tad less sedating by blending them with uplifting and less sedating herbs. They're *not* appropriate for "I can't get out of bed" depression.

▸ Motherwort

Leonurus cardiaca

Availability: G+ C-

Key Properties: Tiny, elaborate pink flowers line this spiky, weedy garden herb, sending the message of tough love in times of need. In spite of its intensely bitter flavor, motherwort quickly brings down anxiety and panic attacks, particularly when stress manifests in the heart with palpitations, pings of pain, and chest tightness. Consider it if you feel overworked, underappreciated, or on the edge of a rampage. Mothers and those who need a little mothering will find it useful. Its Latin name translates to "lion hearted," and indeed, motherwort brings strength during emotional roller coasters.

Additional Benefits: Motherwort brings down hyperthyroid function, eases hot flashes, and induces or increases menstrual flow.

Preparation: Best fresh. Harvest the aerial parts just as the plant begins to flower, though the large, soft leaves in the nonflowering stage will suffice. Once it flowers, it goes from perfect-for-harvest to less-than-ideal within days; you can tell because it suddenly looks less vital and has browning, thinning leaves. Motherwort tastes too terrible for tea; it is most often used as a tincture, glycerite, or vinegar. Standard herb doses (see page 298) apply.

Cautions and Considerations: Do not use during pregnancy. It may (rarely) aggravate hypothyroid disease. High doses can cause nausea.

▸ Kava

Piper methysticum

Availability: G- C+

Key Properties: Think of kava as your herbal benzodiazepine (like Xanax) for acute anxiety, panic attacks, and hysteria; it acts on similar neurotransmitters, including gamma-aminobutyric acid (GABA), a mood booster and nervous system relaxant. Polynesians traditionally drink kava tea before meetings and celebrations to promote happiness, relaxation, and friendship. It begins working within minutes, and modest amounts are unlikely to interfere with daytime functioning.

Additional Benefits: Kava promotes sleep by relieving anxiety. It has an antispasmodic, analgesic, and numbing action that decreases pain on contact and can be useful for headaches and genital-urinary-prostate spasms.

Preparation: Use the root as a fresh or dry tincture, tea, or (less preferred) capsule as needed. Standard herb doses (see page 298) apply. For a panic attack or episode of acute anxiety, try 2 to 4 mL of tincture as needed (each "squirt" from a dropper provides approximately 1 mL).

Cautions and Considerations: Experiencing a numb tongue after drinking kava tea or tincture is normal. Although generally safe with fewer side effects than its drug counterparts, kava is best used as needed. Consider other herbs for daily support. It's less appropriate for children and may interact with psych and pain meds as well as alcohol. Kava overuse causes a scaly rash that goes away after stopping use of the herb. Reports of liver toxicity are primarily due to adulteration with aerial parts of the plant. Use only the root, and purchase it only from reputable suppliers. To be on the safe side, avoid kava in cases of liver disease.

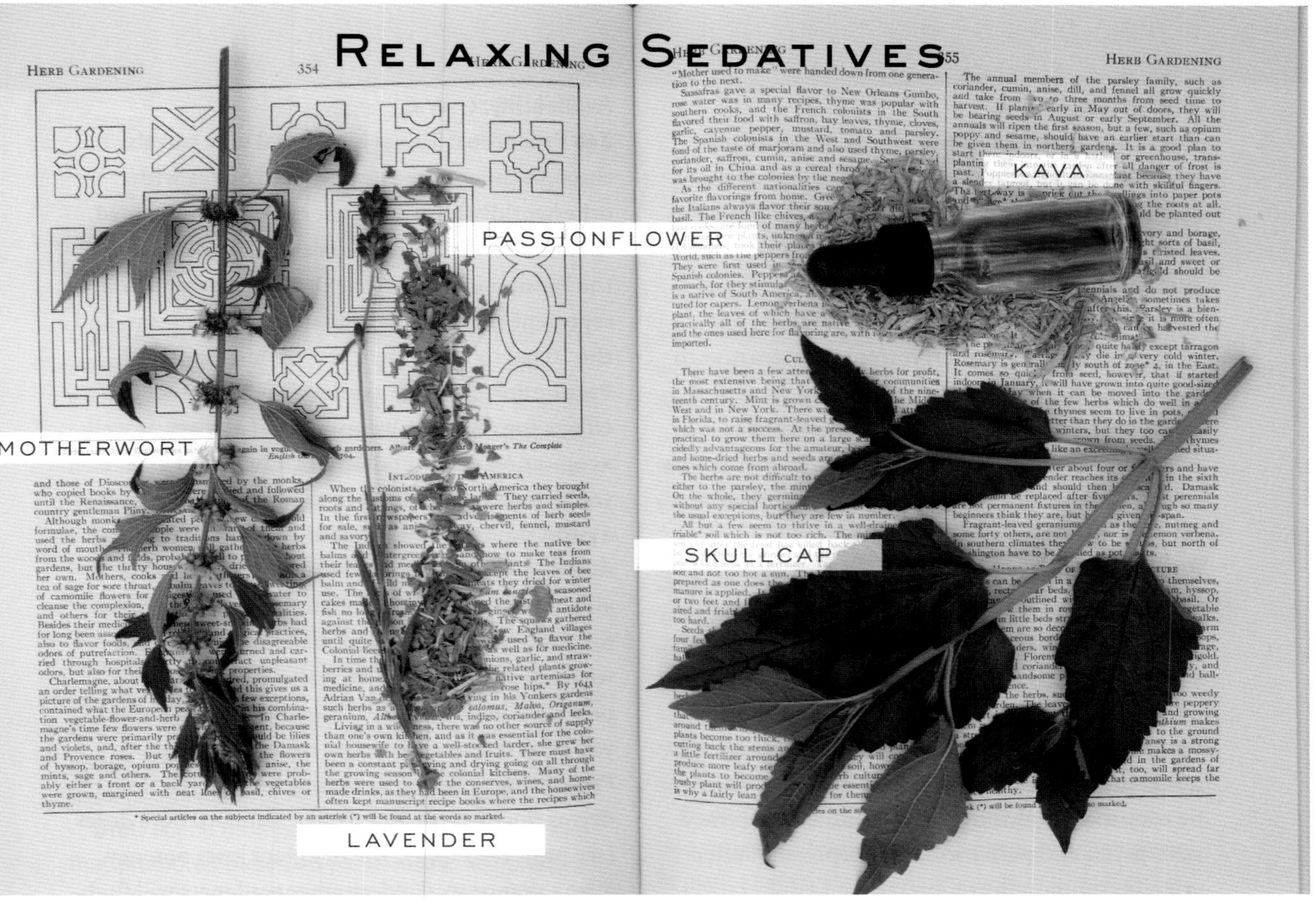

WHAT ARE NERVINES AND SEDATIVES?

Nervines nourish and strengthen the nervous-adrenal system. They may have a calming effect but are not necessarily sedatives. Sedatives slow down the nervous system and have a more depressant action. The two categories overlap.

General Uses: They give your nervous-adrenal system some TLC or bring it down a notch. You can combine nervines and sedatives with other herbs for a range of health issues to make the formula more sophisticated; for example, with more direct blood pressure–lowering herbs for stress-related hypertension. Nervines benefit a range of nervous-adrenal issues, including stress, anxiety, insomnia, depression, and cognitive problems.

Sedatives can help with nervous stimulation, anxiety, and insomnia, but they may aggravate depression and make you sleepy during the day. They support the actions of one another as well as adaptogens and other herbs in formula. Many, but not all, are aromatic.

Examples: Both nervine and sedative: California poppy, passionflower, skullcap, chamomile. More nervine: milky oat seed, lemon balm, damiana, motherwort, St. John's wort, hawthorn, bacopa, gotu kola, mimosa, vanilla, nutmeg, linden. More sedative: valerian, hops, kava, lavender, Jamaican dogwood.

curcumin twice daily alleviated major depression after 2 months. If you take pharmaceutical anti-depressants, seek professional guidance before

anxiety but require different therapies.

► Skullcap
Scutellaria lateriflora

► Passionflower
Passiflora incarnata

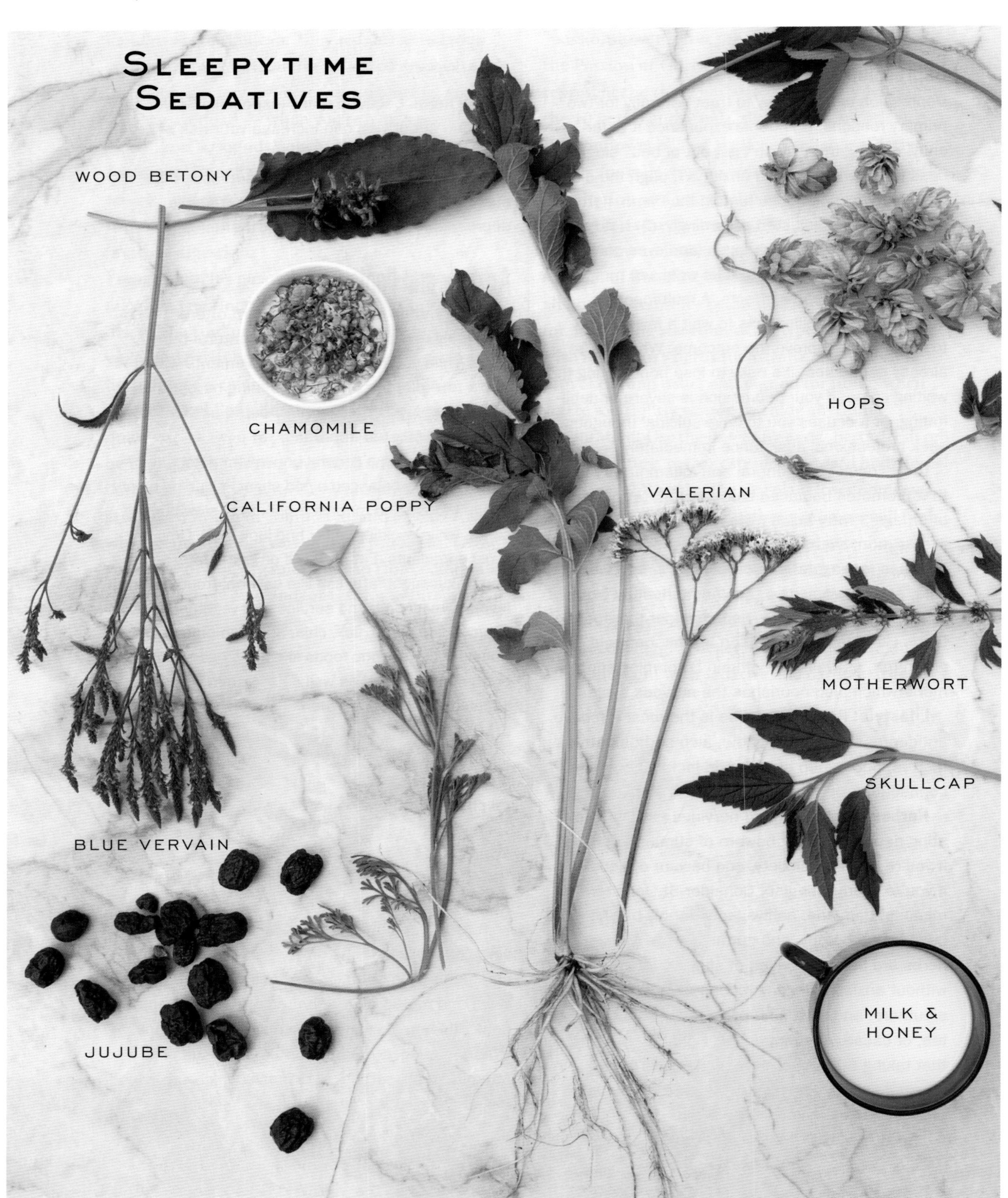

Stronger Sleep Aids

Although most of the nervines and relaxing sedatives mentioned above can help with sleep issues, the following herbs provide more targeted action for relieving insomnia and promoting deep sleep. Think of them as training wheels when your body has gotten into a rut of sleeplessness. They can help balance neurotransmitters, chill out stress hormones, relax muscles, and relieve pain, anxiety, and irritation that may be at the root of your sleep woes. They can be used on an ongoing basis, but you may find that they stop working if you don't also address underlying causes of anxiety, pain, or insomnia.

General Preparations: Take these herbs up to 30 minutes before bedtime. Tinctures act within 15 minutes, while capsules take longer to digest. If you opt for tea, brew it strong and small to prevent nighttime pee breaks. Keep tinctures by the bedside with some water in case you need to redose upon waking.

General Cautions: Sleep herbs are most likely of all our sedatives to interact with psych and pain meds and excess alcohol, and they may aggravate sluggish depression. Try just a little, and then work your dose up as needed. If you feel groggy, take less or try a different herb.

▸ Valerian

Valeriana officinalis

Availability: G+ W C+

Key Properties: The go-to herb for sleep, valerian makes an appearance in almost every insomnia formula on the market. Indeed, it sedates the nervous system while relaxing muscles, making it easier to fall and stay asleep and promoting deeper, more restful sleep. However, it doesn't work for a lot of people. Valerian types tend to be colder, more anxious, and thin. Contrary to a common misconception, valerian has nothing to do with Valium, though the herb and the drug do act on similar receptor sites (like GABA). Valerian's not addictive. Though valerian is our best- researched sleep herb, most of our understanding comes from traditional use. No sleep herbs have been rigorously studied.

Additional Benefits: Valerian's pain-relieving, muscle-relaxing properties make it helpful for pain (especially when it keeps you from sleeping) as well as hypertension (because it relaxes blood vessels). Energetically, this plant warms your body.

Preparation: Fresh root tincture works best, but capsules are also sometimes effective. Standard herb doses (see page 298) apply. Because of the root's skunky-earthy scent, most people would find valerian tea unpalatable. Dig the roots of this easy-to-grow garden herb in spring or fall. It self-seeds rampantly in good soil and pulls up easily. Watch for earthworms!

Cautions and Considerations: A lot of folks (especially those who run hot, have a larger frame, and tend toward anger and frustration) don't like valerian because it either agitates them or makes them groggy. More general sedatives like passionflower and skullcap work better for a broader group of people. Aside from that, just the general sedative cautions apply; see above.

▸ California Poppy

Eschscholzia californica

Availability: G+ W C

Key Properties: This happy golden wildflower self-seeds across open fields of California, Mexico, and the surrounding Southwest and is relatively easy to cultivate. Native tribes relied on this and other local poppies for sleep and treating a range of pain issues. It contains a nonaddictive, nonnarcotic mild opiate "fuzz" responsible for its properties. Consider California poppy for swirling thoughts that prevent sleep, pain that keeps you awake, and bratty moments (for kids and adults).

Additional Benefits: As a milder substitute for opium poppy, California poppy works for all sorts of forms of pain and may also help with colic and crankiness in babies.

Preparation: Use the aerial parts or the whole plant (the roots are a striking translucent orange) as it turns from flower to seed. Fresh is best, and it's most often used as a tincture. Standard herb doses (see page 298) apply.

Cautions and Considerations: California poppy is safe for a range of people but shouldn't be used during pregnancy. Though it may not be an issue, I'd avoid it in cases of opiate addiction, to be safe. It's not likely to give a false positive on a drug test, but declare that you're taking it, just in case.

Other Sedatives and Sleep Aids

So many other herbs can help you sleep better, and it can take some trial and error to find the perfect match for you. **Skullcap** and **passionflower**, mentioned previously, are my favorite all-purpose, reliable sedatives for anxiety, insomnia, and overstimulation. They're particularly nice combined with lemon balm, spearmint, and honey as a bedtime tea for adults and kids. Also consider **chamomile tea**, especially for children and babies. Those who don't respond well to valerian may do better with the flowerlike strobiles of **hops**. Other great sleep herbs to consider include **jujube dates, blue vervain, wood betony**, and **wild lettuce**.

Melatonin supplements at night or a glass of naturally melatonin-rich tart cherry juice in the morning and evening support your body's natural sleep hormone levels. They're particularly useful if your sleep-wake cycles are off or you're experiencing jet lag.

Warm milk with honey has calming action, perhaps due to the low dose of tryptophan in the milk, made more bioavailable by the honey. You can add a pinch of purposeful spices like fresh-grated nutmeg (which has stress-relieving and sleep-promoting properties), natural vanilla (calming) extract, or turmeric (antidepressant!) powder or simmer calming herbs like ashwagandha powder in milk. Delivering herbs in a fatty base (like dairy, nut-based, soy, or other milk) is believed to make them more effective for the nervous system, which is lined with fat. Besides, it tastes good!

PROTOCOL POINTS

Insomnia

While I find insomnia to be incredibly responsive to herbs, they often stop working if you never address the underlying cause, such as stress or poor sleep hygiene, especially in severe or longstanding insomnia problems. Be diligent, and be sure to incorporate nonherbal lifestyle changes (see opposite pages). Not every sleep herb works for everyone: if you notice no improvement after 1 to 2 weeks on an herbal formula, try different herbs or up your dose.

Diet: In general, eat a quality diet that promotes balanced blood sugar, limits stimulants, and avoids late-night meals and snacking. Consider therapeutic foods like tart cherry juice or warm milk with honey, or a pinch of nutmeg in your recipes.

Lifestyle: Find a good sleep ritual and minimize stimulation before bedtime. Address any stress factors. See the sleep tips on the opposite pages for details.

Herbs: Nervine and sedative herbs quell overstimulation while promoting sleep. Top herbs include valerian, hops, passionflower, skullcap, California poppy, and chamomile.

TIPS FOR BETTER SLEEP

IT CAN BE HARD to get out of an insomnia rut. Here are some general tips and common culprits.

De-stress. Stress is a major factor in most cases of insomnia. Sedative herbs at night or stress-relieving herbs during the day can help, but also try to reduce the stressors directly. Maybe you need to back out of stressful situations (bad job or relationship, not saying no when you should) or schedule more R&R time for yourself. Consider regular meditation, yoga, daytime exercise, or an evening wind-down ritual of reading and sipping tea.

Avoid or moderate stimulants. Stimulants of various sorts can make you restless and more apt to wake up.

- **Caffeine:** Coffee, chocolate, yerba maté, soda, and tea are obvious late-night no-nos, but you may be surprised by the effect that morning drink has. Cut down slowly (to avoid withdrawal headaches) to see if sleep improves.
- **Medications, herbs, and supplements:** Even if they don't contain caffeine, many remedies can cause restlessness, especially if you take them later in the day. This includes B vitamins, stimulant adaptogens, blood pressure medications, antidepressants, dementia medications, antihistamines, glucosamine and chondroitin, and statins. Try switching herbs and supplements around or avoid late doses. Talk with your doctor if you suspect medications are the cause; ask if you can try a different medication or change your dose time.
- **Alcohol:** Booze may initially sedate but ultimately makes you restless and prevents restful deep sleep.
- **Late-night eating:** Late dinners and snack binges wreak havoc on a good night's sleep, especially when digestion and liver involvement kick in a few hours after you eat. Try to stop eating at least 4 hours before bedtime and particularly avoid big, heavy dishes and sugar- or fat-laden food.

Exercise. Physical activity is *phenomenal* for insomnia and stress. But not right before bedtime — aim for morning or midday activity instead. That said, late-day exercise is better than none.

Unplug before bed. Light — especially artificial light from TVs, smartphones, tablets, and indoor lighting — messes with the circadian rhythm that governs when you're asleep and awake. Avoid all electronics an hour or so before bedtime, and dim the lights. Keep your bedroom tech-free, and hang curtains or use an eye mask so that you sleep in total darkness. Earplugs help if it's noisy. Stimulate your "wake" cycle during the morning and daytime with exercise, sunlight (or full-spectrum lighting), and exercise, which will improve your overall circadian rhythm.

Develop a sleep ritual. Parents of young children know that consistency and ritual make all the difference. Now that you've unplugged, get ready for bed and get comfy! Enjoy a small cup of relaxing tea or warm milk with honey (but not so much that you'll have to pee at midnight). Good before-bed activities include reading a book (*not* a page-turning suspense novel), journaling (a good time for that gratitude journal!), making love, listening to calming music, cuddling up with loved ones, meditating, inhaling relaxing essential oils or incense, and taking a bath. For me, nonfiction works like a charm!

NERVOUS-ENDOCRINE SYSTEM HERB CONTINUUM

Caffeinated/Very Stimulating		Stimulating		Less Stimulating	Balancing/Neutral	Calming		Most Sedating	
High Caffeine	Low Caffeine	Stimulating Adaptogens	Semi-Stimulating Adaptogens	Balancing Adaptogens	Calm Energy Adaptogens	Calming and Uplifting Nervines	Gentle Nervine-Sedatives	Relaxing Sedatives	Sedatives and Sleep Aids
Guarana*	Black tea*	Red Asian ginseng*	Codonopsis	Maca	Ashwagandha	Lemon balm*	Chamomile	Passionflower	Valerian (warming)
Kola nut *	Chocolate*	White Asian ginseng*	Eleuthero	Schizandra*	Holy basil*	Fresh milky oat seed	Lavender	Skullcap	Hops (cooling
Coffee*	Green tea*	American ginseng*	Cordyceps fungus*	Licorice	Gotu kola*	St. John's wort	Catnip	Blue vervain	Melatonin (sleep cycles)
Yerba maté*	White tea*	Rhodiola*	*Aralia* spp.	Reishi mushroom*	Bacopa*	Damiana	Linden	Wood betony	Wild lettuce
			Jiaogulan*	Chaga	Shatavari	Bay leaf	Hawthorn	Motherwort	Jamaican dogwood (ver strong; use with caution)
						Nutmeg	Tart cherry juice	Jujube	Opium poppy (illegal, addictive)
						Mimosa	Tryptophan and 5-HTP	Kava	
						Vanilla	Warm milk with honey	California poppy (mild opiate)	
						Turmeric		*Pedicularis* spp. (muscle relaxer)	

*These herbs have memory-enhancing, brain-boosting, and/or focus-enhancing properties.

Maria's Sleep Tea

This potent yet tasty sedative tea can be used for all ages, adjusting the dose as needed. You can take it as a daytime anti-anxiety tea, but it may make you sleepy. Using more lemon balm and less passionflower and skullcap will make it less sedating. The formula listed below is for a small cup of tea at just 4 to 6 ounces, so that you're not drinking too much liquid right before bedtime. You can premix a larger batch and keep it on hand.

- ½ teaspoon lemon balm
- ½ teaspoon passionflower
- ½ teaspoon skullcap
- ½ teaspoon spearmint
- 1 heaping teaspoon honey (optional)

Combine the herbs. Pour 4 to 6 ounces of near-boiling water over the herbs and let steep, covered, for 15 to 20 minutes. Strain, then sweeten to taste with honey, if desired.

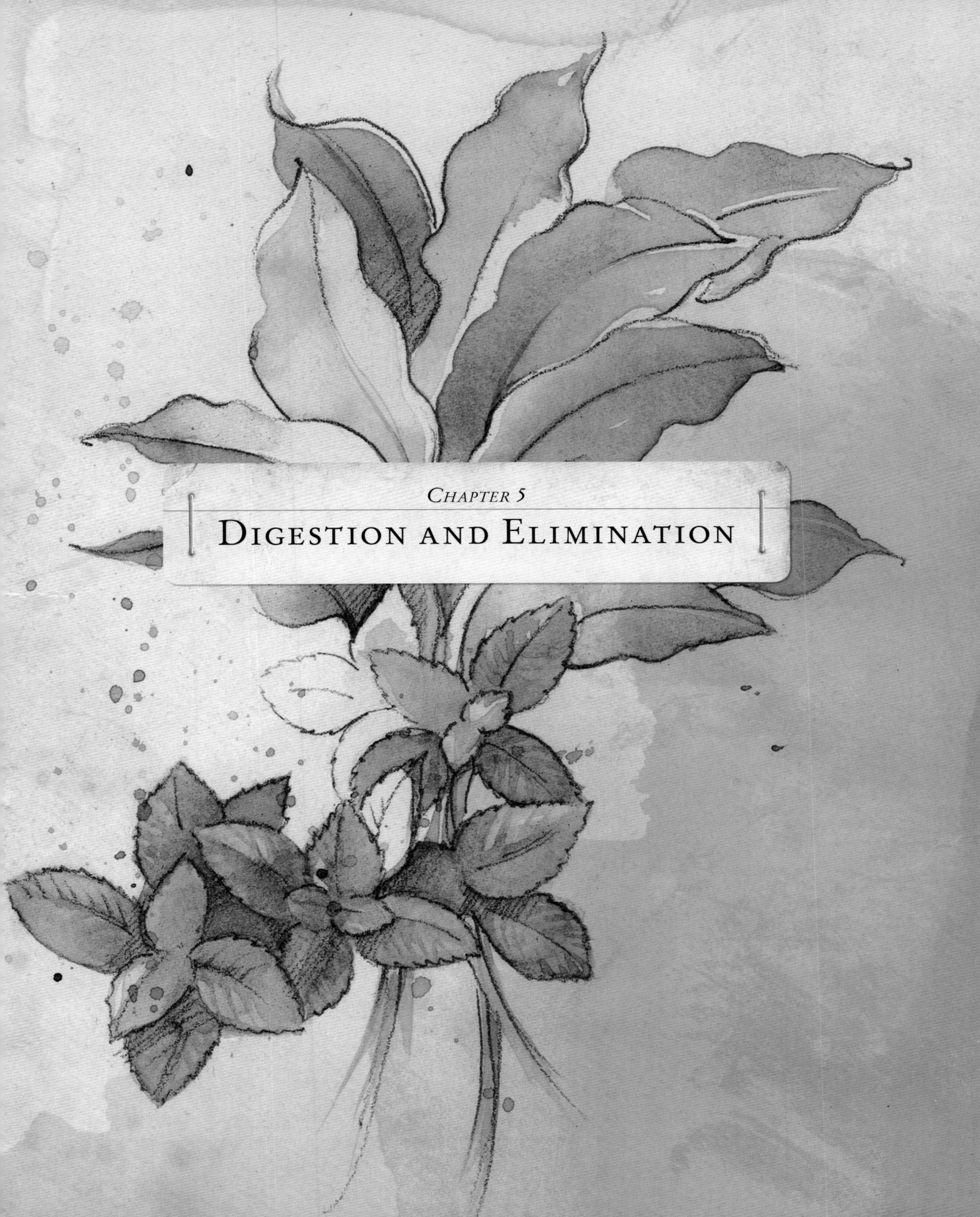

CHAPTER 5

DIGESTION AND ELIMINATION

OPTIMAL DIGESTION PLAYS an *essential* role in your overall vitality and state of balance; it is one of the foundational body systems upon which the rest of your health relies. The upper section of your gastrointestinal (GI) tract focuses on breaking down the food you eat into teeny bits. The lower section of your GI tract absorbs what is needed and eliminates the rest. A perfect diet means nothing if your GI system can't do its job.

An out-of-balance gut is no fun. Indigestion, gas, heartburn, ulcers, bowel irregularity, and the deterioration of your gut can be painful, embarrassing, debilitating, and at times life threatening. Most pharmaceuticals work by suppressing gut function, which resolves the current symptoms, but to the detriment of nutrient absorption and proper gut health. In sharp contrast, the gut responds quickly to herbal therapies and diet changes that heal damage and retrain function, resolving symptoms, supporting health, and bringing balance to the entire system.

The Upper GI Tract: Breaking It Down

Your upper GI tract — from your mouth to your stomach — begins the breakdown of food through mechanics (chewing, churning) and chemistry (enzymes, stomach acid) so that it can be assimilated into the bloodstream later down the pike. But digestion begins before you even put food in your mouth.

Predigestion

You should have a Pavlovian response to food. The sight of a colorful salad or the scent and sizzle of the skillet excite the brain and flip switches in the digestive tract. Saliva pours into your mouth, your stomach pumps out starter acid, and your pancreas gears up to release enzymes, unless your response to food is, for some reason, diminished. A lack of sensory response creates dulled digestive function.

Stress is a major culprit in dulling the predigestive response because the GI tract shuts down when you're in fight-or-flight mode. Try to approach meals in a "rest and digest" state and use digestive herbs that also support and calm the nervous system. If you're simply desensitized to food (common amongst restaurant workers and family head chefs), bring spark back with new ingredients and visually appealing arrangements, as well as bitters, sours, and spices to reawaken your senses.

It's True: Chew Your Food

Putting food into your mouth amplifies the digestive response. Chewing and saliva start the breakdown, but something else important happens as the food moves its way around your mouth. Taste buds and other sensors analyze what you're eating and send signals farther down to alert your body of precisely which kinds of enzymes and chemicals are needed to break down the food. Fats? Get the lipase (fat enzyme) and bile ready! Carbs? Amylase, on deck! Protein? Get moving, protease, hydrochloric acid, pepsin, and trypsin!

MULTITASKING IN YOUR GUT

YOUR DIGESTIVE TRACT plays an important role in seemingly unrelated body systems. Home to hundreds of millions of neurons, your gut (a.k.a. your "second brain") often tells your brain what to do and produces many important neurotransmitters, including mood-boosting serotonin. Your gut also functions as a front line of defense against disease. Germs that you unknowingly ingest (via food or swallowed mucus) meet their doom (you hope!) in the sea of stomach acid. And your gut is the capital city for approximately 100 trillion beneficial bacteria. These "good guys" improve overall digestion and nutrient availability and also play a role in improving immune health and mood, decreasing inflammation, and reducing the risk of chronic disease. (Learn more about probiotics on page 79.)

To support this early digestion and its signals, don't skimp on chewing and tasting your food. This also explains why supplements in pill form (especially omega-3 fish oil) can cause indigestion and are poorly absorbed. (The solution? Take fish oil in liquid form or with a fatty food.) Herbal remedies like teas and tinctures have a distinct advantage over pills because they engage all your senses, including taste and the signals it engenders, and as liquids they may begin to enter the bloodstream before they even hit the stomach.

▸ Artichoke Leaf

Cynara scolymus

Availability: G C

Key Properties: A classic, basic bitter, artichoke leaf stimulates all aspects of digestive function — enzymes, stomach acid, peristalsis, elimination, fat digestion — as well as liver detoxification, bile production, and bile excretion. It is useful in cases of weak digestive function and can be helpful in some cases of heartburn/reflux, Crohn's disease, indigestion, and irritable bowel.

Additional Benefits: Artichoke also protects and regenerates the liver, decreases cholesterol and blood sugar levels, reduces the glycemic effect of food, and is rich in antioxidants.

Preparation: Use the fresh or dry leaf as a tincture, infused vinegar, elixir, oxymel, or cordial, and take with or just before meals. Standard herb doses (see page 298) apply, although you may find lower doses suffice. Most find it unpalatable as tea, and it doesn't work as well if you don't taste it (i.e., in capsule form). Artichoke's immature flowers, commonly eaten as a vegetable, have a similar but weaker effect.

Cautions and Considerations: Generally safe, though the fresh leaf can irritate the skin of sensitive people.

▸ Other Bitters to Consider

Other favorite bitters include **dandelion** (the leaf or root), **burdock, turmeric, schizandra,** and **citrus peel** or the gentler relaxing bitters like **lemon balm, chamomile, holy basil,** or **catnip.** (For a more comprehensive list of bitters, see below.)

WHAT IS A BITTER?

Bitters are those herbs and foods that literally taste bitter. Sour and pungent herbs and foods can have similar actions. "Relaxing bitters" tend to be a bit milder and more aromatic; they also relax or normalize the stress response.

General Uses: Bitters single-handedly turn on your GI tract: peristalsis (the wavelike motion that moves everything through), saliva, enzyme production and excretion, stomach acid production, bile production and excretion, and (thanks to peristalsis) bowel movements. Indirectly, bitters also benefit liver function and detoxification, lower blood sugar, reduce cholesterol, alleviate skin conditions, and fix some cases of heartburn or reflux. They have a remarkable ability to modulate weak or excessive appetite and weight, as needed, stimulating a weak appetite, curbing cravings (especially for sweets), and making healthy food more appealing. Think of bitters for sluggish digestion and elimination, constipation, indigestion, excess fullness, poor nutrient absorption (especially fat indigestion), and high cholesterol. Bitters work best when you *taste* them. Use teas, vinegars, cordials, tinctures, and elixirs — not pills — with meals.

Examples: Artichoke leaf, gentian (organic only), dandelion leaf and root, burdock, turmeric, ginger, schizandra, citrus peel, tamarind, bitter salad greens. Sour foods that function like bitters include vinegar, fermented or pickled produce, and citrus juice. Relaxing bitters include chamomile, catnip, lemon balm, and holy basil. Because most bitters are cooling by nature, complement them with warming carminative herbs (ginger, cinnamon, cardamom) for balance.

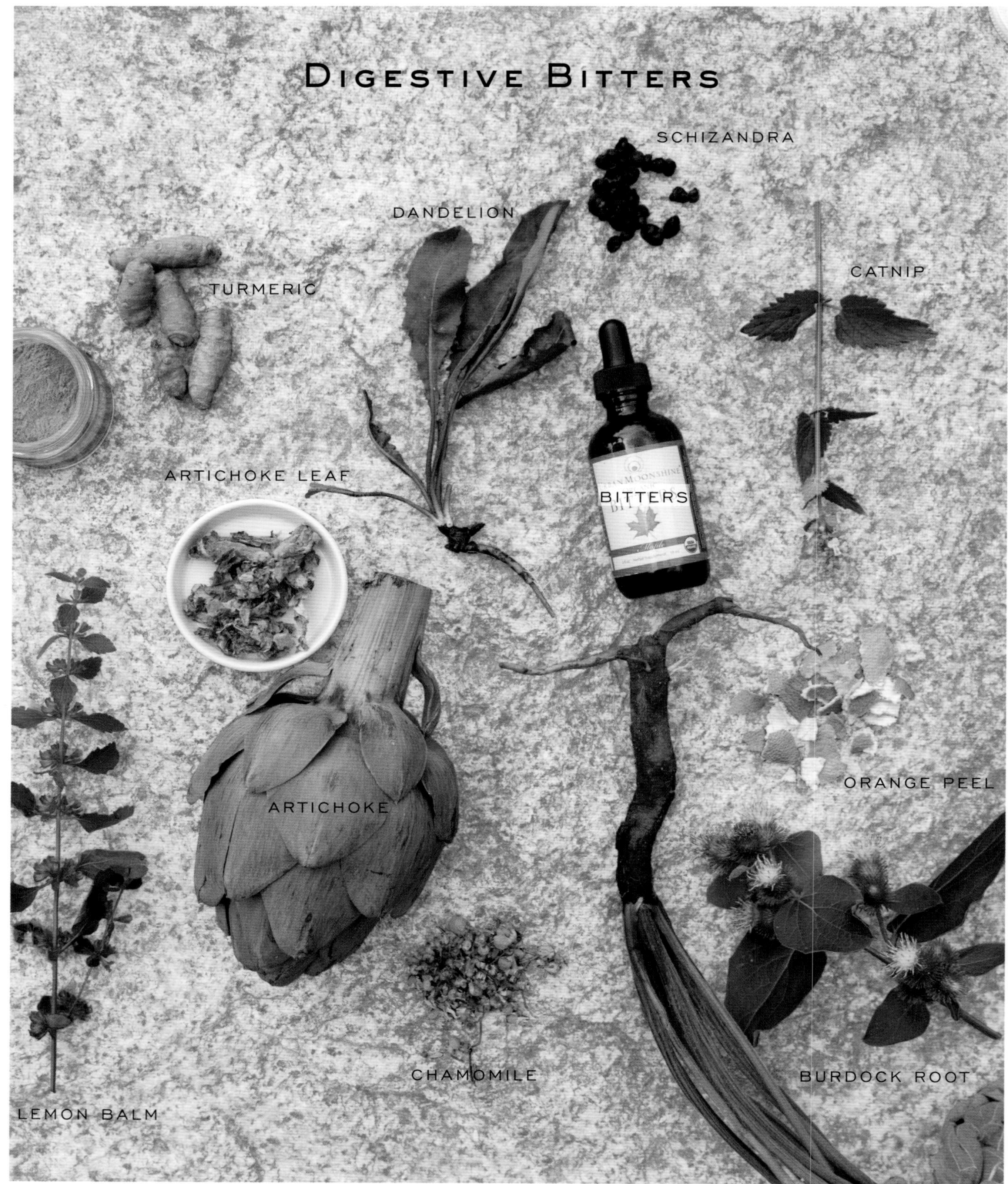
Digestive Bitters
Schizandra
Dandelion
Turmeric
Catnip
Artichoke Leaf
Bitters
Orange Peel
Artichoke
Chamomile
Burdock Root
Lemon Balm

Bitters Spray

This bitters recipe combines bitters, sours, and warming carminative spices, plus a little something sweet for palatability. Although lemon balm, ginger, and citrus work and taste best fresh, and the others are more commonly available dried, technically, you can use either the fresh or dry form of any of these herbs.

- 2 parts dandelion root
- 2 parts fresh lemon balm
- 1½ parts fennel seed
- 1½ parts schizandra berry
- 1 part artichoke leaf
- 1 part fresh ginger
- 1 part fresh grapefruit or orange (entire fruit, chopped)
- A few cardamom pods
- 100-proof vodka
- Maple syrup or honey

Combine the herbs, and loosely pack enough of them into a glass jar to fill it about three-quarters full. Cover with a mix of 75 percent vodka and 25 percent maple syrup or honey. Shake to combine. Let sit on your counter for 2 to 4 weeks, shaking every day or two. Then strain out the herbs through a fine-mesh strainer, squeezing the herbs to get as much liquid out as possible. Pour the liquid into a spray bottle. Take two or more sprays in your mouth before meals.

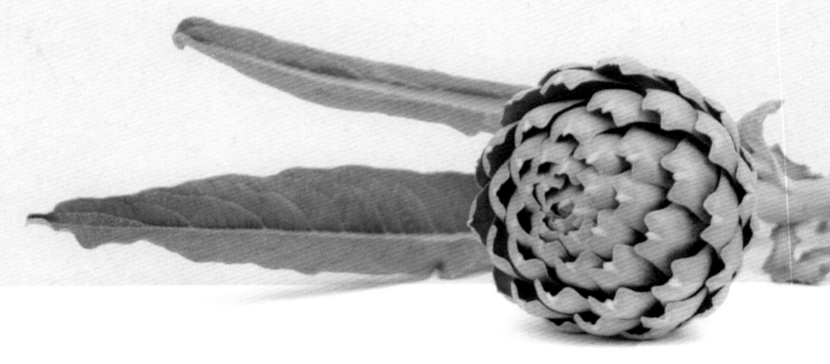

Sphincter Issues — Fire in the Hole!

Your stomach deals in strong chemicals. Its hydrochloric acid can burn a hole through the floor, but a thick mucosal lining protects your stomach as the acid does its job (breaking down protein, boosting nutrient absorption, and killing pathogens). The rest of your digestive tract has far less protection, so sphincters at the top and bottom of the stomach cinch shut when stomach acid levels rise and it's time to churn away.

Those who eat a standard American diet tend to have a hard time with the little sphincter above the stomach, known as the lower esophageal sphincter (LES), or cardiac sphincter. When it doesn't shut properly — due to malfunction or damage — your digestive juices churn up into your esophagus, causing reflux and heartburn, irritating and damaging tissue. Repeated damage causes scarring and ultimately increases your risk of esophageal cancer. Americans' use of proton pump inhibitor drugs like Prilosec to treat reflux, heartburn, and other digestive issues is staggering. These drugs nearly shut off stomach acid production — but is that really a good idea? Sure, we need to stop the damage and give the body a chance to heal. But we *need* stomach acid to properly digest our food, and these meds come with a host of side effects. Studies show that regular use of these drugs can even *create* a reflux problem, and when they're stopped withdrawal reflux can result, because they weaken digestive function.

If you suffer from heartburn or reflux, instead of reaching for pharmaceuticals that shut down stomach acid production and may, in the end, have a host of unpleasant side effects, try to figure out the root cause of the problem. Different things cause heartburn and reflux in different people. Common causes include the following:

- **Low stomach acid.** That's right, when stomach acid levels are too *low*, the lower esophageal sphincter fails to shut properly when your stomach fills with food. You should notice immediate improvement by taking a bit of bitters, sours, or raw apple cider vinegar with meals. Also look at the common underlying causes of low stomach acid: poor or highly processed diet, stress, and excessive carbs and sweets. Stomach acid production also tends to decrease with age; however, natural remedies and a good diet will help counteract that decline.
- **Stuffed stomach.** Eating too much or not letting gravity work for you puts pressure on the sphincter, pushing it open. Eat smaller meals, more frequently if needed.
- **Stomach irritants.** Acid and irritation can result from eating acidic or personal trigger foods, hyperacid secretion in the GI tract, stress, and some medications, including many pain relievers. Avoid your personal irritants (which may include bitters, vinegar, citrus, tomatoes, and hot spices), and make good use of demulcent herbs that soothe and heal the gut, like licorice (especially the deglycyrrhizinated form, known as DGL) and marshmallow root. Also limit foods that cause excessive acid production, including meat, fried foods, alcohol, coffee, tea, and dairy products.

PROTOCOL POINTS

Acid Reflux, Heartburn, Gastritis, and Ulcers

These digestive woes plague many Americans, and the holistic approach is quite simple: stop the irritation, soothe and heal the gut, improve the diet, reduce stress, and then slowly restore proper function and digestive juice production.

Diet: Eat smaller, more frequent meals with more plant-based whole foods, including plenty of fiber (whole grains, starchy vegetables, legumes, seeds), water, and green veggies. Avoid or limit coffee, alcohol, and meals with a lot of protein and fat (e.g., steak, dairy). Sleuth out your personal triggers — green or black tea, citrus, spices, tomatoes, vinegar, bitters, sours, and spicy flavors like ginger and peppermint are common — and avoid those that seem problematic.

Lifestyle: Let gravity work for you — don't recline, lean over, go to bed, or do bouncy exercises shortly after eating. Sit upright, stand, or take a gentle walk after meals. Address stress if that's a factor. Avoid or limit NSAIDs (aspirin, ibuprofen, naproxen, et cetera). Ask your doctor if your meds could be making your condition worse and if you can reduce, eliminate, or change offending drugs.

Herbs: Bitters, sours, aromatics, spices, and vinegar can *help* heartburn/reflux caused by low acid but *worsen* high-acid states and are never recommended in cases of acute ulcers. Soothing, demulcent, wound-healing herbs are always appropriate: licorice, plantain, marshmallow, slippery elm, gotu kola, and maybe comfrey leaf (see the cautions on page 78). Gentle astringents like rose petals, calendula petals, and cinnamon can aid healing by tightening, repairing, and toning the mucosal lining of the digestive tract. Ulcer cases relating to *Helicobacter pylori* (*H. pylori*) infection must also be treated with antibiotic drugs or herbs (see page 75); otherwise the ulcer will just come back.

Ulcers and Gut Wounds

Gastric inflammation (gastritis) and thinning mucosal lining spells trouble for your gut, in and out of the stomach. As acid and inflammation eat through that protective mucosal lining, wounds (ulcerations) open. Gastritis and ulcers of the stomach (gastric, peptic) and intestines (duodenal) cause gnawing pain. Most aspects of holistic treatment are identical to the treatment for heartburn and reflux: soothing, demulcent, healing herbs; stress reduction; and a diet free of gastric irritants. However, the causes can differ and must be addressed to resolve the issue and avoid recurrence. Common factors include the following:

- **NSAIDs.** These pain relievers (full name: nonsteroidal anti-inflammatory drugs), including ibuprofen and aspirin, reduce inflammation throughout the body, but they actually *increase* inflammation in the gut. That's because NSAIDs decrease prostaglandins. Prostaglandins cause inflammation throughout most of the body; however, they paradoxically decrease inflammation in the gut. Frequent use of NSAIDs shuts down this protective prostaglandin effect, aggravating inflammation in the stomach and gut, thinning the mucosal lining, and making it prone to wounds (ulcers). Wean yourself down or off these meds if you can. Taking them with DGL licorice tablets and plenty of food buffers the damage.

- ***H. pylori.*** *Helicobacter pylori* infection is closely linked to gut inflammation and ulcers, especially episodes that come and go. Ask your doctor to test for the bacteria. Drinking licorice tea, chamomile tea, green or black tea, and cranberry juice and eating garlic and olive oil regularly will discourage future bacteria proliferation. Stronger antimicrobial herbs like goldenseal (preferably organic), similar berberine-rich herbs (Oregon grape root, barberry, coptis) or isolated berberine supplements, usnea lichen, or mastic gum may resolve an acute infection, but they're not always as reliable as antibiotic drugs.

- **Stress and dietary irritants.** Other gastric aggravators include stress, a history of chronic vomiting, and an irritating diet — especially involving excessive alcohol, coffee, refined food, fried fare, red meat, and sometimes dairy. Foods that you're allergic or sensitive to, such as gluten or dairy, can also worsen gastritis and gut lining. See the dietary recommendations in the discussion of acid reflux and other gastric ailments on page 74.

WHAT IS A DEMULCENT?

Demulcent herbs (a.k.a. "slimers") are mucilaginous, which means they become mucus-like on contact with water and form a protective coating on mucosal tissues that soothe and promote healing.

General Uses: Use demulcents when the gut lining is compromised, irritated, or inflamed. They act similarly on the respiratory and urinary tracts and can be applied topically for skin irritation. Great for heartburn, reflux, ulcers, gastritis, leaky gut, inflammatory bowel disease (IBD), diarrhea, constipation, and dysbiosis, including small intestinal bacterial overgrowth (SIBO); for coughs, dry irritated lungs, asthma, and sore throat; for urinary irritation, infection, and cystitis; and for dry, irritated skin and rashes. Note that demulcents don't generally fight infections but can be combined with antimicrobial herbs. They're best in a water base: tea, food, bath.

Examples: Marshmallow and related *Malva* and *Althaea* species, slippery elm, aloe inner gel/juice, licorice, comfrey (note cautions on page 78), violet leaf, fenugreek, oatmeal, flax gel, and corn silk. Wound-healing (vulnerary) and soothing — but less slimy — herbs include plantain, yarrow, gotu kola, St. John's wort, and calendula.

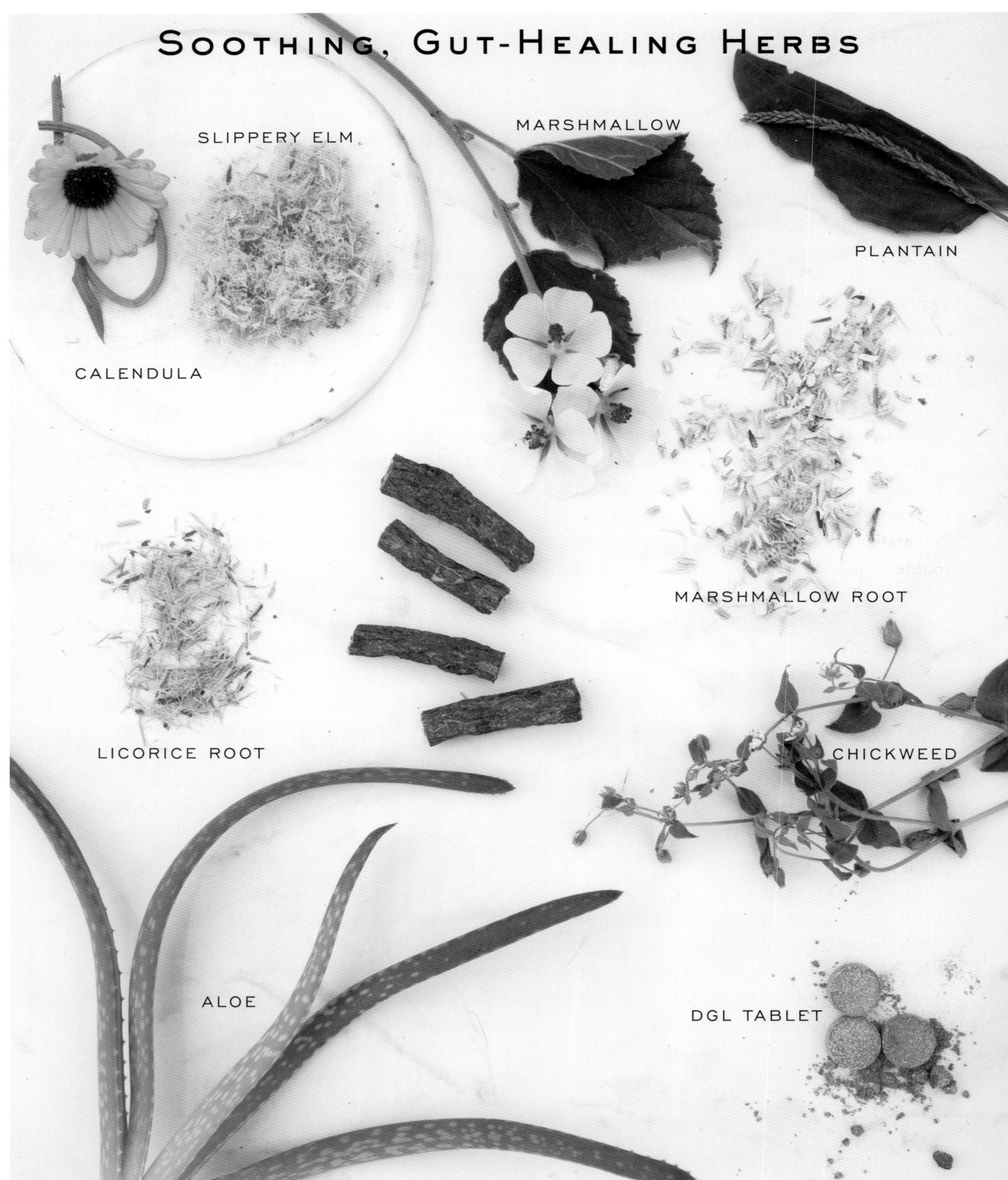
Soothing, Gut-Healing Herbs
Slippery Elm
Marshmallow
Plantain
Calendula
Marshmallow Root
Licorice Root
Chickweed
Aloe
DGL Tablet

▸ Licorice Root

Glycyrrhiza glabra

Availability: G- W- C+

Key Properties: Licorice root has an incredible affinity for healing wounded, inflamed gut tissue while also addressing the root of imbalance. Demulcent, soothing, and slimy, licorice immediately coats the digestive tract, forming a temporary protective lining and quelling acidity and inflammation. Regular use fends off bad gut microbes like *H. pylori* and heals wounds while encouraging the production of a healthier, thicker gut mucosal lining. And it tastes good!

Additional Benefits: In Ayurveda and traditional Chinese medicine, small amounts of licorice are added to formulas to harmonize the herbs and improve overall flavor. Licorice contains steroid-like compounds that support adrenal function and suppress inflammation. It also contains phytoestrogens.

Preparation: Add dried licorice root to your teas to soothe the gut (make it 5 to 20 percent of the formula). Original Throat Coat tea from Traditional Medicinals works in a pinch, as will plain licorice tea and real licorice candy. Deglycyrrhizinated licorice (DGL) chewable tablets are best for regular use — this "dumb" licorice retains the soothing, healing properties and lacks the safety concerns of regular licorice. Chewing two or more tablets before meals and at bedtime can provide instant relief and prevent anticipated problems.

Cautions and Considerations: Long-term, high-dose licorice can raise blood pressure, irritate the kidneys and liver, and interact with some medications due to the compound glycyrrhizin. Some people become hypertensive with even small amounts of licorice, though this is rare. The DGL form is unlikely to pose any risk.

▸ Marshmallow Root

Althaea officinalis

Availability: G W C

Key Properties: A simple "slimer" (a.k.a. a demulcent that gets mucilaginous when it comes in contact with water), marshmallow root coats and soothes inflamed or damaged tissue, creating a temporary mucus-like lining that promotes healing. It tastes pleasant and blends well with other digestive herbs.

Additional Benefits: Marshmallow performs similar feats in the respiratory and kidney-urinary tracts and topically for the skin. It gently stimulates immune function, quells spasms, and decreases inflammation.

Preparation: Best as a tea, whether a long-steeped cold or hot infusion or a decoction. Standard herb doses (see page 298) apply. You can also add marshmallow root to broth or soup, and the powdered root to oatmeal or gruel. Once it gets really slimy, you may not be able to strain it.

Cautions and Considerations: Generally very safe. High doses may delay the absorption of drugs if taken at the same time — separate them by an hour or so. The snot-like consistency can be off-putting; mixing it in slimy food (oatmeal, yogurt) or preparing lighter brews with the cut/sifted (not powdered) root can help.

▸ Other Gut-Healing Herbs

Licorice and marshmallow roots are the classic remedies for ulcers and gastritis, but there are other herbs that can help. **Marshmallow** (leaf and flower) offers similar effects, as does **slippery elm bark** and most ***Malva*** and ***Althaea*** species. Drinking **aloe gel or juice** may also heal and soothe the gut, but beware of whole-leaf preparations that include a harsh irritant laxative from the inner rind.

Other healing herbs include **plantain**, **calendula**, **gotu kola**, and **chickweed** (best fresh), all of which you can incorporate daily into tea blends, soup broth, pesto, or other kinds of food. These plants soothe inflamed tissue and promote the wound-healing process. They're better known as topical wound healers — same concept!

Gut-Healing Tea

This tasty recipe is easily adapted, based on the individual and herb availability. It's appropriate for gastritis, ulcers, heartburn, reflux, leaky gut, acid indigestion, and any condition involving digestive irritation where soothing, healing action is needed. If licorice's side effects are a concern, you can skip it.

- 1 teaspoon marshmallow root
- 1 teaspoon plantain
- ½ teaspoon cinnamon chips or 1 cinnamon stick
- ½ teaspoon licorice root
- ½ teaspoon rose petals
- 3 cloves
- 1 star anise (optional)
- Pinch of freshly grated nutmeg (optional)

Combine the herbs in a small pot. Add 2 cups water, bring to a boil, then reduce the heat and let simmer, covered, for 20 minutes. Remove from the heat and let sit overnight. Strain. Reheat as desired before serving.

Alternatively, if you don't want to wait overnight, you can prepare the tea as a basic decoction or, though weaker in action, an infusion (steep for 60 minutes or longer, preferably in an insulated thermos).

COMFREY: FRIEND OR FOE?

COMFREY LEAF SOOTHES, slimes, and heals, and the allantoin in comfrey *rapidly* heals tissue on contact by encouraging cell proliferation. Small amounts in a tea blend, consumed for up to 1 week, can work miracles in healing ulcers and GI damage. However, comfrey's variable levels of pyrrolizidine alkaloids (PAs) make it one of our most controversial herbs. PAs pose a rare but real risk of accumulating and causing severe liver damage (veno-occlusive disease) when ingested for a long period. The United States bans the internal use of comfrey leaf. You will find varying recommendations (and rampant misinformation) among herbalists. See www.comfreycentral.com for a research summary. Never use comfrey internally if you're pregnant, nor give it to children. If you use comfrey, choose large, older leaves, which have fewer PAs than young leaves (the roots have even higher PA levels).

The Lower GI Tract: Absorption *and* Elimination

Digestion breaks food into the smallest parts possible and then assimilates (absorbs) them into the body where they can be reassembled into new things. Your GI system is like a conveyor belt in a factory, with twists and turns and points at which different components come squirting in or are absorbed up and shuffled elsewhere.

Food exits your stomach in a liquid state called chyme and enters your small intestine, the start of your lower GI tract. Your liver, meanwhile, has been storing bile — a waste product from its work cleansing the blood — in your gallbladder, and your pancreas has been busy making digestive enzymes. The bile and enzymes squirt out of the common bile duct to combine with the chyme as it enters the intestines. Bile acts like soap on a dirty dishpan, breaking up fat molecules into tiny particles that are easier for the body to deal with. Enzymes break compounds into simple forms. Protein becomes amino acids, carbs become simple sugars, fats break down into fatty acids, and so on.

Now the chyme moves through the 20-plus-foot-long meandering, narrow tube of the small intestine. Little fingerlike villi and microvilli increase the surface area and "grab" key nutrients to be directed into the body, primarily via the bloodstream. By the time the chyme reaches your large intestine, most nutrients have been removed. As the chyme passes through the large intestine, the muscular structure of the colon wrings most of the liquid out of it, much like you would wring out a wet towel. The rectal sphincter opens, and peristalsis moves the waste out of your body as feces. This last act of elimination is often triggered by a new meal stimulating peristalsis along the GI tract.

Good Bugs, Bad Bugs, and Probiotics

Intestinal health depends largely on beneficial bacteria, or probiotics. Good gut flora — part of your "microbiome" — discourage pathogens, help break down fiber and complex sugars, help your body make essential vitamin K, folic acid, and vitamin B_{12}, keep your bowel movements regular, decrease inflammation, modulate immune health (helping to ward off allergies, cancer, and autoimmune disease), and support healthy metabolism. But the typical overprocessed American diet tends to starve good bugs while feeding the bad. If your lower GI tract isn't behaving properly, boosting beneficial bacteria can bring it back into balance. To begin, try adding traditional fermented foods like kimchi, sauerkraut, yogurt, and kefir to your diet, a little every day. Fermented foods are full of beneficial bacteria and a host of essential nutrients. Simultaneously and slowly increase your consumption of fiber, plants, and complex carbohydrates to feed the beneficial bacteria: honey, leeks, cabbage, beans, onions, garlic, and pretty much everything on the FODMAP list (see page 85).

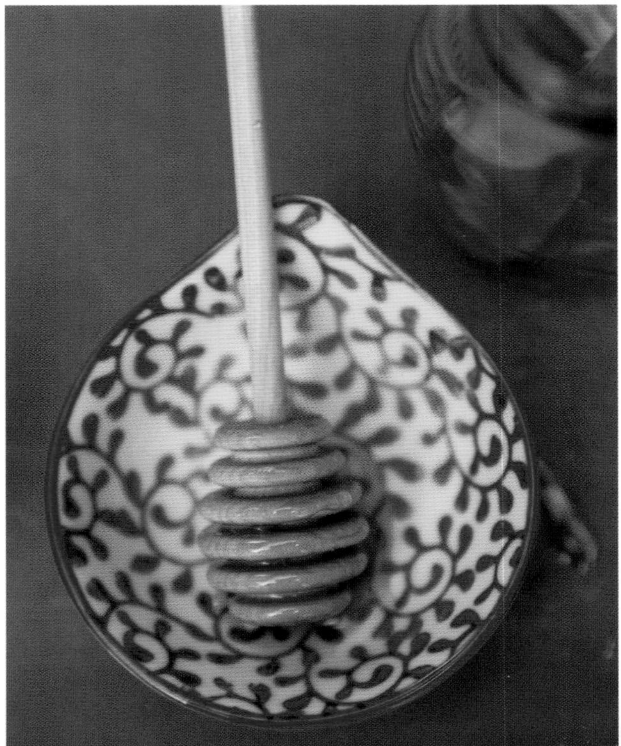

Rose petals and ginger discourage pathogens while encouraging probiotics — add them to digestive tea blends. Probiotic dietary supplements can do quick work to correct an imbalance — look for products that contain a variety of species, particularly those from the *Lactobacillus* and *Bifidobacterium* genera. Choose one with more than 1 billion live bacteria per pill and a coating to help the pill bypass stomach acid to release in the intestines.

Probiotics correct many cases of chronic diarrhea, constipation, and irritable bowel syndrome (IBS). They are an important part of a larger protocol for more serious conditions, including inflammatory bowel disease (IBD), small intestinal bacterial overgrowth (SIBO), dysbiosis, dysentery, and acute gut damage, as well as complex issues like autism and hyperactivity. Commercial probiotic supplements are a convenient option, but you can easily make your own fermented foods at home. Check out the books *Fermented Vegetables* by Kirsten and Christopher Shockey and *Wild Fermentation* by Sandor Katz for more information and recipes.

Gas, Pain, and Bloating

An unbalanced digestive system will often produce gas, pain, and bloating. Common culprits include dysbiosis (lack of beneficial bacteria and/or influx of bad bacteria/yeast), poor diet, stress, food allergies/sensitivities, and physical damage to the gut (from celiac disease, inflammatory bowel disease, diverticulitis, leaky gut).

Fiber and complex starches feed good bacteria while modulating gut motility. If you've been eating a more refined, processed diet, you'll probably find the addition of fiber and certain foods (beans, garlic, onions, cruciferous vegetables) uncomfortable because your body and gut flora aren't accustomed to them. Work them in gradually while simultaneously boosting good gut flora with probiotic supplements and/or fermented food.

Carminative herbs and spices like fennel, ginger, and peppermint relax cramped intestines to move gas through and help it dissipate. Almost any GI blend should include at least a carminative or two, which often adds great flavor, because carminatives include our most beloved culinary and tea herbs. If you have reflux, though, sip with caution; carminatives sometimes relax the lower esophageal sphincter and worsen symptoms. (And sometime they relieve reflux, so try it out and see.) Carminatives tend to be warming — they're a nice complement to "cold" digestive bitters, but go easy on them with "hot" GI issues including inflammation and tissue damage. Your body will let you know whether or not carminatives are right for you.

WHAT IS A CARMINATIVE?

Carminatives improve digestion, dispel gas, ease bloating, and act as antispasmodics to relieve cramps.

General Uses: Carminatives provide almost immediate relief for GI distress and work well as tasty synergists in GI blends. They tend to be warming in nature, and many have antimicrobial properties that encourage good gut flora while inhibiting pathogens. They are primary herbs for indigestion, gas, pain, bloating, colic, IBS, and intestinal cramps and supportive herbs alongside bitters and in herbal blends to heal the gut or address diarrhea/constipation, IBD, or dysbiosis. Also use them for other muscle cramps and tension, including menstrual cramps and headaches. Use them in cooking to make other ingredients easier to digest.

Examples: Many aromatic culinary seed spices: fennel, cardamom, anise, cumin, coriander, caraway, dill, juniper, nutmeg, black pepper. Also cinnamon, ginger, turmeric, peppermint, chamomile, catnip, lemon balm, holy basil, savory, oregano, bee balm, angelica root, and elecampane.

▸ Fennel

Foeniculum vulgare

Availability: G+ W C+

Key Properties: Fennel seeds — and to a lesser extent the bulb, fronds, and flowers — provide almost instantaneous GI relief. Chewing on just a few seeds can bring folks up off the floor within minutes after writhing in pain from intestinal gas. Fennel also stars in many "gripe water" recipes for babies with colic and can be similarly used for these symptoms in adults.

Additional Benefits: Fennel offers sweet, licorice-like flavor to blends and may also aid coughs due to its antispasmodic properties. A small taste of the seeds can ease nausea.

Preparation: Chew the fresh or dry seeds (easy and fast), or use them in tea, cordials, tinctures, and elixirs. Use the low end of standard herb doses (see page 298). Try the fronds and bulbs for cooking, or infuse them in seltzer (see page 312).

Cautions and Considerations: Fennel is one of our safest carminatives in low to moderate doses, especially as food or tea, even for pregnant and nursing women and infants. High doses (tinctures, capsules, several cups of tea daily) may be less appropriate.

Similar Herbs: Closely related **anise** and **dill** offer very similar benefits. Also consider other carminatives like **cardamom**. Mint-family garden herbs **anise hyssop** and **Korean licorice mint** also have a fennel-like flavor and benefits for the digestive system. Because fennel's flavor is so similar to that of anise, star anise, and licorice, there is sometimes confusion and mislabeling. Star anise and licorice are unrelated and offer different healing properties. Candy, extracts, and other flavored products labeled "licorice" or "anise" may include different herbs or even artificial flavors; read the ingredients list.

▸ Peppermint

Mentha × piperita

Availability: G+ W C+

Key Properties: Peppermint leaves are another classic carminative tonic. The oil extracted from the leaves is rich in menthol, which acts as a potent antispasmodic, and enteric-coated peppermint oil capsules perform well for gas, pain, and IBS — though they can be minty fresh on the way out. The tea offers milder action, and you can also dilute a drop of peppermint essential oil in some olive oil and rub it onto your belly.

Additional Benefits: Peppermint invigorates the mind and spirit, clears the sinuses, relieves coughs, eases some types of pain (like headaches), and quells nausea.

Preparation: Peppermint enteric-coated capsules target lower GI spasms and pain. Tea works better for the upper GI tract. Standard herb doses (see page 298) apply. Dilute the essential oil in vegetable oil for topical use (too much burns the skin). Peppermint candy or gum works in a pinch.

Cautions and Considerations: Peppermint often aggravates reflux (though spearmint may not), and the essential oil should always be diluted.

Similar Herbs: Other mint-family culinary and tea herbs provide similar benefits even though their essential oil profiles and strength vary, including **lemon balm, oregano, rosemary, savory, thyme, bee balm, holy basil, anise hyssop, Korean licorice mint,** and **lavender.**

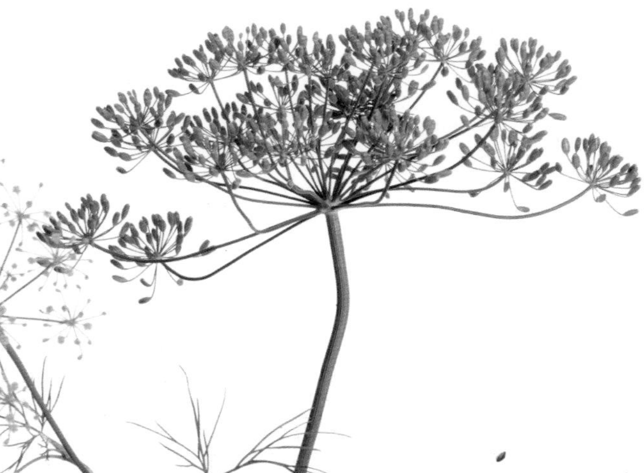

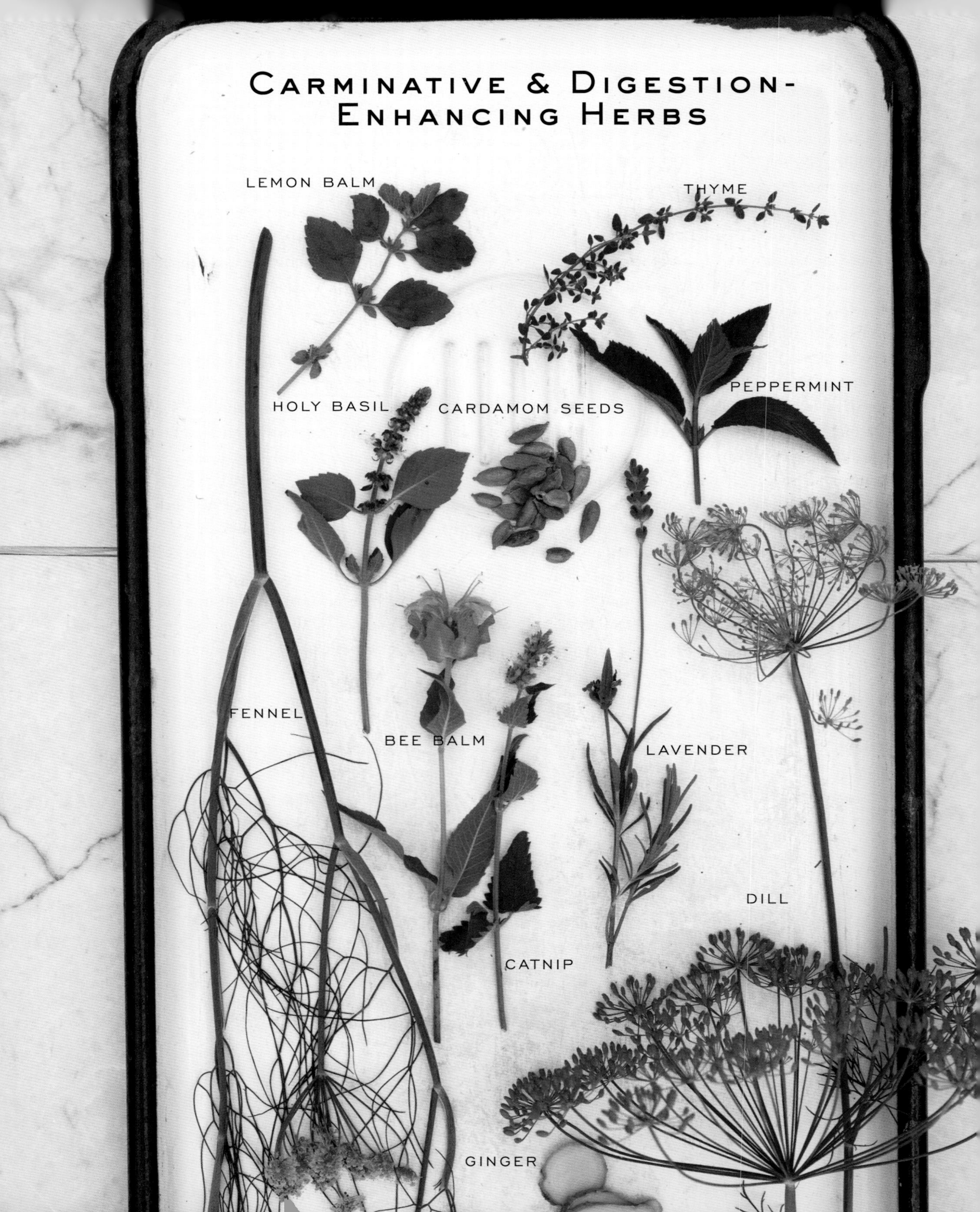
CARMINATIVE & DIGESTION-ENHANCING HERBS
LEMON BALM
THYME
PEPPERMINT
HOLY BASIL
CARDAMOM SEEDS
FENNEL
BEE BALM
LAVENDER
DILL
CATNIP
GINGER

▸ Ginger

Zingiber officinale

Availability: G C+

Key Properties: This zingy root is a carminative and a whole lot more! Employ it like a digestive bitter. The fresh root contains protein-digesting enzymes. Its spicy nature warms up a sluggish digestive system, promotes beneficial bacteria, kills gut pathogens, and relieves gas, pain, bloating, and — ginger's biggest claim to fame — nausea.

Additional Benefits: Ginger also decreases inflammation, boosts detoxification, reduces blood sugar, improves insulin sensitivity, increases circulation, breaks down fibrin and makes blood less sticky, fights respiratory infections, and eases the painful symptoms of a range of ailments, from a sore throat to rheumatoid arthritis and osteoarthritis.

Preparation: Fresh works best. Thinly slice or grate the root to simmer or infuse (i.e., in a thermos for an hour or longer) it for tea, or prepare it as a tincture. Standard herb doses (see page 298) apply, but feel free to use ginger generously in all sorts of food preparations, and also consider ginger-infused honey, ginger juice, pickled ginger (skip the pink dye), and strong ginger candy.

Cautions and Considerations: Generally very safe, even in pregnancy, but ginger can be too hot and spicy for some, especially in its dried form or excessive doses. Opt for weaker forms (candy, honey, mild tea) during pregnancy. Use caution when combining it with medications, especially blood thinners.

Similar Herbs: Closely related **turmeric** offers similar benefits but acts more like a bitter/liver herb and isn't quite so hot. It blends well with ginger.

Killer Chai

Consider this tasty blend for support during dysbiosis; it discourages pathogenic bacteria and fungi in the gut. It's best served without cream or sugar.

- 1 teaspoon cinnamon chips or 1–2 sticks
- 1 teaspoon pau d'arco
- 1 (½-inch) piece ginger, sliced thin
- 6 whole cloves
- 3 cardamom pods
- 1 star anise pod (optional)
- Few rose petals (optional)
- Pinch of nutmeg (optional)
- Pinch of black pepper (optional)

Combine the herbs with 2 cups water in a saucepan. Bring to a boil, then reduce the heat and let simmer, covered, for 20 minutes. Strain and serve. That's the best method. Alternatively, you can put the herbs in a thermos, pour 2 cups boiling water over them, and let steep for 30 to 60 minutes or longer.

COMMON FOOD ALLERGENS AND SENSITIVITIES

FOOD ALLERGIES AND SENSITIVITIES tend to play a major role in chronic digestive woes, including indigestion, gas, pain, bloating, irritable bowel syndrome, inflammatory bowel disease, and dysbiosis. In contrast to the swift, severe allergic reaction caused by IgG antibodies, the IgE antibodies associated with most food sensitivities and mild allergies cause low-level inflammation and irritation, as can other forms of food intolerance. This can create immediate discomfort as well as long-term degradation of the digestive tract structure and function. Food sensitivities may also create or worsen other health concerns, including depression, impaired cognitive function, inflammation and pain, seasonal allergies, and autoimmune disease. While herbs help, they're unlikely to fix the problem unless the aggravating food is removed. It is possible to be allergic or sensitive to any food, and allergies and sensitivities change over time. The information below should serve as a guide, not as rules.

Gluten and/or Wheat

Common sources: Wheat (including varieties and ancient forms: spelt, kamut, einkorn, emmer, durum, semolina, triticale, freekeh, farro, farina), barley and bulgur, rye, seitan, malt, brewer's yeast. Wheat and gluten are in many processed foods. (Note: Oats and corn don't contain gluten, but some people with gluten issues also react to them due to cross-contamination or grain allergies beyond gluten.)

Possible reasons: Reaction to gluten, reaction to more recent breeds of wheat, celiac disease, difficulty digesting starches in grains (including poor gut health, dysbiosis), reaction to herbicides (such as Roundup) used in nonorganic grain production. Because most gluten/wheat-based foods are also high carbohydrate, negative reactions (like brain fog, bad mood, inflammation, cravings, and weight gain) may simply be due to the blood sugar roller coaster.

Common symptoms: Many digestive issues (gas, pain, bloating, diarrhea/constipation, IBS, IBD, leaky gut, dysbiosis, gastritis), poor nutrient absorption, whole-body inflammation, chronic pain, skin rashes/issues, autoimmune disease (particularly celiac disease, IBD, thyroid disease, rheumatoid arthritis), attention/brain/memory issues, autism spectrum disorders, insulin resistance, diabetes, heart disease, obesity

Dairy

Common sources: Milk, cheese, cream, butter, ghee, yogurt, kefir, et cetera. Many processed foods contain dairy ingredients.

Possible reasons: Reaction to casein (a protein in milk), difficulty digesting lactose (milk sugar), reaction to the damp/cool nature of dairy, reaction to processed dairy (some people who don't normally tolerate dairy do fine if it's raw, fermented, unpasteurized, or nonhomogenized). Note: People whose ancestry derives from cultural groups that rarely ate dairy tend to have a more difficult time digesting it.

Common symptoms: Many digestive issues (gas, pain, bloating, diarrhea/constipation, IBS, IBD, leaky gut, dysbiosis, gastritis), poor nutrient absorption, whole-body inflammation, chronic pain, chronic congestion (respiratory issues, cough, ear infections, sinus infections, weak immune health, allergies), autism spectrum disorders

Soy

Common sources: Soy, soya, soybeans, tofu, tempeh, miso, natto, soy milk, edamame, soy nuts, isolated soy protein, soy isoflavones, soy flour, soy sauce, lecithin, soy nut butter, tamari/soy sauce/liquid aminos, textured vegetable protein. Soy is found in many processed foods as well as vitamin E.

Possible reasons: Reaction to soy protein, reaction to phytoestrogen activity of soy, difficulty with highly processed soy products/ ingredients, difficulty digesting soy. Note that raw soy is hard on the pancreas, soy can interfere with thyroid function, and most nonorganic soy is genetically modified.

Common symptoms: Allergy responses (including rashes, inflammation, anaphylaxis), digestive issues, autoimmune disease, thyroid disease, hormone/reproductive issues

Eggs

Common sources: Eggnog, mayonnaise, meringue, and egg-derived ingredients like albumin, ovalbumin, and lysozyme. Eggs may also be found in egg substitutes, lecithin, marzipan, pasta, nougat, marshmallows, and many baked goods, desserts, and processed foods. They're found in some vaccines.

Possible reasons: Reaction to egg protein or difficulty digesting eggs. Egg allergies are more common if you have atopic dermatitis, are a child (in which case you may outgrow the allergy over time), or have a family history.

Common symptoms: Digestive issues (especially diarrhea/loose stools), skin reactions (rashes, hives, atopic dermatitis redness, scaly skin), overall inflammation, chronic pain

FODMAPs

Common sources: FODMAPs = fermentable oligo-, di-, and monosaccharides and polyols. This group encompasses a wide range of carbohydrate-based foods that may be difficult to absorb. They include oligosaccharides and fructans (wheat, rye, barley, onion, garlic, sunchokes, asparagus, beets, chicory, dandelion, cruciferous vegetables, and other prebiotics including fructooligosaccharides and inulin), galactans (beans and legumes), polyols (stone fruits, watermelon, sugar alcohols like xylitol), fructose (high-fructose corn syrup, agave nectar, honey, and fruits like pears, apples, raisins), and lactose (dairy).

Possible reasons: Lack of beneficial gut bacteria, which would normally feed on these ingredients; dysbiosis and overgrowth of pathogenic bacteria or fungi in the gut, which react poorly to FODMAPs; damage and inflammation in the lower GI lining

Common symptoms: Digestive issues (especially lower GI complaints like gas, pain, bloating), poor nutrient absorption, inflammation. You may find that only certain FODMAP foods are triggers for you. Reactions to FODMAP trigger foods generally are a symptom of poor gut health and dysbiosis (including SIBO); the foods are not themselves the cause of disease. To treat, avoid large quantities of FODMAPs, introduce beneficial bacteria, support gut health, and gradually reintroduce/increase FODMAP foods to feed good bacteria as gut health begins to normalize. While sugar may not cause digestive distress, it feeds pathogens.

Sugar and High-Glycemic Foods

Common sources: Sugar, flour, potatoes, "white foods," processed/refined carbohydrates, honey, maple syrup, grains, starchy vegetables

Possible reasons: Sugars and high-glycemic foods can aggravate cases of high blood sugar, insulin resistance, or diabetes; create a hospitable environment for pathogenic bacteria and fungi; take the place of healthy, nutrient-dense whole foods in the diet; cause inflammation; and irritate the nervous-endocrine system.

Common symptoms: Poor mood, stress, memory issues, hyperactivity, fatigue, dysbiosis (including SIBO), yeast infections, blood sugar issues, insulin resistance, diabetes, hormone/ reproductive issues, weight gain/fat storage (especially abdominal obesity), inflammation, heart disease, high triglycerides/high bad cholesterol/low good cholesterol

Moving Things Along: Smooth Elimination

Excessive bowel movements — or a lack thereof — are a significant source of stress and debility for many. Here's a basic overview of what sets you up for good bowel health:

- **Hydrate.** Water keeps your GI tract functioning properly. Dehydration aggravates constipation and makes fiber less effective. In diarrhea, excessive water loss can cause dangerous dehydration. Increase fluid intake and restore electrolytes with special formulas, soup, miso, or a pinch of salt and dash of juice. (Dehydration due to acute diarrhea can be lethal and may require immediate medical treatment.)

- **Reduce stress.** Stress slows gut motility for most, leading to constipation, and can also aggravate chronic diarrhea due to IBS and IBD. Meditation, breathwork, and relaxing digestive herbs (such as chamomile, catnip, holy basil, or lemon balm) can help.

- **Address food allergies and sensitivities.** These particularly aggravate chronic diarrhea, IBS, IBD, leaky gut, gas, pain, and bloating. Keep a food diary and consider having a blood test or trying an elimination diet to identify the source of the problem. (See page 84.)

- **Eat a whole-foods diet and fiber.** Processed and sugary foods aggravate constipation and diarrhea. Slowly switch over to a whole-foods diet rich in vegetables, whole grains, seeds, fruit, and beans, which will naturally provide fiber. Or take ground flax or psyllium seed mixed with water, though a naturally high-fiber diet works best. Insoluble fiber soaks up water to act as a bulk laxative in constipation and pull together loose stools. It also encourages good gut bacteria.

- **Add probiotics and fermented foods.** Good gut flora help push out gut pathogens and normalize bowel movements. Start with small amounts; diarrhea may occur initially (especially if bad bugs flourish in your gut) but should pass with time. Be cautious with fermented dairy — even though it's the most popular fermented food, many people with lower GI issues are sensitive to dairy. (For more on probiotics, see page 79.)

WHAT IS AN ASTRINGENT?

Astringent herbs generally contain tannins, which tighten and tone tissue by binding together the proteins that are present in the gut lining (think: tanning hides to make leather).

General Uses: Astringent herbs heal tissue while counteracting conditions like bleeding, diarrhea, leaky gut, inflammation, and infection. They tend to have a dry feel on the tongue but aren't truly drying; they hold fluids in. Many also discourage pathogens. Use them for diarrhea, bleeding, leaky gut, wounds, varicose veins, weak skin, IBD, gastritis, ulcers, dysbiosis, menstrual bleeding, excessive vaginal discharge, pregnancy preparation, fungal infections.

Examples: A continuum of astringent herbs are available to us. White oak bark, witch hazel, and other tree barks are best used topically and short term for acute conditions. Gentler rose-family astringents like rose petals, raspberry leaf, blackberry root, and wild strawberry leaves are appropriate for daily or long-term use. Aerial parts of common weeds in the *Bidens* genus, Canadian fleabane, and purple loosestrife are also astringents. Somewhere in the middle lies cinnamon bark. It's tasty, carminative, and strongly antimicrobial. Also consider fresh yarrow and dry alder bark.

- **Obey the urge.** Going poo can seem so . . . inconvenient, but ignoring the urge makes your gut cranky and dulls peristalsis and digestive signals. If you're constipated, bitters and some practice listening to your body will help you avoid long stretches between bowel movements and unsuccessful throne visits. Diarrhea-prone folks already know that holding back is a bad idea, and living off Imodium just masks underlying imbalance. As you sit, relax by reading, doing breathing exercises, slowly breathing out through your mouth (which helps relax your rectal sphincter), and doing abdominal massage (up the right, across, down the left).
- **Use modulating herbs.** If all else fails, yellow dock root and the Ayurvedic blend triphala contain small amounts of laxative compounds called anthraquinone glycosides, which irritate the colon and stimulate peristalsis, but they also contain some tannins, which tone and strengthen the colon. Modest doses aid constipation *and* diarrhea. They're relatively safe and can be taken short- or long-term as capsules, tincture, tea, or powder. Don't go nuts on the dose, though — you're likely to end up with explosive diarrhea followed by terrible constipation.

PROTOCOL POINTS

IBS and IBD

Irritable bowel syndrome (IBS) and inflammatory bowel disease (IBD) are completely different conditions — the first is a malfunction of the gut that can be uncomfortable but not generally dangerous, while the second is an autoimmune disease that results in the gradual disintegration of the gut lining and an increased risk for colorectal cancer. Yet their symptoms overlap, as do many of the diet, lifestyle, and herbal remedies that help restore gut vitality and address these two conditions.

Diet: Sleuth out and avoid your personal food allergens and sensitivities, which often include dairy, wheat/gluten, eggs, corn, and soy. A food diary can be a helpful place to start — these allergens are hidden in *lots* of processed food. This is important! No matter how many herbs you take, your gut will never be 100 percent right if you eat foods that you're allergic or sensitive to. (Leaky gut increases food allergies via the immune response. Once you've avoided all problem foods for a while and healed your gut, you may find that some "allergies" go away and that some foods you were sensitive to are now tolerable in small amounts in rotation.) Also temporarily limit personal triggers for gas and bloating, which often include legumes, fiber, garlic/onions, and members of the cabbage family — these prebiotics feed good bacteria but cause gas and bloating when bad gut bacteria proliferate. Add in probiotic supplements and/or fermented foods, and then slowly work in the prebiotic foods. Avoid refined foods and excess carbs. (For more on identifying and managing food allergies and sensitivities, see page 84.)

Lifestyle: Address stress, a major trigger for all causes of gas and bloating, including IBS and IBD. Incorporate stress-relieving herbs (see chapter 3), and take part in mindfulness activities like breathwork or meditation. Set aside relaxing time to eat. Be nice to your intestines: avoid tight clothing and stand and walk more. Abdominal massage (up the right side, across, and down the left, following the path of the large intestine) can help move things along.

Herbs: Carminatives for immediate spasm and gas relief: fennel, cardamom, anise, dill, ginger, peppermint (ideally enteric coated), or add a few drops of carminative essential oil to olive oil and rub it on your belly. For stress-related colic-type symptoms, use relaxing digestive herbs like holy basil, lemon balm, chamomile, or catnip. In IBD and other cases where the gut lining is physically damaged, use the healing, soothing herbs recommended for ulcers and gastric wounds (see page 75), and rely on easily digested foods like broth, soup, and tea; stronger medications and surgery may also be necessary for IBD.

PROTOCOL POINTS

Diarrhea

Diarrhea is more complicated than constipation. Short bursts of diarrhea during an infection provide your body with an easy way to eliminate pathogens before they can do too much damage. Generally you just want to stay out of its way, rest, and keep hydrated (including replacing electrolytes). However, diarrhea that persists or is chronic requires medical attention and proper diagnosis. Severe diarrhea can be life threatening. If the situation is recalcitrant or chronic, get tested for parasites or other pathogens, dysbiosis, food allergies and sensitivities, and IBD.

That said, you can use herbs to slow down chronic diarrhea or curb infection-related diarrhea that has outlived its purpose while also discouraging pathogens and healing inflamed, irritated, and even damaged gut tissue. Even in serious conditions like Crohn's disease and ulcerative colitis (types of IBD), holistic therapies can often be used alongside conventional care, but it's important to know what you're dealing with first. In addition to the general tips on page 87, especially hydration, consider the following:

Diet: First and foremost, hydration plus electrolytes. Food therapies include the BRAT diet (bananas, rice, applesauce, toast) and broths made with nutritive herbs, animal bones, mushrooms, seaweeds, or miso to rehydrate while providing useful electrolytes and easy-to-absorb nutrients. A digestive system in a constant state of diarrhea and inflammation is likely doing a poor job absorbing nutrients from typical food. Probiotics and fermented foods will help pave the road to recovery.

Herbs: In acute diarrhea, white oak bark or its gentler leaves, dry alder bark, blackberry root tincture, or a full teaspoon of cinnamon or carob (the unimpressive chocolate substitute) powder mixed in water or applesauce can help staunch the flow. Most of these herbs also address pathogens. For chronic diarrhea, cinnamon can still be helpful, as can gentle astringents like rose petals, smaller doses of alder bark, and aerial parts of common weeds beggar's-ticks, Canadian fleabane, and purple loosestrife; take them as tea or tincture. Depending on the situation, antimicrobial, demulcent, and gut-healing herbs may also be appropriate.

The demulcent, soothing, healing herbs mentioned earlier for ulcer and reflux (see page 74) are equally valuable in the lower GI for damage control, as are probiotics for repopulating the colon with good bacteria that can restore digestive function while pushing out the bad guys. Be particularly aware of foods that aggravate digestive wellness — particularly any food allergies/sensitivities. They are *often* at play in chronic diarrhea as well as other forms of lower gut imbalance. Even if you didn't have food issues to begin with, inflamed gut tissue may occasionally become "leaky," which means that food particles may float out of the GI tract where the immune system encounters the out-of-place particles, deems them intruders, and marks them with antigen status. You might find that once the gut is back in working order, food reactions diminish.

For diarrhea related to infection or dysbiosis, antimicrobial digestive herbs often help. Some of the best include cinnamon, bee balm, oregano, chamomile, ginger, rose petals, pau d'arco, usnea, alder, and cloves. Consider making a strong herbal chai with added pau d'arco or alder, for example. One of the best-researched plant-based compounds for killing gut microbes is berberine, a bitter yellow alkaloid found in goldenseal, barberry, Oregon grape, and *Coptis* species. Berberine offers stellar antibacterial and antifungal action when it comes into contact with pathogens in the gut or elsewhere. (Take note: It works locally, not systemically.) It's also a bit of an antihistamine, it is incredibly bitter, and it increases digestive secretions, yet is drying by nature. Due to berberine's strength and ethics surrounding the overharvesting of most of its plant sources, seek organically cultivated sources and use berberine only for short-term, acute needs. Finally, limit or eliminate sugar in the diet, including refined foods and flours, because these tend to stress the GI while feeding pathogens.

Dysbiosis

Dysbiosis occurs when pathogens like harmful bacteria and fungi outcompete your good gut flora. Poor digestion, gut inflammation and damage, gas and bloating, and wonky elimination get worse as it progresses. Though this is sometimes called "candida," this term may be myopic and inaccurate. Small intestinal bacterial overgrowth (SIBO) is a form of dysbiosis. Dysbiosis can cause FODMAP food reactions, leaky gut, malnutrition/malabsorption, and more food allergies and sensitivities over time.

Diet: Reduce or eliminate sugar and white foods like flour, potatoes, refined carbs, juice, alcohol, and sweeteners. (Some people go a step further and remove all starchy vegetables, all grains, and most beans and fruit for several months, though it may not be necessary.) Slowly increase fermented foods such as kimchi, fermented veggies, and miso. Also take fermented dairy (yogurt, kefir) if you tolerate it. Focus on foods and spices that discourage gut pathogens: garlic, oregano, thyme, cinnamon, cloves. Eat a nutrient-dense diet emphasizing nourishing broths, lean protein, vegetables and leafy greens, nuts, and seeds. As your symptoms subside, slowly reintroduce small amounts of whole-food carbohydrates like beans, grains, and starchy vegetables. As your beneficial bacteria increase, slowly introduce prebiotic foods (foods that feed gut flora) such as sunchokes, dandelion roots, burdock roots, chicory roots, garlic, onions, leeks, and asparagus. If you've previously had a hard time digesting cruciferous vegetables (broccoli, cauliflower, cabbage), beans, and grains, you may find that this gets better as your gut health improves.

Lifestyle: Aim for a general healthy lifestyle, especially stress management and adequate sleep. Treat yourself in other ways — a massage, relaxation time, creative projects — if you find that limiting your diet and former comfort foods provokes anxiety.

Herbs: Emphasize antimicrobial herbs that target gut pathogens, including cinnamon, bee balm, oregano, cloves, ginger, chamomile, rose petals, pau d'arco, usnea, licorice, garlic, and alder. Berberine-rich herbs may be used short term as well. Support the health of your gut lining with demulcent and vulnerary herbs. Consider a high-dose probiotics supplement.

Constipation

Yes, you have several laxative herbs at your disposal. But before you even think about dipping that bag of Smooth Move into your teacup, try some more holistic approaches first. See the tips on page 87, and try those first. Especially look at stress, obeying the urge, hydration, and fiber intake.

Phase 1 Herbs: Digestive bitters can indirectly stimulate peristalsis and bowel movements while retraining gut health. Consider artichoke, schizandra, dandelion, turmeric, lemon, grapefruit, and so on; see page 71.

Phase 2 Herbs: Try yellow dock or triphala; both of these colon tonics are safer, gentler, and more appropriate for the long term than more potent stimulant laxatives.

In Acute Cases: In acute situations, a stronger stimulant laxative may be helpful for short-term use. Senna leaves and pods, cascara sagrada bark, turkey rhubarb root, buckthorn bark, and aloe latex are quite effective. They should be blended with soothing and carminative herbs to ease the irritation and cramping that they cause. Even though these herbs are natural and commonly used, they are not holistic. Over time, they weaken the body's ability to induce peristalsis, atrophy the colon, and are quickly habit forming (not emotionally but physically — you can't go without them).

AT A GLANCE

Herbs for Digestion and Elimination

UPPER GI TRACT: Enhancing Digestion

Bitters and Sours

- Artichoke leaf
- Dandelion leaf and root
- Burdock root
- Yellow dock root
- Turmeric
- Schizandra
- Citrus peel
- Gentian*
- Wormwood** (low dose)

Bitter Berberines

- Goldenseal*
- Coptis/goldthread
- Oregon grape root
- Barberry

Relaxing Bitters

- Catnip
- Lemon balm
- Chamomile
- Blue vervain
- Skullcap
- Motherwort
- Wood betony
- Holy basil

Sialogogues

- Echinacea (fresh, all parts)
- Spilanthes

Other Digestive Stimulants & Aids

- Ginger
- Apple cider vinegar
- Digestive enzyme supplements
- Papaya
- Pineapple/bromelain
- Carminatives (e.g., ginger, cinnamon, cardamom, cayenne)

UPPER AND LOWER GI TRACT: Healing Inflammation and Damage (Ulcers, Reflux, Gastritis, IBS, IBD)

Demulcents ("Slimers")

- Licorice
- Comfrey leaf and root**
- Slippery elm*
- Marshmallow
- Mallow leaf and flower
- Violet leaf
- Aloe inner gel
- Flax gel (steeped in cold or hot water, flaxseeds form a mucilaginous gel)

Vulneraries

- Plantain
- Gotu kola
- Cabbage juice (raw)
- Calendula
- Yarrow
- St. John's wort
- Astragalus
- Glutamine (an amino acid supplement)

Muscle Toner

- Bitter orange peel extract

LOWER GI TRACT: Promoting Healthy Elimination

Insoluble Fiber

- Psyllium
- Flaxseeds
- Hemp and chia seeds

Soluble Fiber

- Apple pectin
- Pears
- Beans and lentils

Demulcents

- Slippery elm
- Marshmallow root

Mild/Tonifying Laxatives

- Triphala
- Yellow dock root
- Aloe inner gel

Stimulant Laxatives

- Aloe latex/whole leaf**
- Senna**
- Cascara**
- Buckthorn bark**
- Turkey rhubarb root**

Antidiarrheals

- Tonic/gentle astringents listed for healing the lower GI tract (page 79)
- Cinnamon

Stronger Astringents (for short-term or low-dose use)

- Blackberry root
- Carob
- White oak bark

LOWER GI TRACT: **Healing Damage, Repairing Dysbiosis**

Tonic/Gentle Astringents

- Rose family (raspberry leaf, rose petals, lady's mantle, wild strawberry leaf, cinquefoil leaf, agrimony)
- Yarrow
- Canadian fleabane
- *Bidens* spp.
- Purple loosestrife
- Alder bark and twigs (dry)

Sources of Good Gut Flora

- Probiotics
- Fermented foods

Supports for Good Gut Flora

- Ginger
- Inulin (good sources include chicory, dandelion, burdock, elecampane, and sunchoke roots)
- Leek, onion, garlic
- Asparagus
- Oligosaccharides (fructooligosaccharides, inulin, etc.)
- Fiber
- Rose petals

Antimicrobials

- Pau d'arco
- Bitter berberines (goldenseal,* coptis/goldthread, Oregon grape root, barberry)
- Chai spices (clove, cinnamon, cardamom, ginger, licorice)
- Mint family (oregano, bee balm, thyme, savory, holy basil)
- Garlic and onion
- Rose petals
- Chaga
- Probiotics
- Black walnut leaf
- Fireweed
- Spilanthes
- Usnea
- Alder bark and twigs (dry)
- Elecampane

Antiparasitics

- Clove
- Garlic
- Black walnut hull
- Wormwood**

UPPER AND LOWER GI TRACT: **Stimulating Function, Relaxing Spasms**

Antispasmodics and Carminatives

- Peppermint and other mint-family herbs (oregano, bee balm, thyme, savory)
- Anise and fennel seeds (also the bulb and fronds)
- Cardamom pods
- Dill seeds (also the fronds)
- Angelica root
- Caraway, coriander, and cumin seeds
- Relaxing bitters (catnip, lemon balm, holy basil, chamomile, holy basil, etc.)
- Chai-like spices (cinnamon, cloves)
- Oregano, bee balm, thyme, savory
- Ginger and turmeric
- Elecampane root

Antimicrobials

- Mastic gum
- Bitter berberines (goldenseal,* coptis/goldthread, Oregon grape root, barberry)
- Usnea
- Licorice (preventive)
- Chamomile (preventive)
- Black tea (preventive)

**These plants are at risk in the wild. Use responsibly or find an alternative herb to use.*

***Though of course you should always research the plants before you use them, the plants marked with a double asterisk can have more significant side effects than others. Understand the cautions associated with them before using them.*

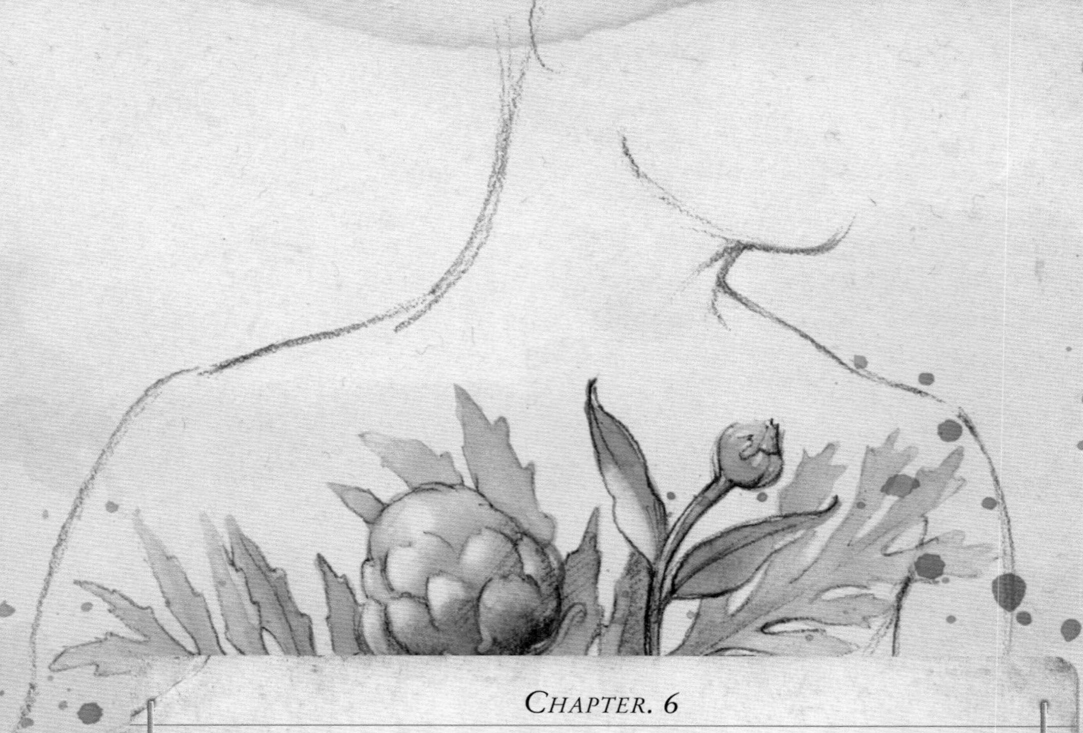

Chapter. 6

Detoxification: Cleanup Time!

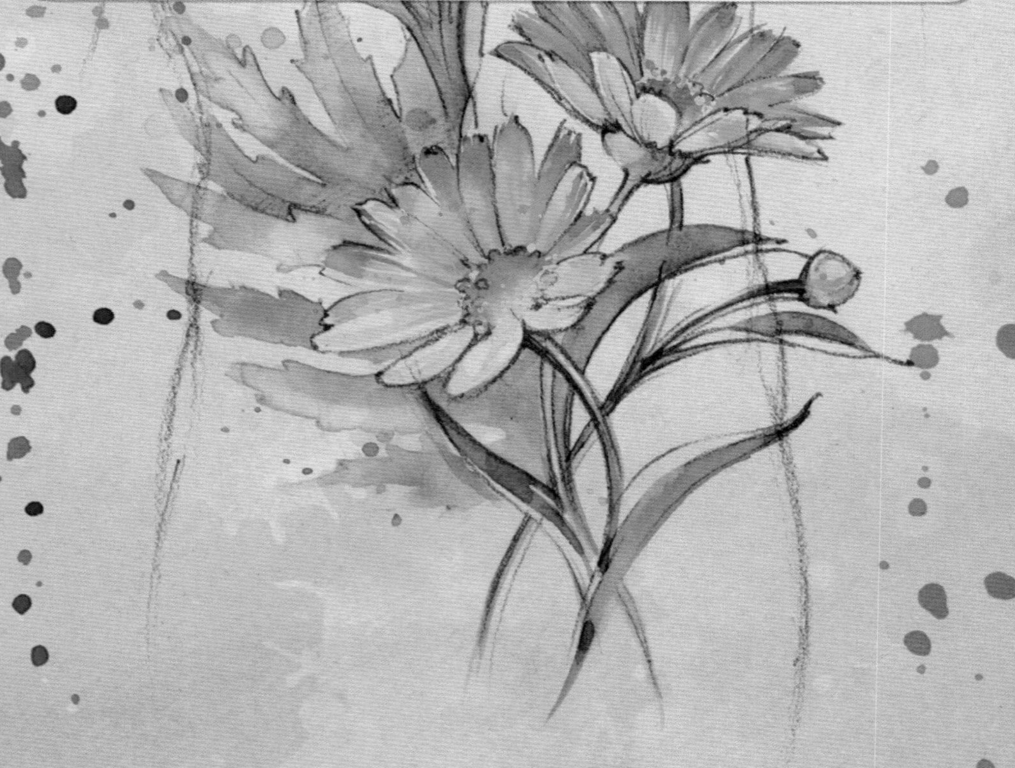

A HEALTHY DETOXIFICATION system is critical for good health, but it is often overlooked in conventional medicine. Many herbalists and holistic practitioners, on the other hand, consider a happy liver and open detoxification channels a top priority for overall well-being. Many disease patterns are connected to subpar detoxification, including skin problems (acne, rashes, liver spots), asthma and allergies, migraines, autoimmune disease, and cancer. In fact, the potential warning signs that the detoxification system is compromised or overburdened with day-to-day toxins are many:

- Dull skin tone
- Skin issues: acne, rashes, eczema, sensitive skin
- Dark circles under the eyes
- Chronic pain, arthritis, migraines
- Poor digestion, especially of fats
- High cholesterol
- Hypertension
- Bad breath
- Constipation
- Overly stinky bowel movements
- Reproductive issues
- Lingering infections
- Poor wound healing
- Food and seasonal allergies (highly reactive)
- Asthma
- Fatigue, sluggishness
- Brain fog
- Depression
- Anger and frustration
- Gout
- Edema, water retention
- Dark, scanty urine
- Frequent urinary tract infections

Most body systems have a "center of the universe" organ around which they revolve, and your liver is your sun in the galaxy of detox. However, no organ works in isolation, and detoxification primarily takes place via the intricate interconnection of the liver, gallbladder, kidneys, lymphatic system, colon, and skin. The liver, kidneys, and lymphatic system each filter different toxins in different areas of the body while also performing other crucial duties. Your skin isn't the most efficient detoxification organ; however, it is the largest, and it may pick up the slack if other organs are overburdened.

Many of the classic "detox" herbs taste bitter and work primarily by encouraging your liver to clean the blood more efficiently, creating and excreting more bile. However, you'll also find among them lymphagogues that improve lymph flow and drainage, laxatives that keep the bowels moving so that bile and other waste is cleared out promptly, and diuretics that keep fluid moving through your kidney filters. As a whole, all these different types of detoxifying herbs are often called alteratives and sometimes "blood cleansers." Together, they work to keep the body's detoxification channels open and moving, so that we have less waste and fewer toxins floating around in the blood and the rest of the body. This can mean less inflammation and less irritation, with things running more smoothly.

Your Liver: Detox Superstar

Your liver is one of the largest organs in your body, second only to your skin (*also* a detox organ), and it resides near your stomach in the upper right section of your abdomen. It acts as a gatekeeper, tirelessly filtering toxins in the blood coming from your GI tract before allowing it to enter the rest of the body. Later, it filters old blood to clean it of metabolic waste. The filtered waste and toxins are turned into bile, stored in your gallbladder, and then released into your digestive tract as the next meal flows into your intestines. (If your gallbladder has been surgically removed, bile trickles out slowly throughout the day.) Some of bile's compounds get reabsorbed into your bloodstream as it gets processed and waits for elimination in the gut, but most bile waste is excreted in your feces. Your liver isn't *just* focused on detoxification. It also plays a key role in the metabolism of various compounds — sugar, vitamin D, iron, cholesterol, fats, and much more — shuffling things to and from storage and inactive to active states, creating them, and breaking them down. Bitter- and sour-tasting herbs stimulate your liver to produce and excrete more bile.

Liver Movers

"Liver movers" are herbs that encourage bile production (choleretics) and bile excretion (cholagogues), which improve the liver's ability to clear waste from the blood and your body and help pull toxins from storage in fat cells so that they can be eliminated. As liver action increases, you may experience an initial "healing crisis" — your symptoms (skin woes, headache, fatigue, brain fog) may get worse before they get better. This happens when the liver pulls toxins from storage and releases them into the bloodstream, which makes the body a bit cranky until they are then removed as bile and excreted in the feces. It should pass within a day or two. Going slowly limits this ill effect.

▸ Dandelion

Taraxacum officinale

Availability: G+ W+ C+

Key Properties: This ubiquitous weedy ally has earned superstar status for encouraging detoxification via the liver, colon, and kidneys. All parts do a little of everything; however, the roots have a particular affinity for the liver and the leaves for the kidneys. You'll get more of a volume diuretic effect from the leaves, whereas inulin from the roots acts more like a sodium-leaching diuretic.

Additional Benefits: Dandelion is also a terrific nutritive; see page 37 for more on that front. It's a classic herb for skin issues and allergies (especially the fresh tinctured root or slurry). Some people find dandelion leaf and root extract effective for hypertension due to the diuretic effect. Oddly, it tends to work better as a hypotensive for folks of Mexican and Central American descent than the average gringo, but for its other uses it's helpful for everyone regardless of ethnicity.

Preparation: Use both the leaf and the root (preferably fresh) tinctured or infused in vinegar. Also enjoy the dried or roasted roots for coffeelike tea and the leaves in food (like pesto; see page 274). Actually, dandelion does well in any form. Standard herb doses (see page 298) apply.

WHAT IS AN ALTERATIVE?

Often called "blood purifiers," alteratives improve the body's detoxification processes and efficient removal of metabolic waste. They often encourage detoxification of the blood and interstitial fluid via the liver, lymphatic system, and kidneys. Many different categories of herbs come under the heading of "alterative": lymphagogues (lymph movers), choleretics and cholagogues (liver movers, including bitters and sours), and diuretics (which increase urine output) are all considered alterative and are often combined for a more whole-body detox action.

General Uses: Alteratives "clean" the blood and interstitial fluid, which improves overall body function and vitality. They have a major role in detoxification and are crucial for treating skin issues, edema, and other signs of subpar detoxification. They can play a supportive role in addressing allergies, respiratory problems, reproductive issues, chronic pain, cancer, and much more.

Examples: Dandelion leaf and root, burdock root and seed, cleavers, chickweed, turmeric, schizandra, echinacea, nettles, red clover blossoms, sarsaparilla, red root, yellow dock, ocotillo, alder, celery, parsley, violet, and bitter berberine-rich herbs like Oregon grape root

Cautions and Considerations: Dandelion leaf is a supremely effective diuretic; don't take it right before bedtime, and exercise caution with medications that interact with diuretics. If you have an intestinal, bowel, or bile duct blockage, don't try to fix it with dandelion — call your doctor. Be sure to properly identify dandelion using a field guide, because many plants look similar.
Similar Herbs: Dandelion's close cousin **chicory** can be used similarly but is not quite as medicinal. Most bunches of "dandelion leaves" sold by farms and grocers are actually a variety of chicory, but that's okay. For those who find dandelion too strong, **burdock** root may work better.

▸ Burdock

Arctium lappa, A. minus
Availability: G+ W+ C+
Key Properties: Where burdock takes hold as a weed, it quickly proliferates, with huge rhubarb-like leaves that, in its second year, give way to tall thistle-like blooms and brown burrs that were literally the inspiration for Velcro. The mildly bitter, slightly sweet roots encourage liver and lymph detoxification. While incredibly effective, burdock root is also a gentle, nourishing tonic that's appropriate for a broad range of people (for whom other alteratives may be too strong). It blends well in many formulas and takes the edge off dandelion's bitter taste.
Additional Benefits: Consider burdock root for general detox support, nutrition, skin issues, digestive woes, dysbiosis, arthritis, gout, reproductive issues, hypertension, and possibly cancer; it has also been shown to help prevent pre-eclampsia (but use only with supervision during pregnancy). The inulin fiber in burdock root (as well as dandelion and chicory roots) helps feed beneficial bacteria in the gut. Like dandelion, burdock makes good food. Use the fresh, peeled root in soups and stir-fries. You can buy it in well-stocked natural food stores and Asian markets (where it's sometimes called *gobo*).
Preparation: Dig up the plant in the fall of the first year or spring of the second — basically, before it flowers, because the root loses vitality as the plant puts up flower stalks and begins to rot after flowering. The taproot loves to work its way around rocks and can be quite a bugger to dig. Try a digging stick or "cobra," some muscle, and a lot of patience. Burdock that grows in wild, rocky soil will be more potent medicinally than plush cultivated counterparts. Use the fresh root as food, dry it for tea and capsules, or use it fresh or dry to make tinctures, vinegar, and similar extracts. Don't be alarmed by a cloudy white substance at the bottom of your burdock root tincture; it's just the inulin. Standard herb doses (see page 298) apply.
Cautions and Considerations: Quite safe. It's one of the safest herbs discussed in this chapter for use during pregnancy, though in that case it would be used preferably in modest doses with professional supervision.

Bitter Brew

This blend tastes a bit like coffee and delivers a good dose of liver-moving herbs. You can add a cinnamon stick for flavor (but it slows the colon) or ½ teaspoon yellow dock root as a gentle laxative.

- 2 teaspoons burdock root
- 1 teaspoon roasted chicory root
- 1 teaspoon dandelion root

Combine the roots with 2 cups water in a small pot. Bring to a boil, then reduce the heat and let simmer, covered, for 20 minutes. Strain and enjoy hot or iced.

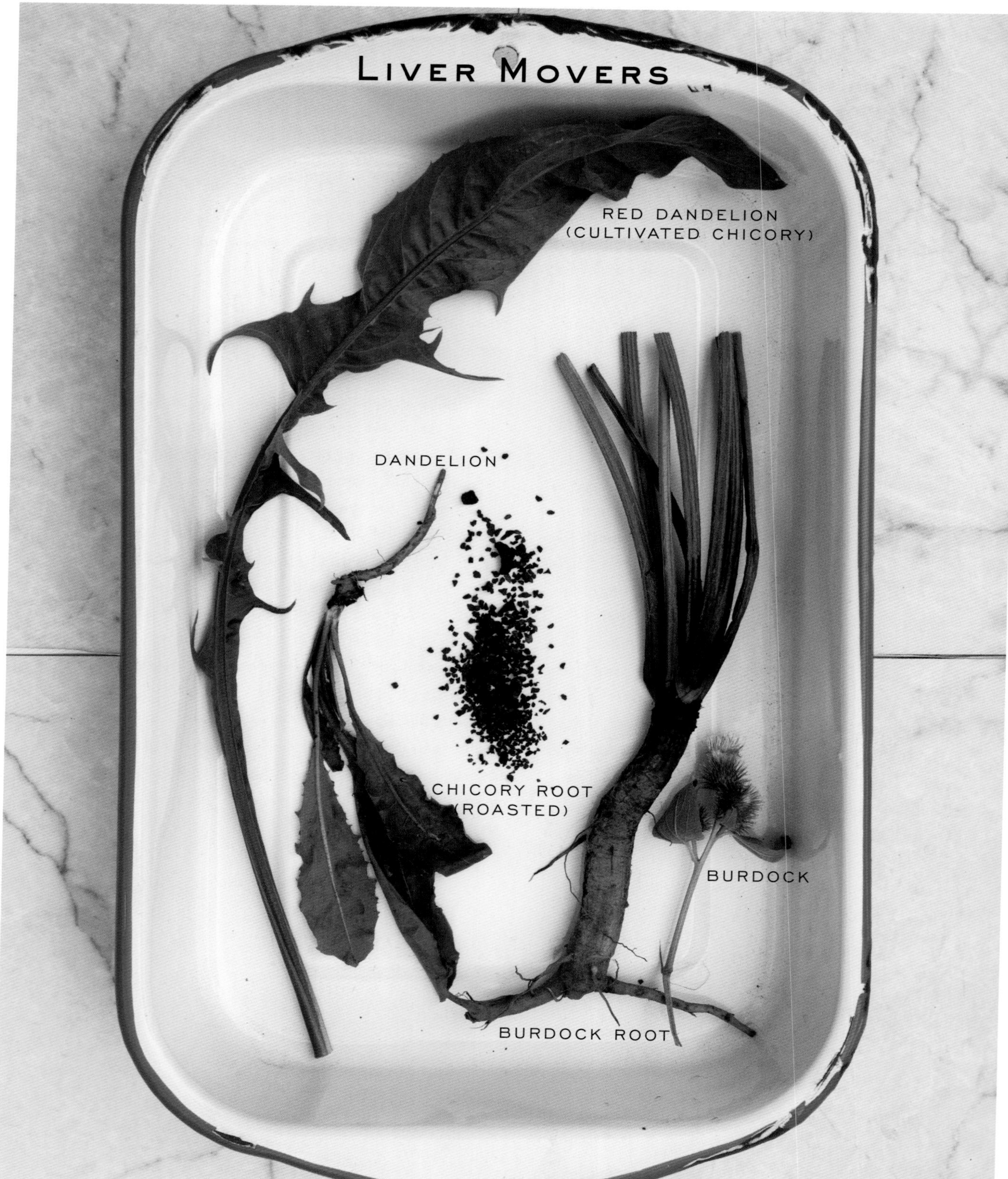
LIVER MOVERS
RED DANDELION
(CULTIVATED CHICORY)
DANDELION
CHICORY ROOT
(ROASTED)
BURDOCK
BURDOCK ROOT

THE DETOX DIET

MUCH HOOPLA AND WHOLE BOOKS are devoted to "cleansing" and the detox diet. The three typical goals of a cleanse or detox diet are: (1) to remove potentially "toxic" foods, (2) to eat a simple diet so that detox organs like the liver can focus less on digestion and more on detoxification, and (3) to increase your consumption of water and foods that encourage the detoxification organs to do their job more efficiently.

A detox diet generally involves eating a simple diet with ample amounts of detox-friendly foods and herbs, along with plenty of water, detoxifying herbal teas (dandelion, burdock, nettle, red clover, et cetera), vegetables, low-sugar fruits, and plant foods in general. Raw, juiced, steamed, soup, and broth forms are preferred. Avoid processed food, sugar, alcohol, caffeine, common food allergens, dairy, and red meat, at least for a limited period of time. Don't skimp on protein, though — it's important for adequate liver function. Get it from beans, nuts, seeds, wild-caught salmon/seafood, chicken (preferably free-range or organic), or a high-quality protein powder.

The length of a cleanse can range from 1 day to a full month depending on personal preference and how limited the diet is. For example, a juice/water/tea/broth fast is usually not sustainable for more than a few days. You're likely to feel terrible for the first few days of a cleanse as you adjust to caffeine withdrawal, sugar withdrawal, less food, and the release of toxins from storage — but after that, you should feel fabulous!

Talk with your doctor before embarking on a strict cleanse, especially if you have an eating disorder, heart disease, diabetes, liver or kidney disease, or are overly thin. Pregnant and nursing women should not cleanse.

Detox-Friendly Foods

Although a plant-based diet rich in vegetables and fiber supports healthy detoxification in general, certain foods play detox superstar by encouraging bile production, containing glutathione (which is good for the liver), or acting as diuretics. Aim to eat lots of the following foods during a detox, and extend the benefits by enjoying them regularly in your daily diet.

- Bitter veggies (artichoke, lettuce, escarole, radicchio, arugula, bitter greens, bitter melon)
- Diuretic veggies (dandelion, parsley, burdock, celery)
- Cruciferous veggies (broccoli, kale, watercress, cabbage, bok choy, Brussels sprouts)
- Asparagus
- Avocado
- Beets
- Berries
- Sour citrus
- Cranberries
- Pomegranate
- Garlic and onions
- Mushrooms (cooked or in broth)
- Green tea
- Flax and chia seeds
- Walnuts
- Water
- Culinary herbs and spices, especially turmeric

For detox-friendly lifestyle tips, see Clean and Green Living, page 26.

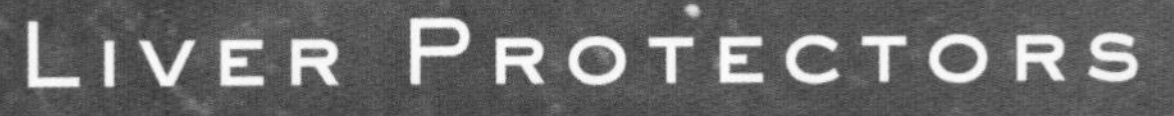
Liver Protectors

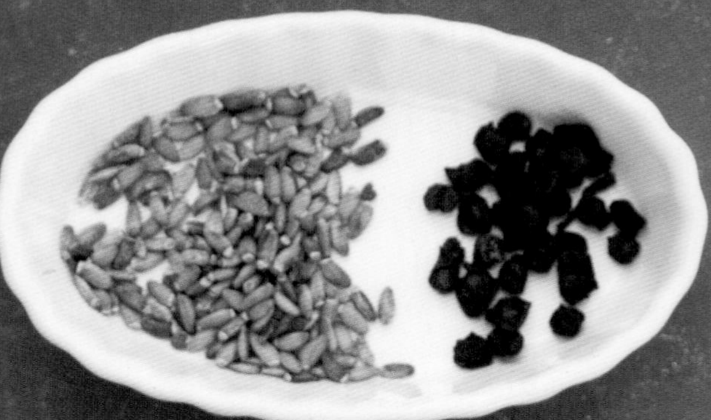
MILK THISTLE SEED
SCHIZANDRA

GINGER
TURMERIC

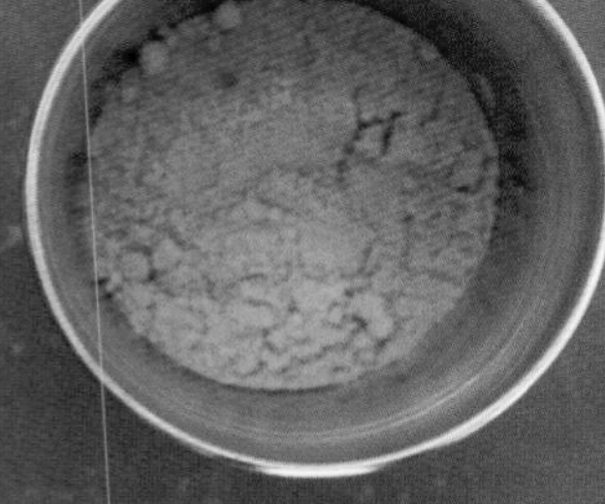
GROUND TURMERIC

ARTICHOKE

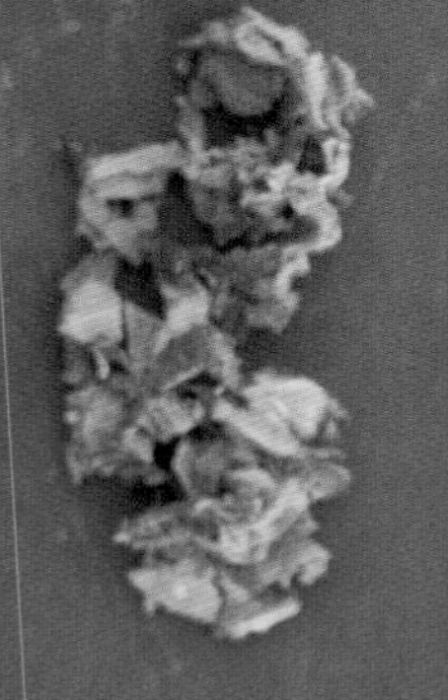
ARTICHOKE LEAF

Liver Protectors

Hardworking organs need some TLC now and then, and your liver is no exception. "Liver protectors" safeguard your liver from damage due to toxins and encourage regeneration after damage. These herbs are sometimes described as "hepatoprotective" ("hepato-" means "liver").

▸ Turmeric and Schizandra

Curcuma longa and *Schisandra chinensis*

Availability: G- C

Key Properties: Turmeric root and schizandra berry are incredibly useful herbs that come from the distant lands of India and China, respectively, and have the unique ability to both stimulate liver detoxification ("liver movers") while also protecting and healing the liver itself ("liver protectors").

Additional Benefits: These herbs have so many "side benefits" that they find their way into formulas for a wide range of ailments. You'll find more details about them in other chapters. I turn to turmeric root when I also want its anti-inflammatory, antioxidant, cholesterol-lowering, and/or digestion-enhancing properties. Schizandra berry is a favorite balancing adaptogen for stress that also supports respiratory and immune health, libido, and the mind.

See page 188 for more on turmeric and page 51 for more on schizandra.

▸ Milk Thistle

Silybum marianum

Availability: G- W- C+

Key Properties: While I don't consider milk thistle seed a proper detox herb, it may be the best liver protector and regenerator. Both milk thistle seed and its primary constituent, silymarin, protect the liver from being damaged by toxins (even those of the deadly amanita mushroom) while also preventing and possibly treating a range of liver conditions including fatty liver, hepatitis, and cirrhosis. Studies suggest it can promote liver regeneration by up to 20 to 30 percent while also encouraging the presence of liver-supportive antioxidants like glutathione and superoxide dismutase (SOD). It is a good herb to consider for individuals who are or have been exposed to solvents and chemicals via lifestyle choices (drugs, alcohol) or their job (hairdressers, mechanics, factory workers).

Additional Benefits: Milk thistle may also lower blood sugar levels.

Preparation: Unfortunately, milk thistle seed's properties do not extract well in traditional remedies. This is one of the few herbs I recommend as a standardized extract in pill form with approximately 80 percent silymarin. Follow the manufacturer's dosage recommendations. If you prefer to use milk thistle seed in its whole form, grind it up and eat it. The flavor is not unlike that of its relative sunflower seeds. Keep it refrigerated to prevent rancidity.

Cautions and Considerations: Very safe, though it may interact with medications.

Similar Herbs: Fellow thistle-like herb **artichoke leaf** offers some liver-protective properties as well as classic bitter-alterative action. See page 71 for more on artichoke. **Blessed thistle** is sometimes used similarly, too.

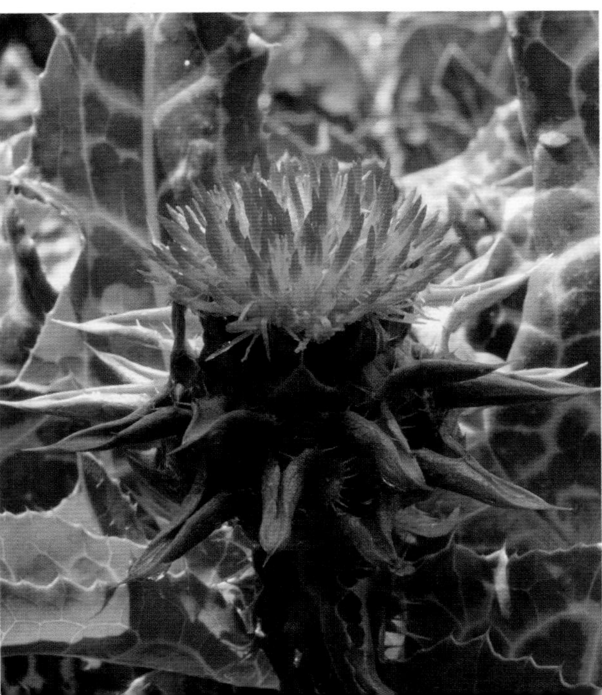

Your Colon: Keep Those BMs Going

Your colon in the lower gastrointestinal tract functions as both a digestion and a detoxification organ; it's one of the easiest ways to get things out of your body. Your liver has dutifully dumped its detoxification waste into the digestive tract so that the colon can eliminate it. If bile and waste hang around too long in a constipated colon, they risk being reabsorbed into your bloodstream. So steady bowel movements are an important part of a functioning detoxification system. In fact, most "cleanse kits" sold in natural food stores are basically fiber plus laxatives and *sometimes* other detoxifying herbs. (You can do better with diet and herbs.) How often should you go? One to three bowel movements (BMs) a day is ideal.

Bitter alterative herbs (like dandelion root and leaf, burdock root, artichoke leaf, turmeric root) not only serve as digestive tonics and blood cleansers but also indirectly act like laxatives by triggering peristalsis, while insoluble fiber (psyllium, flaxseeds, whole grains, most veggies and fruit) bulks up the stool and helps pull toxins out of the body. The combination of fiber plus the gentle laxative effect help encourage healthy elimination. A fiber-rich whole-foods diet works better than fiber supplements, but any fiber is better than no fiber. Start slowly to give your body the chance to adjust, and be sure to drink plenty of water. Stimulant laxatives (senna, cascara, aloe latex, rhubarb, and buckthorn) are usually *not* necessary and can be habit forming. Nonetheless, most store-bought cleanse kits contain them. If you feel that you really *need* a laxative, try the gentler, tonifying action of yellow dock root or the Ayurvedic formula triphala. For more on addressing constipation, see page 89.

▸ Yellow Dock

Rumex crispus

Availability: G W+ C

Key Properties: Yet another weedy bitter alterative detox ally! Yellow dock root offers similar benefits to dandelion and burdock roots; however, it brings a few extra attributes to the plate. The root supports balanced lower GI function with dual action as a gentle laxative *and* a gentle astringent that tightens and tones the colon, effectively treating both diarrhea and constipation. In detox blends, add yellow dock for liver support, skin support, and its gentle laxative action.

Additional Benefits: Yellow dock root also supports healthy iron levels both by providing some iron and by encouraging the liver to release iron from storage into the bloodstream.

Preparation: Dig yellow dock in poor, rocky soil for stronger medicine — the yellow inner root hue indicates potency. Yellow dock doesn't taste great, but small amounts in tea aren't bad. Also try a decocted yellow dock syrup (great for the iron benefits), or take it as tincture or capsule. Blending yellow dock with blackstrap molasses synergizes the iron-rich, blood-building properties. Standard herb doses (see page 298) apply.

Cautions and Considerations: Generally quite safe, but more is *not* better: taking too much yellow dock causes explosive diarrhea followed by massive constipation. If you have iron overload issues, try triphala instead. Due to yellow dock's naturally high level of oxalic acid, use caution if you have a history of calcium oxalate kidney stones. Laxatives are not recommended during pregnancy because they can stimulate the uterus to contract; yellow dock is gentler and often effective for pregnancy-related constipation but should still be used with professional supervision if you are pregnant.

Similar Herbs: Closely related **broad dock** is often misidentified as yellow dock but is almost identical in use. **Triphala**, a blend of three Ayurvedic herbs, offers similar colon-toning laxative action. Mixing triphala powder in water works best, but you can also take it in capsules.

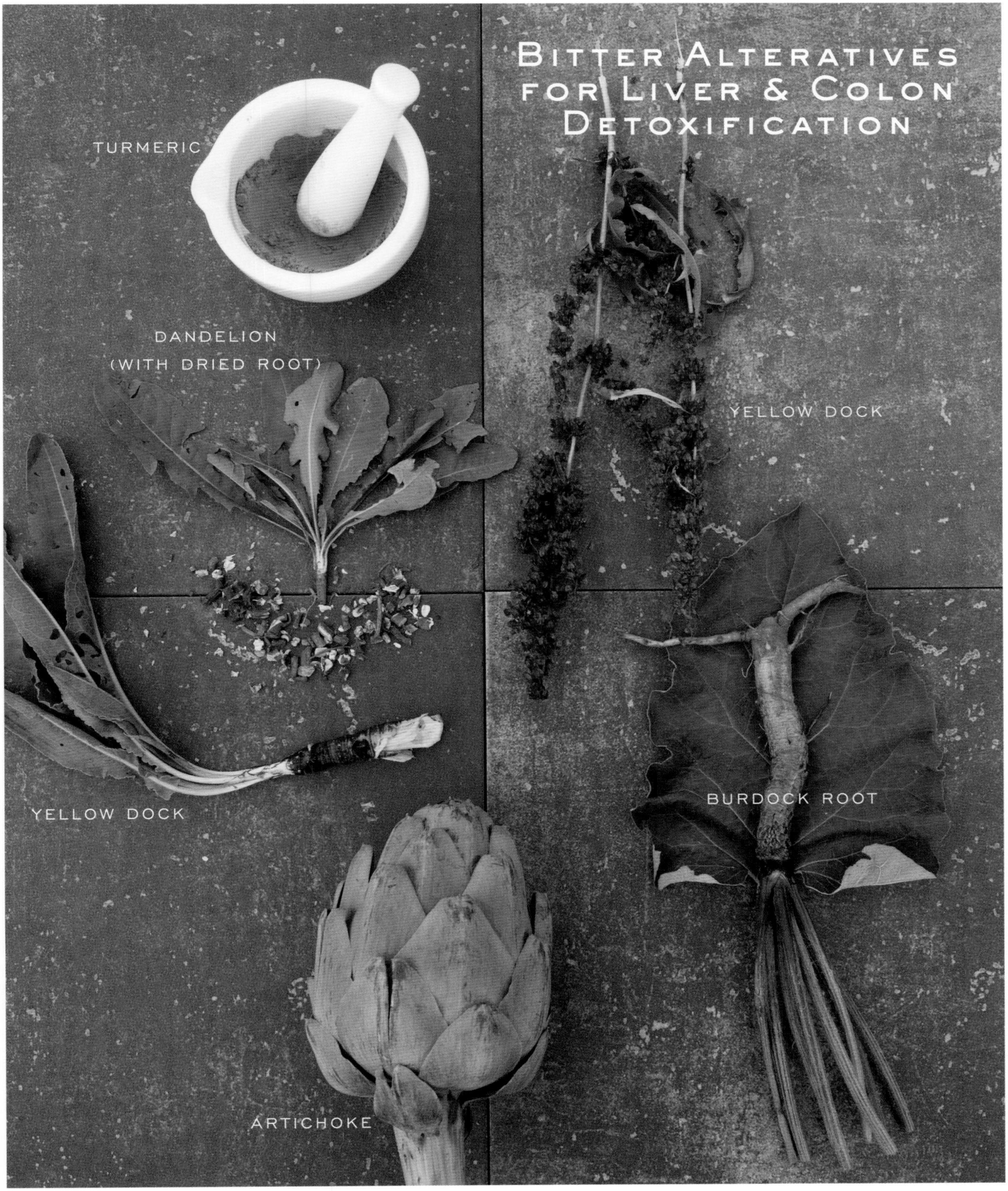

Bitter Alteratives for Liver & Colon Detoxification

TURMERIC

DANDELION
(WITH DRIED ROOT)

YELLOW DOCK

YELLOW DOCK

BURDOCK ROOT

ARTICHOKE

DETOX CAUTIONS AND CONSIDERATIONS

WHEN WE TALK ABOUT DETOXIFICATION and supporting your detoxification organs, we are not talking about treating liver failure, kidney failure, hepatitis, and other potentially life-threatening conditions that demand medical attention. Herbal and holistic care may play an adjunct role in the care of these serious conditions, but they are beyond the scope of this book and usually require a skilled health-care practitioner's assistance.

The detoxification herbs discussed in this chapter are generally very safe. However, some folks should tread carefully into the land of detox. Most detox herbs — particularly those that taste bitter — stimulate digestion. While this is good for most people, it may aggravate stomach problems (e.g., ulcers or gastritis) and lower blood sugar, so seek the advice of your health-care practitioner first if you have diabetes or hypoglycemia. Taking bitters with food may help, delivering the bitters' healing actions exactly when you need them. Bitters also stimulate bile and act as indirect laxatives — which is generally good, but check in with your practitioner first if you have gallbladder or bowel issues. Also seek professional guidance first if you are taking medication, because detox herbs and detox diets may alter various pharmaceuticals' effectiveness. Pregnant and nursing women generally shouldn't detox. You may experience a "healing crisis" at the beginning of a detox — it's normal to see increased skin breakouts and feel fatigued for a few days before things get better.

Deep Cleanse Tea

This blend is inspired by a Flora tea available (at least as a special order) at most natural food stores. It tastes pleasant and provides general detoxification support, particularly for skin conditions.

- 1–2 sticks cinnamon, or 1 teaspoon cinnamon chips
- 1 teaspoon burdock root
- 1 teaspoon dandelion root
- ½ teaspoon ginger, or 1 slice fresh root
- ½ teaspoon licorice root
- ½ teaspoon nettles
- ½ teaspoon oat straw
- ½ teaspoon yellow dock root
- ¼–½ teaspoon fennel seeds

Combine all the herbs. Pour 1 to 2 cups boiling water over the herbs, cover, and let steep for 1 hour. (Alternatively, simmer the herbs in the water, covered, for 20 minutes.) Strain and enjoy.

Your Secondary Cleanup Crew: Lymph *and* Skin

Your lymphatic system and skin are separate yet closely interconnected detoxification organs, and many of the therapies that work for one also aid the other. The lymphatic system is an intricate network of tiny lymphatic vessels and groups of nodes that lie alongside your circulatory system, cleaning the interstitial fluid in your body and dumping the waste into your bloodstream for removal. It is also home to a variety of immune cells and assists in the transportation of fatty acids. Nothing "pumps" the lymph, so it moves very slowly in one direction (thanks to a system of valves) as muscles outside the system press against the vessels. Gentle movement, light lymphatic massage, and skin brushing all encourage better lymph movement, as do certain lymph-moving herbs, or lymphagogues.

Your skin is another important secondary detoxification organ — possibly the least effective detox organ in the bunch but also the largest. It picks up the slack when the body gets overburdened with sluggish detoxification, and you can often gauge the vitality of detoxification in the body by looking at how happy your skin is. Baths (especially when infused with lymph-moving herbs), steams and saunas (sweating), exfoliation, and skin brushing help the skin with detoxification.

Lymph Movers: Lymphagogues

The following are some of my favorite lymph-moving herbs. Not only do they aid lymph flow and detoxification, but most also work well for skin issues related to toxin burdens, acne, rashes, insect bites, and poison ivy.

▸ Red Clover

Trifolium pratense

Availability: G+ W+ C

Key Properties: Red clover blossom's lymph-moving action earned it a top spot in alterative, "blood purifying," and controversial cancer treatment formulas including Hoxsey's blend and Flor-Essence. I can't speak to its ability to treat cancer; however, red clover is a worthy addition to your detox blend. Try the flowers internally and externally for a range of skin conditions connected to the body's toxic load, such as eczema, psoriasis, and acne. Consider it for autoimmune disease, rheumatoid arthritis, and swollen lymph glands, too.

Additional Benefits: Red clover blossom is perhaps most popular as a nutritious herb, rich in minerals, including calcium. As a member of the legume family, it also contains weak phytoestrogens (less potent than soy) that support hormone, cardiovascular, and bone health.

Preparation: Pinch off vibrant blossoms, including the top leaves, once the morning dew has dried, and dry them quickly in the dehydrator to prevent fermentation. Use the flowers in tea — they taste quite nice! — tincture them, use capsules, or add them to the bath. Standard herb doses (see page 298) apply.

Cautions and Considerations: Red clover thins the blood and should be avoided if you have a bleeding disorder or are on blood-thinning medications. It may not be safe during pregnancy. Dried red clover tends to be poor quality: if you're buying red clover, look for vibrant shades of purple and green — not brown dust. Red clover and other legumes may contain coumarins — which can be toxic (especially to grazing livestock and people with coumarin allergy) — especially if the plants are allowed to ferment during the drying process.

▸ More Lymph-Moving Herbs

Calendula improves lymph flow and detoxification. It is also rich in carotenoids, which boost vitamin A levels. Use in combination with echinacea in mouthwash and lymph-moving blends. Tincture, tea, and infused broth are popular. Calendula also decreases inflammation and itching, improves wound healing, and acts as a mild

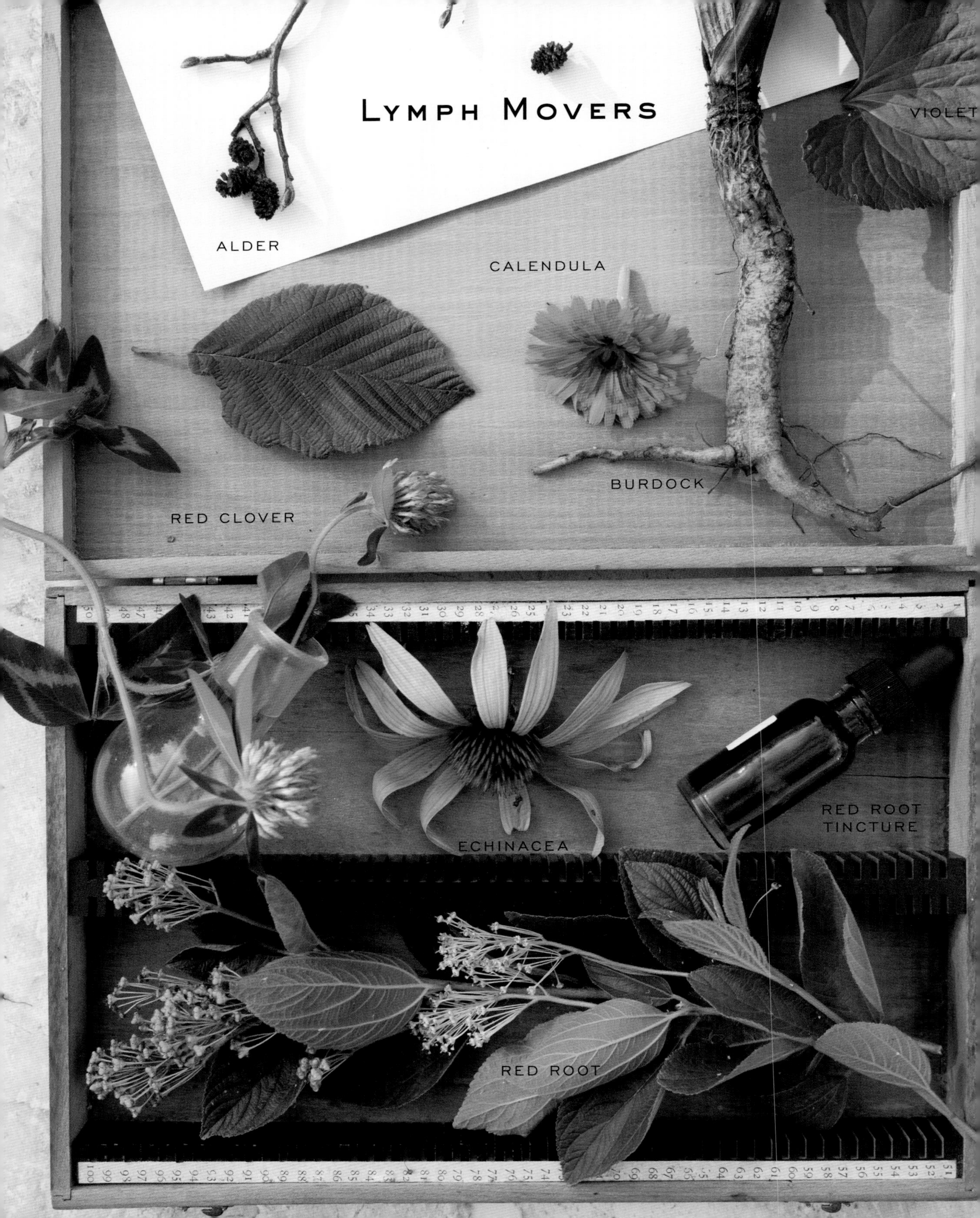
LYMPH MOVERS
ALDER
VIOLET
CALENDULA
BURDOCK
RED CLOVER
ECHINACEA
RED ROOT TINCTURE
RED ROOT

antimicrobial on contact for the skin, gut, and other tissues for conditions like itchy skin rashes and irritations, wounds, hemorrhoids, ulcers, ear infections, and conjunctivitis. (Learn more about calendula on pages 41 and 219.)

Though it may be more famous for its liver-detoxifying properties, **burdock root** is also valuable as a lymph-moving herb. It blends well in many formulas, whether as a tea, tincture, infused broth, or capsules, and is among our safest and most well-tolerated lymph herbs. (Learn more about burdock on page 95.)

Echinacea has achieved star status for its ability to stimulate immune function; however, it was traditionally best known for its potent alterative, lymph-moving action and ability to treat sepsis and blood poisoning. Native Americans used the root of *E. angustifolia* for poisonous snakebites and other venomous injuries because it inhibits hyaluronidase (a damaging enzyme found in snake and bee venom and certain bacteria, including *Streptococcus*) while helping to flush residual toxins from the body via the lymph. It's equally valuable for sore throats. Apply topically and internally — fresh mashed roots or fresh root tincture is preferred, but all parts of the plant have some benefit. Combine echinacea with red root and/or calendula for immune-related lymphatic congestion and swollen glands. Don't use echinacea in cases of autoimmune disease due to its immune-stimulating nature. (Learn more about echinacea on page 118.)

Red root is the queen lymphagogue and a tonic for the spleen, a blood-filtering organ associated with your lymphatic and immune systems. Red root can be added to general detox formulas, but it's most often used for blends that relate to lymph or spleen congestion in infections, including the common cold, sore throats and tonsils, swollen lymph nodes, mono, syphilis (a traditional use), Lyme disease (a modern use), and spleen enlargement. It also makes blood less sticky, which improves circulation. Many local species can be used interchangeably as a tea or tincture.

Thanks to popularization by traditional folk herbalists, including Michael Moore and Kiva Rose, **alder bark and twigs** are seeing more use in modern herbalism. Alder's astringency tightens and tones structures of the body (e.g., the gut lining), while other components improve fluid movement and circulation. It also acts as a lymph mover and alterative while simultaneously strengthening immune function and helping to clear stubborn infections, swollen lymph nodes, sore throat, fungal issues, et cetera.

Violet leaf and flower have a gentle yet profound lymph-moving action, taste pleasant, and offer a nice array of nutrients. In contrast to other herbs in this chapter, violet has a more moistening, soothing property that makes it more broadly useful. It's used internally and externally to help dissolve fatty cysts, cystic breasts, and fibroids.

Fellow weeds **chickweed** and **cleavers** also have lymph-moving, detoxifying, and cooling properties and are commonly used both internally and externally. They both work best fresh —fresh-plant tincture, poultice, bath, or infused oil/salve — though quality dried herb may suffice. Try juicing them or making them into pesto.

Fluid Balance, Homeostasis, *and* Your Kidneys

When it comes to detoxification, your kidneys deal in water and fluid balance. They filter specific toxins, including nitrogen-based compounds (think: protein, meat, cured foods), and excrete them via your urine, and they also maintain fluid homeostasis, including blood pressure, electrolytes, sodium-potassium, and acid-base balance. The kidneys can be a complicated system to work with herbally, and it's important to know your goals and understand these sensitive organs. In their function, your kidneys are all about balance — and balance is important to keep in mind when choosing herbs. Many kidney-urinary remedies can help or harm, depending on the situation. See your doctor *immediately* if you develop a kidney infection or symptoms that indicate that the organ itself is damaged (lower-back pain, fever, flu-like aches, cloudy urine). Treating kidney disease is best left to the doctor and is outside of the scope of this book. Instead, we'll focus on ways to support overall kidney health, gentle kidney detoxification, and kidney-related conditions that respond favorably to herbs, like gout and urinary tract infections.

Two categories of herbs, in particular, are essential for supporting kidney health:

- **Gentle diuretics.** For general kidney support, think hydration and diuretics. Together, they help flush out toxins through the kidneys and urine. Look no further than classic diuretics, including parsley leaf, celery stalks, dandelion leaf, burdock root, and nettle leaf. The preferred delivery system to the kidneys is water: tea, broth, juice. Or you can just eat these herbs with your food. (Parsley seed and celery seed are more potent diuretics but also more apt to irritate the kidneys.)
- **Demulcents.** With their soothing, slimy, healing properties, demulcent herbs are a welcome addition to kidney formulas. In addition to the classic demulcents like marshmallow root (page 77) and slippery elm (page 283), try corn silk, a simple, safe demulcent specific to the kidney-urinary system. You can easily harvest your own during corn season: pick up some organically grown corncobs and save the golden silk, discard the black/brown tops, and then dry the silk for tea or tincture it fresh (an exception to the water-based rule).

PROTOCOL POINTS

Urinary Tract Infections

Urinary tract infections (UTIs) and cystitis affect many women and often respond quickly to natural remedies. However, if your UTI gets worse or doesn't improve within a few days of natural therapies, go see your doctor. Infections that move up into the kidneys (symptoms include lower-back pain, fever, cloudy urine) require immediate medical attention. Most herbal UTI remedies irritate the kidneys, especially uva ursi, which shouldn't be used for more than 1 week.

Diet: Most important, ditch sugar in all its forms. This includes carbs that break down quickly into sugar such as pasta, bread, white rice, crackers, bananas, flour, and most types of juice. Pathogenic bacteria thrive in a high-sugar environment. Also drink plenty of water and take a probiotics supplement to help "push out" the bad bacteria while recolonizing the good guys.

Lifestyle: Practice good hygiene — wipe from front to back, wear breathable cotton undies, pee after sex, and go commando when you sleep.

Herbs: Cranberries prevent bacteria from sticking to the bladder, which can prevent and sometimes treat UTIs, particularly in the early stages. Most cranberry research has been done on Ocean Spray's original cranberry cocktail (sugar and all), though you can also seek out pure cranberry juice. (Avoid cranberry juice that is sweetened with other juices, though, as they tend to have less actual cranberry juice present.) If you can't stand cranberries, try their close relative, blueberry. Unfortunately, once the infection has taken hold, the berries may not be sufficient. Blueberry leaves and the leaves of their more potent relative uva ursi will better address the bacterial overgrowth and can be used for approximately 1 week to treat a UTI.

AT A GLANCE
Herbs for Detoxification

Liver

Bile Movers/Alteratives
- Dandelion root (and leaf)
- Burdock root
- Yellow dock root
- Turmeric
- Schizandra
- Ginger
- Artichoke leaf
- Bitter berberines (goldenseal,* coptis/goldthread, Oregon grape root, barberry)

Protectors
- Milk thistle seed
- Schizandra
- Turmeric
- Ginger
- Artichoke leaf

Lymph

Movers/Alteratives
- Red root (and aerial parts)
- Burdock root and seed
- Red clover blossom
- Calendula flowers
- Alder bark and twig (dry)
- Cleavers and chickweed
- Echinacea root (and aerial parts)
- Violet leaf (and flower)
- Sarsaparilla root*
- Ocotillo bark*
- Poke root*

Activities to Support Lymph Movement
- Lymphatic massage
- Skin brushing
- Physical activity/movement

Colon

Bulk Laxatives (Insoluble Fiber)
- Psyllium seed
- Flaxseed
- Hemp seed
- Chia seed

Supportive Foods Soluble Fiber
- Apple pectin
- Pears
- Beans
- Lentils

Mild/Tonifying Laxatives
- Triphala
- Yellow dock root
- Turkey rhubarb root
- Aloe inner gel

Stimulant Laxatives
- Aloe latex
- Senna
- Cascara
- Buckthorn bark

Soothing Mucilages
- Slippery elm
- Marshmallow root

Kidneys/Urinary Tract

Soothing Diuretics
- Corn silk
- Marshmallow root
- Slippery elm bark
- Kava root (pain relieving)

Volume Diuretics/Tonics
- Dandelion leaf
- Nettle leaf
- Parsley greens
- Celery greens, stalks, root

Sodium-Leaching Diuretics
- Dandelion root
- Burdock root
- Chicory root

Skin

Exfoliants and Toxin Pullers
- Skin brushing
- Gentle skin exfoliation
- Sauna, bath, sweating
- Clay, topically/bath
- Juniper, topically/bath
- Seaweed bath
- Epsom salt bath
- Ginger, topically/bath
- Plantain poultice
- Aloe leaf or prickly pear pad poultice
- Water (lots!)

**Be particularly aware of cautions and/or ecological status before using plants marked with an asterisk.*

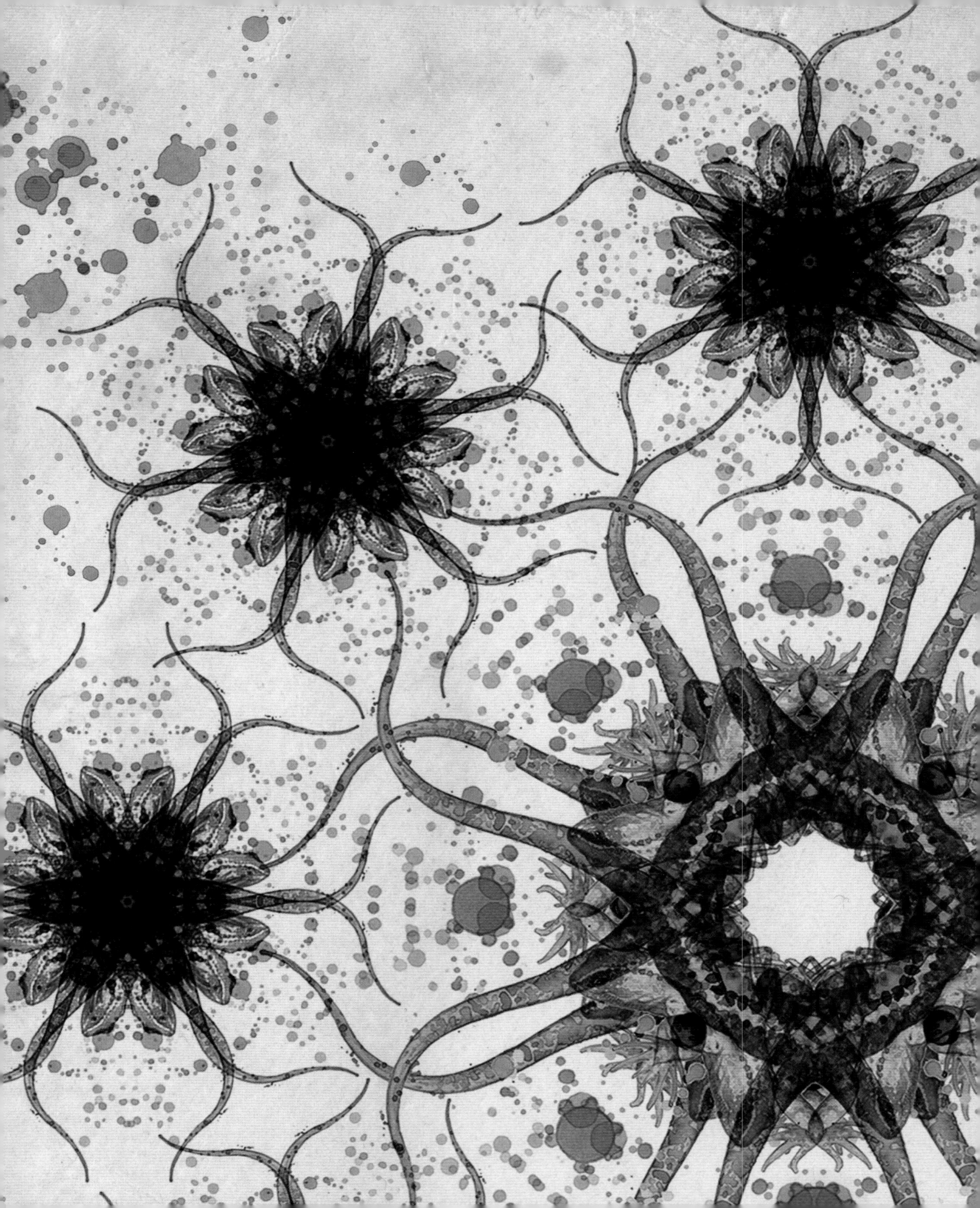

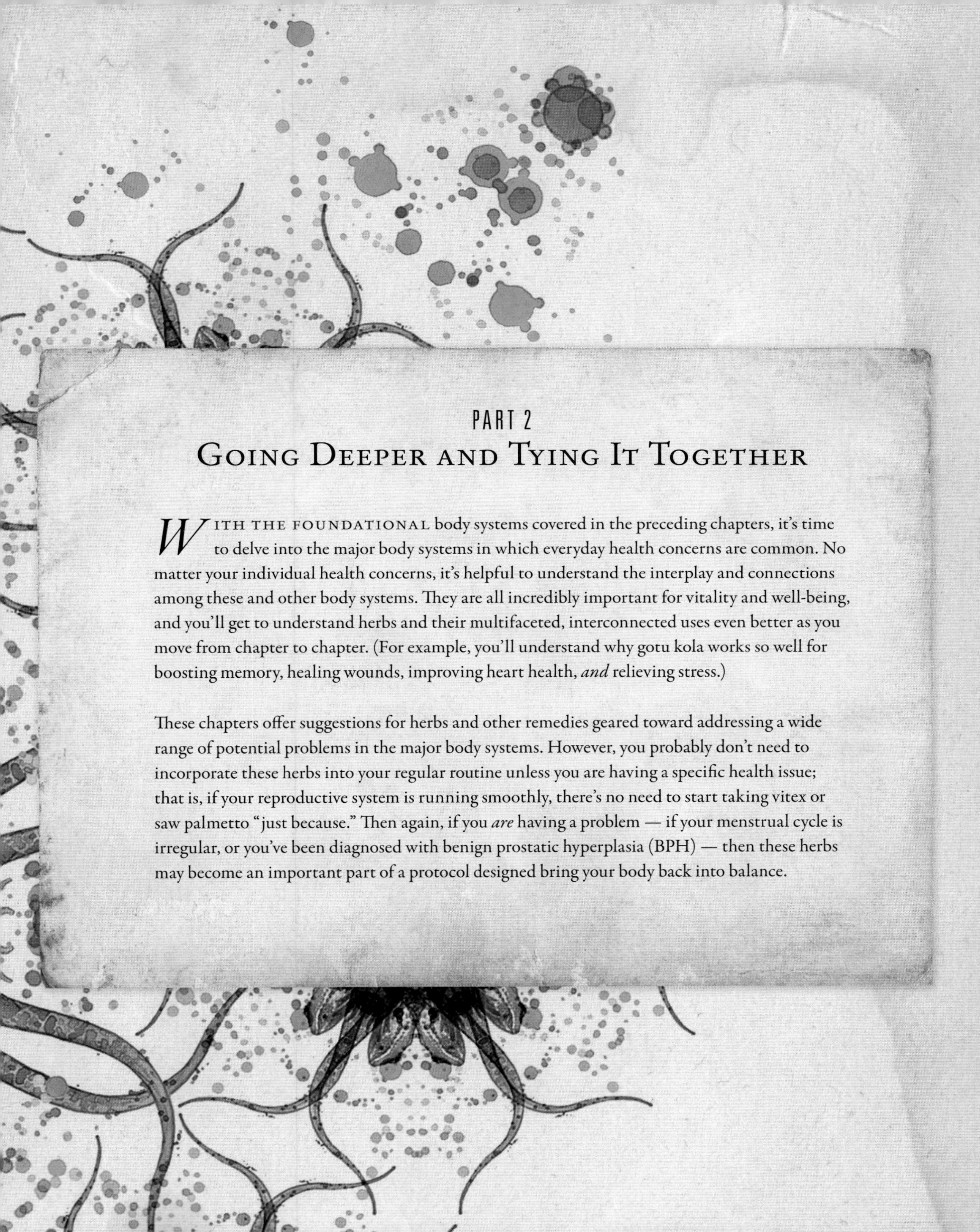

PART 2
Going Deeper and Tying It Together

With the foundational body systems covered in the preceding chapters, it's time to delve into the major body systems in which everyday health concerns are common. No matter your individual health concerns, it's helpful to understand the interplay and connections among these and other body systems. They are all incredibly important for vitality and well-being, and you'll get to understand herbs and their multifaceted, interconnected uses even better as you move from chapter to chapter. (For example, you'll understand why gotu kola works so well for boosting memory, healing wounds, improving heart health, *and* relieving stress.)

These chapters offer suggestions for herbs and other remedies geared toward addressing a wide range of potential problems in the major body systems. However, you probably don't need to incorporate these herbs into your regular routine unless you are having a specific health issue; that is, if your reproductive system is running smoothly, there's no need to start taking vitex or saw palmetto "just because." Then again, if you *are* having a problem — if your menstrual cycle is irregular, or you've been diagnosed with benign prostatic hyperplasia (BPH) — then these herbs may become an important part of a protocol designed bring your body back into balance.

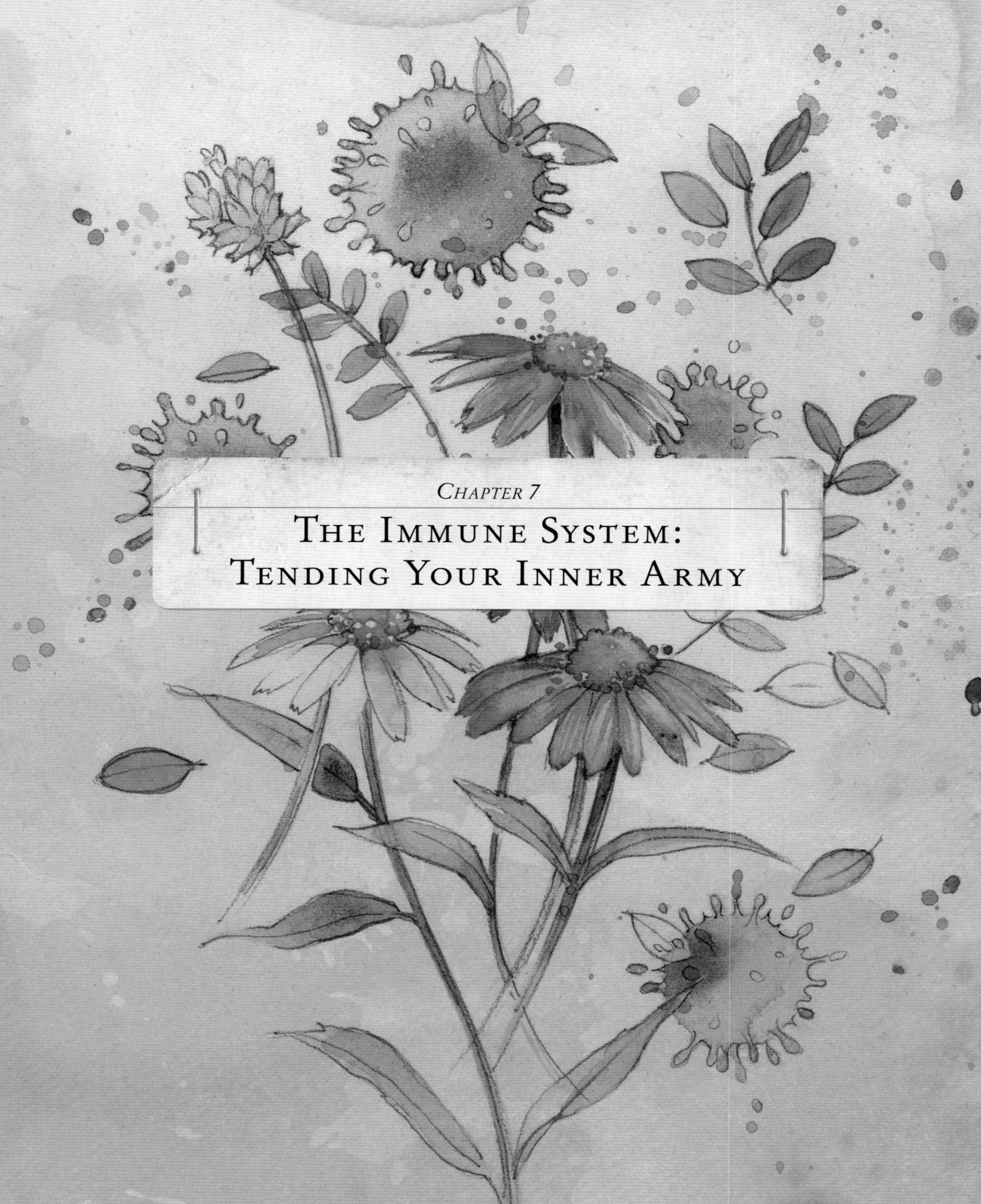

Chapter 7

The Immune System: Tending Your Inner Army

A HEALTHY IMMUNE SYSTEM serves as your personal smooth-running militia, with the number one goal of protecting your body from pathogenic invaders. Infections and immune issues may seem inevitable, but you can do a lot to train your army so that it can fight swiftly and effectively when you need it — and switch into "peacetime" mode when you don't.

Meet Your Immune Army

The human body is amazingly intricate and interconnected, and your immune system is no exception. Unlike most other body systems, which have a clear base of operations (the cardiovascular system in your heart and blood vessels, for example, or your digestive system in your digestive tract), your immune system needs to be anywhere and everywhere. A complex hierarchy of immune cells sends signals — communicating the status quo, setting off invader alerts — and swoops in to do battle when pathogens invade. Your immune cells can be found throughout your body, including your skin, blood, bone marrow, and intestines. However, many immune cells are concentrated in your lymphatic system, with its lymph nodes, your spleen, and the thymus acting as central intelligence offices and training grounds where new immune cells are created.

Much like the branches of a country's military, your immune system is a layered defense system, ready to fight wherever a pathogen tries to enter, with each "branch" specialized to various terrain. Your digestive system, nasal passages, and skin serve as your front line of defense, and the vitality of these areas (e.g., good mucus production and lubrication and plenty of stomach acid) should block or kill invaders at the border before they can truly enter your body. When a pathogen enters your body, your inner immune "army" steps up to deal with it. It has two different arsenals, or types of immune responses, at its disposal: the innate and the acquired.

You're born with the innate immune system, which has a reliable, nonspecific response, including stomach acid, fever response, mucus, beneficial bacteria, and certain types of immune cells. When your innate immune system is fighting a major battle, you feel it! It's best to simply rest as much as possible, stay hydrated, and let your immune system do its job.

Your other immune response is the acquired or adaptive response, and it's what we refer to when we say that you can "develop an immunity" to something. This more sophisticated immune response is built over time as you are exposed to various infections, and its job is to prevent the innate immune system from having to wage full-fledged war every time a germ comes your way. During the first battle with a new pathogen, the immune system "catalogs" the germ by identifying a specific compound in it (an antigen). If a similar antigen later enters the body, the immune system "remembers" it and takes swift, specific action to destroy it. The battle may be fought and won without your ever realizing you were sick.

Modern medicine *is* sometimes necessary to prevent or fight off infections, but often a totally holistic approach works quite nicely, and it builds long-term immune system health to boot. It is important to know your limits and when to call the doctor, however — for example, when you suspect that you have a serious infection, such as strep or pneumonia, or you have an illness that lags or causes intense symptoms (dehydration, listlessness). But remember that herbal therapies can often be used alongside conventional care with improved results. And not just for colds, flu, and the like; the evidence is preliminary but promising for cancer and antibiotic resistance.

What Could Go Wrong? Allergies *and* Autoimmune Disease

Allergies and autoimmune disease stem from poorly trained and weak (or agitated), trigger-happy soldiers. Your acquired immune system begins to mark otherwise harmless compounds like food, pollen, dander, or your own cells as antigen invaders. It becomes obsessed in fighting a long-term futile attack. The inflammation associated with fighting an ongoing "infection" ultimately wreaks havoc on your body and sense of vitality. This is a common scenario in many health concerns, including allergies, asthma, Crohn's and other forms of inflammatory bowel disease, rheumatoid arthritis, certain forms of thyroid disease, the onset of type 1 diabetes, and a complication of Lyme disease.

Why on earth would your body decide to attack otherwise harmless cells and compounds? Two theories seek to explain the situation.

The Hygiene Hypothesis

Any well-tended army does best when it gets a practice run now and then. Studies suggest that we have done *such* a good job keeping common pathogens under control that the immune system gets an itchy trigger and starts looking elsewhere for things to fight. *Some* low-level germ exposure can actually be good! It's the ol' "what doesn't kill you makes you stronger" idea. Kids who grow up in environments where they come into contact with more germs, like farms and pets, and get sick with common infections more often when they're young are less likely to be afflicted with allergies and autoimmune disease later in life. Some studies have also found that introducing benign pathogens into the body takes its attention off autoimmune disease: for example, swallowing parasitic worms to treat Crohn's disease. Research is still preliminary, but you may do well to relax a bit when it comes to common germs, spend more time out in the dirt, and eschew all the antiseptic products in favor of plain soap and water. Medicinal mushrooms and polysaccharide-rich herbs like astragalus modulate immune function and can help retrain your inner army to fight the right battles.

The Cascade Theory

Another approach to autoimmune disease and allergies looks at the layering of inflammation, stress, and other irritants like food allergies/sensitivities. Like a filling bucket, it doesn't seem too bad until it overflows into a big mess. By controlling what you can, you can often avoid or reduce the frequency of flare-ups. Control stress (yoga or meditation, perhaps?), limit exposure to toxins, get enough sleep, avoid eating foods you're sensitive to, support gut health (very important!), get enough nutrients through diet and supplements, and amp up anti-inflammatory food, herbs, spices, and omega-3s in your regular routine. Then you can also consider specific remedies for allergies (e.g., herbal antihistamines) or autoimmune disease (immune modulators). Often, once you get your body into balance for an extended period of time, a few irritants here and there are less likely to pose a reaction.

The Germ *vs.* the Host: Which Matters Most?

Louis Pasteur's germ theory of the 1800s made a major breakthrough in understanding infections when it identified the source of illness: invading viruses, bacteria, and other pathogens. Forthcoming vaccines and antibiotics promised to wipe infectious disease off the planet. Two centuries later, these interventions have surely saved lives, but the germs have gotten smarter, too, leading to our current arms race with drug-resistant supergerms.

Pasteur's friend and colleague Claude Bernard had an opposing theory: the "terroir" or overall health of the person (or host) plays an important role in whether or not that person actually gets sick from the germ. We're *always* surrounded by pathogens, and yet some folks get sick while others don't.

Stressed and run down? Didn't get a good night's sleep? Wham! That's usually when you're most susceptible.

Rumor has it that Pasteur conceded on his deathbed, "Bernard is right. The germ is nothing. The environment is everything." In holistic herbal medicine, we borrow from *both* theories and take a *three-pronged* approach to infections. First, we strengthen overall health using immune-tonic herbs, nutritious food, and a good lifestyle. Second, in the early signs of infection, we boost immune function so that it can act more swiftly to fight germs and clear away the battle debris so that we feel better faster. (Conventional medicine usually ignores these first two approaches, even though they make such a huge difference!) Third, we use herbs that have direct antimicrobial action. Our most popular immune herbs do at least two and often all three of these tasks. Natural antimicrobials may not have the kick of antibiotic meds, but they contain a wider range of antimicrobial compounds that makes it more difficult for germs to become resistant.

Surefire Ways *to* Zap Your Immunity

Do what you can to keep these things in check, especially if you know your immune system is already being challenged.

- Sleep deprivation
- Stress
- Dehydration
- Poor diet
- Smoking
- Excessive alcohol
- Excessive sugar
- Exposure to virulent germs (wash your hands!)

THE FOOD AND GUT CONNECTION

A WEAK IMMUNE SYSTEM — indicated by such ailments as autoimmune disease, chronic asthma, recurring infections — often coincides with poor gut health and food choices. A healthy digestive system and good levels of stomach acid help prevent germs from entering your body and doing damage. So poor digestive health automatically puts you at an immune disadvantage. In addition, reactive foods (those you're allergic or sensitive to, as well as junk food) create a low-level state of inflammation that upsets everything else, including immune function and the balance of beneficial bacteria in your body. Long term, this leads to overreactive immune function, with concomitant allergies and autoimmune disease. For example, gluten reactivity may create a cross-reaction with the thyroid in thyroid autoimmune disease. Milk and dairy issues can aggravate mucus buildup, ear infections, and sinus problems. If you suspect that gut health is affecting your overall health, scrutinize your diet — could something be irritating your system? If you suspect a particular food, try avoiding that food for a month (do your symptoms get better?), then reintroduce it (do they get worse?). Also, key in on herbs that help soothe and heal gut tissue, including demulcents (licorice, marshmallow, slippery elm), soothing wound healers (plantain, calendula, gotu kola), gentle astringents (roses, bidens), and probiotics and fermented foods. For more details, see chapter 5.

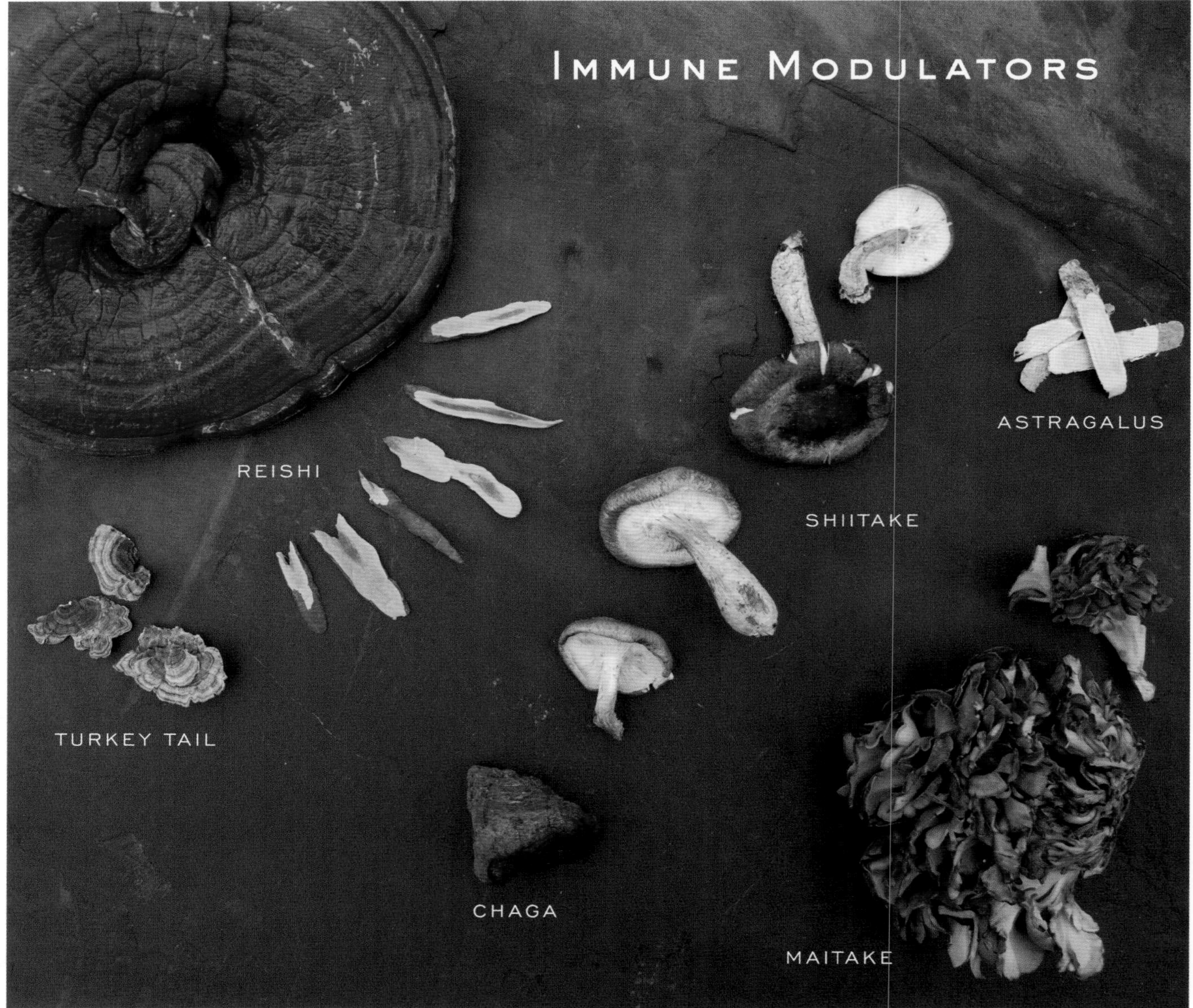

WHAT IS AN IMMUNE MODULATOR?

Immune modulators tend to balance and strengthen immune system function rather than simply up-regulating or down-regulating it. They usually create a healthy challenge to the immune system and improve cell signaling, making it less fragile (antifragility).

General Uses: A wide range of immune issues, including prevention of colds and the flu, cancer prevention and adjunct cancer care, respiratory ailments, asthma, allergies, autoimmune disease, mononucleosis, and weak immune function (i.e., constantly getting sick)

Examples: Medicinal mushrooms, including reishi, shiitake, maitake, chaga, and turkey tails, along with astragalus and adaptogens, including codonopsis, schizandra, ashwagandha, and holy basil

Strengthening *(and Modulating)* the Immune System

Medicinal mushrooms and adaptogenic herbs can play an important role in strengthening and modulating immune function, which makes them useful for preventing illness, balancing autoimmune and allergic conditions, and even potentially fighting cancer and other diseases relating to your immune system. Thank traditional Chinese medicine for introducing most of these amazing tonics to the Western world.

▸ Medicinal Mushrooms

Availability: G W C

Key Properties: Medicinal mushrooms, including reishi, maitake, shiitake, turkey tail, cordyceps, and chaga, improve your immune function by challenging it. They contain complex starches (polysaccharides), including glucans, that your body perceives as a threat, and so the body mounts an immune system response even though the mushrooms themselves are harmless. This might sound like a bad thing, but it actually benefits your immune system. In a sense, these glucans give your immune system a training run, which improves the function of a range of immune cells and pathways and takes attention off allergies and autoimmune disease. Your stronger, smarter immune cells become more adept at fending off true pathogens like the common cold as well as dispatching rogue cells that cause cancer. Some mushrooms, particularly reishi and cordyceps, also have compounds that strengthen lung structure and function and improve oxygen utilization, which helps those who are prone to asthma, bronchitis, pneumonia, chronic obstructive pulmonary disease (COPD), and so on. (See page 133 for more on these mushrooms and lung health.)

Additional Benefits: Medicinal mushrooms offer a range of benefits beyond the immune system, depending on the mushroom. Some are heart tonics, hypoglycemics, or anti-inflammatories; others are excellent edible sources of fiber, protein, and vitamin D. See books by Greg Marley, Paul Stamets, Christopher Hobbs, and Robert Rogers for more details.

Preparation: Get the most out of mushrooms by cooking them. Eat more tender and tasty medicinals like shiitake and maitake in stir-fries and soups. Tougher reishi, chaga, and turkey tails can be simmered for a few hours to make broths, teas, or decoction tinctures. You can also use dried mushroom powders, which you can add to soups, broth, and stews, or take specially made capsules. To specifically strengthen the immune system, medicinal mushrooms are best taken daily or for an extended period; standard herb doses (see page 298) apply.

Cautions and Considerations: Generally safe, though some people don't tolerate mushrooms or are allergic to them. Avoid eating mushrooms raw; cooking makes the beneficial starches more digestible and usable to the body and inactivates potential toxins.

▸ Astragalus

Astragalus propinquus, syn. *A. membranaceus*

Availability: G- C+

Key Properties: This polysaccharide-rich root acts much like the medicinal mushrooms. Consider it to strengthen a weak immune system function, to prevent infection, or if you're always getting sick. Preliminary research also suggests that astragalus helps with autoimmune disease and cancer. It's energetically warming and nourishing and best for cold, stagnant states.

Additional Benefits: Although it's primarily used for immune health, astragalus may also be considered an adaptogen. It aids the healthy function of many body systems and supports the cardiovascular system, liver, and kidneys.

Preparation: This sweet, earthy-tasting root blends easily into teas like chai as well as soup broth. It blends well with adaptogens and mushrooms. You

Treating Common Infections

Most viral infections can be traced back to stress, overextending yourself, and not getting enough sleep. If you start to get sick, take it as a signal to take a break and get as much rest and sleep as possible, until you are feeling a *lot* better. Pushing through a cold or flu, or trying to bounce back too quickly, puts you at a greater risk of a secondary infection — bacterial infections, sinus infection, bronchitis, and pneumonia — because your immune system is weak and a cold body full of stagnant phlegm is the *perfect* breeding ground for more germs.

Bump up your elderberry syrup — taking it as often as you can remember — and keep up with all the previously mentioned immune-boosting foods, especially raw garlic, ginger, and broth.

▸ Echinacea

Echinacea spp.

Availability: G+ W- C+

Key Properties: Echinacea turns on immune system function, activates immune cells for swifter battle action, interferes with a virus's ability to spread (in part by inhibiting the hyaluronidase that viruses use to hijack cells), kills bacteria, and keeps your lymph flowing to help clear the battlefield of debris so you feel better faster. Though today it's often touted for its ability to combat the flu, echinacea actually has a much longer history of use for bacterial infections and septicemia (not to mention venomous snakebites!) than for viruses. All parts of most echinacea species (garden variety *E. purpurea* and harder-to-grow wild *E. angustifolia*) have medicinal value, though some feel *E. angustifolia* root works best.

Additional Benefits: Echinacea treats sepsis, numbs on contact, and also increases saliva output (it's a natural sialagogue). It may help prevent infections, too.

Preparation: The roots tend to be the strongest medicinally, but most herbalists use a combination of all parts, often as a tincture of the fresh plant. Take ½ to 1 teaspoon (2 to 5 squirts from the dropper) as often as you can remember (every waking hour or so), starting at the first tickle of infection or anticipation of exposure. A good-quality extract will numb your tongue. Teas and capsules may suffice but tend to be weaker. Because echinacea is energetically cold, consider adding a warming herb like ginger or a pinch of cayenne.

Cautions and Considerations: Echinacea is generally safe, but some people are allergic to it (especially the flower and aboveground parts, if you're allergic to other daisy-family flowers), and its immune-boosting activity may cause an autoimmune flare-up. Watch for potential drug interactions.

Similar Herbs: Some echinacea relatives offer similar benefits: **spilanthes**, certain species of **wild black-eyed Susan**, and **balsam root**. Though rare commercially, they grow abundantly in some locales, and some are easily grown in the garden.

WHAT IS AN IMMUNOSTIMULANT?

Immune stimulants activate the immune system so that it can more swiftly and effectively fight an infection. They may also have direct antiviral, antibacterial, or antifungal effects.

General Uses: Best taken short term at the first sign of a cold, flu, or other infection in frequent high doses until the infection passes. With some exceptions, they tend to be less appropriate if you have an autoimmune disease and for long-term use.

Examples: Echinacea, spilanthes, garlic, usnea, elder, boneset, elecampane

Immune Stimulants & Antimicrobials

ECHINACEA

ECHINACEA ROOT

THYME

OREGANO

ELDERBERRY SYRUP

BEE BALM

▸ Garden-Variety Antimicrobials

Availability: G+ W C+

These include oregano (*Origanum vulgare*), thyme (*Thymus vulgaris*), and bee balm (*Monarda fistulosa*). Although you will often just see oregano or thyme mentioned as "immune herbs," *all* the oregano- and thyme-flavored mint-family herbs can be used interchangeably. Bee balm is rarely found on the commercial herb market, but it's a darling of backyard herbalists because it's gorgeous, grows abundantly, and often provides more potent and easy-to-harvest medicine than its more famous relatives.

Key Properties: These mint-family herbs do double-duty as immune tonics and kitchen seasonings. The more bite, the better. As aromatic antimicrobials, they fight germs directly and have an affinity for the lungs and sinuses, helping to open airways and disinfect. Thyme has particular affinity for opening the lungs and relieving asthmatic issues.

Additional Benefits: These herbs also stimulate healthy digestion. They target gut pathogens and yeast infections, and they can be applied topically to fight many types of germs.

Preparation: Use strongly flavored leaves, with or without the flowers. Consider them as strong tea infusions or in soup broth (added at the end), steams, tinctures, vinegars, oxymels, and infused honey. Some people turn to the concentrated oregano essential oil (just a drop or two internally); however, this may be more potent than necessary, and less safe. I prefer more traditional forms of the crude herbs. Standard herb doses (see page 298) apply.

Cautions and Considerations: As long as the herbs agree with you, they're generally safe. Do not use therapeutic doses during pregnancy due to their emmenagogue effects. Use caution with the essential oils; they are significantly more potent and can be dangerous if used internally (in doses of more than a drop or two) or long term.

Fresh Ginger Thermos Tea

This is my go-to tea when I start to get that achy feeling and a tickle in my throat. It feels good (and tastes delicious) just sipping it. Fresh ginger offers significantly more antiviral protection than dry. Brew it strong or even consider juicing it. Feel free to play around with additional ingredients like cinnamon sticks, star anise pods, or thyme sprigs in place of, or in addition to, the lemon and honey.

- 1 (1-inch) piece ginger, sliced thin or grated (no need to peel)
- 2 lemon wedges (optional)
- 1–2 tablespoons honey (optional)

Place the ginger in a thermos. Squeeze the juice from the lemon wedges (if using) into the thermos, and drop in the rinds. Pour in 2 cups boiling water, add the honey (if using), and stir. Let steep for 30 to 60 minutes, or longer. (Lemon's bioflavonoid-rich rind is good for you but can get unpleasantly bitter after an hour or more of steeping. You can remove it or just refrain from tossing the rind in, if you'd like.)

WHAT IS AN ANTIMICROBIAL?

Antimicrobials directly (and sometimes indirectly) kill germs, such as viruses, bacteria, and fungi. They generally have disinfectant and antiseptic properties and are often strongly flavored or scented. Most have broad action but may work best against specific types of pathogens.

General Uses: Infections of the respiratory and digestive tracts, skin, or other areas of the body

Examples: Elderberries, echinacea (best fresh), goldenseal and berberine-rich herbs (on contact, whether on the skin or in the throat, gut, or sinuses), elecampane, usnea, bee balm, oregano, thyme, sage, holy basil, garlic (especially raw), ginger (fresh), onions, thuja (externally or drop-dose internally), chaparral (external use only), spilanthes, lemon balm, licorice, calendula, myrrh, yarrow, and many others

PROTOCOL POINTS

Cold and Flu

Although almost every herb in this chapter — and many more — could be used to address a cold or flu, here are some of the key herbs and therapies to consider. The earlier you catch an oncoming infection, the easier it will be to lessen its severity or duration. You can also employ these tactics in anticipation of exposure (when you're around others who are sick or traveling by plane) to reduce your risk of infection.

Diet: Focus on fluids, especially broth, clear soups, water, and tea. Eat ample amounts of pungent, warming antimicrobials, including ginger, garlic, onions, curry, and cayenne. Limit or avoid junk food, alcohol, and sugar. Drink green tea, unless it interferes with sleep.

Lifestyle: Rest and sleep as much as possible! If you're coming down with an infection, take it easy. Keep up with hand washing and hygiene to prevent infecting others.

Herbs: Consider elderberry syrup, medicinal mushrooms, and astragalus for prevention. At the first sign of an infection, hit it hard with frequent (approximately every waking hour) doses of elderberry syrup, echinacea tincture, or strong tea made with fresh ginger and honey.

Targeted Care: Infections tend to settle into "weak spots" that vary from person to person. Do what you can to target those areas to keep them healthy.

- **Sinuses:** Neti pot/nasal irrigation with warm salt water (add goldenseal/berberine as an antimicrobial if needed), herbal antihistamines, and remedies that help thin mucus and promote drainage, including goldenrod and horehound tinctures and eating wasabi or horseradish
- **Throat:** Demulcent soothers (licorice, slippery elm, marshmallow, plantain, honey), antimicrobials (propolis, goldenseal, echinacea, oregano, bee balm), and numbing agents (echinacea, cayenne) as tea, soup/broth, or throat spray
- **Lungs:** Aromatic antimicrobials (oregano, bee balm, thyme, elecampane, pine), mucus-thinning expectorants (grindelia, horehound), and antispasmodics for cough (honey, cherry bark for dry cough, horehound for wet cough, peppermint or evergreen cough drops), particularly as syrups, cough drops, steams, tea, and soup; also helpful are tonic mushrooms (reishi, cordyceps) as soup, decoction, tincture, or capsules
- **GI tract:** Demulcent soothers (see the recommendations for the throat), gentle astringent toners (rose petals, cinnamon), antimicrobials (goldenseal/berberine, oregano/bee balm, cinnamon, bidens, short-term oak bark/tannins), and fermented foods (miso, kimchi), especially as tea, food, soup

AT A GLANCE

Herbs for the Immune System

The herbs listed here are grouped by their beneficial action for the immune system, with my favorite, most effective, safest, and most common herbs listed first. Herbs that support the respiratory system can also help support immune function; for more on them, see page 133.

Antimicrobials

- Echinacea
- Bitter berberines (goldenseal, coptis, oregon grape root, barberry)
- Elecampane
- Usnea
- Bee balm
- Oregano
- Thyme
- Sage
- Garlic (raw)
- Ginger (fresh)
- Onions
- Thuja (drop dose)*
- Spilanthes
- Calendula
- Myrrh
- Yarrow
- Alder
- Evergreens (balsam fir, white pine, hemlock tree)
- Balsam root
- Yerba mansa
- Propolis

Immune Boosters & Antivirals

- Echinacea
- Elderberry (black)
- Andrographis (bitter!)
- Umcka
- Ginger (fresh)
- Lemon balm (fresh)
- Licorice
- Baptisia*
- Thuja*

Immune Boosters & Modulators

- Astragalus
- Medicinal mushrooms
- Elderberry
- Adaptogens (codonopsis, ashwagandha, holy basil)

Lymph Movers

- Echinacea root (and aerial parts)
- Red root (and aerial parts)
- Burdock root and seed
- Red clover blossom
- Calendula flower
- Alder bark and twig (dry)
- Cleavers and chickweed
- Violet leaf (and flower)
- Movement
- Massage
- Skin brushing

Diaphoretics

- Boneset
- Peppermint
- Yarrow
- Elderflower
- Ginger (best fresh)

**Be particularly aware of cautions and/or ecological status before using plants marked with an asterisk.*

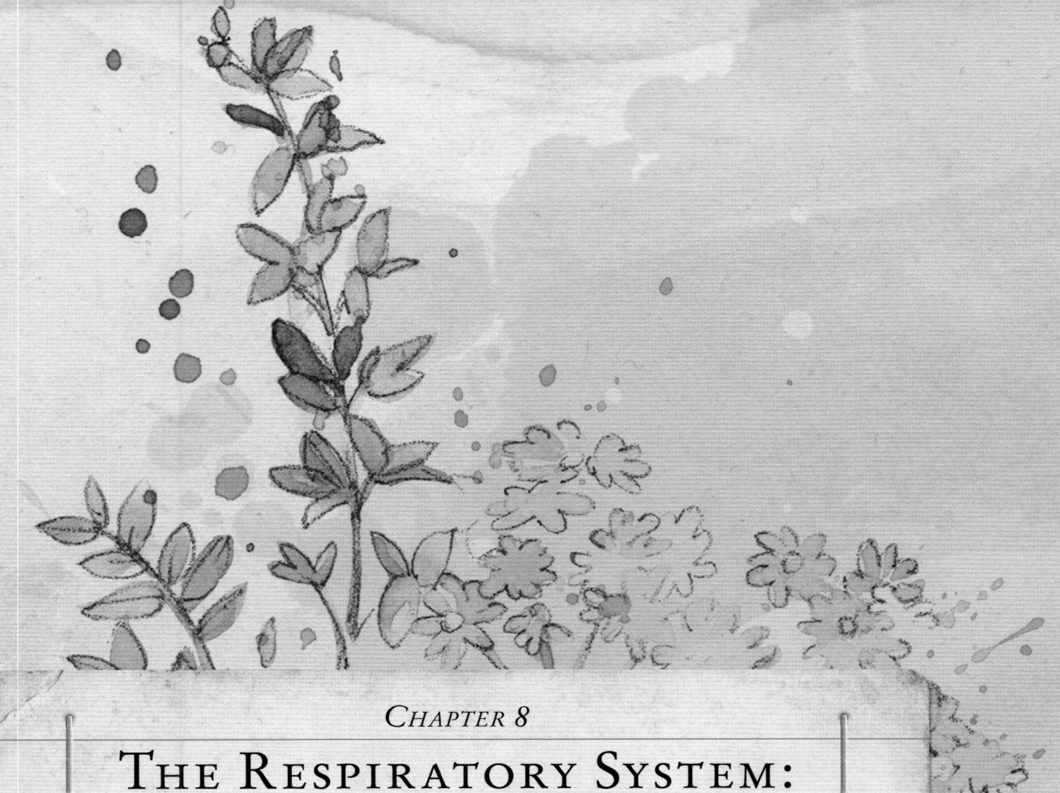

Chapter 8

The Respiratory System: Breathing Deeply

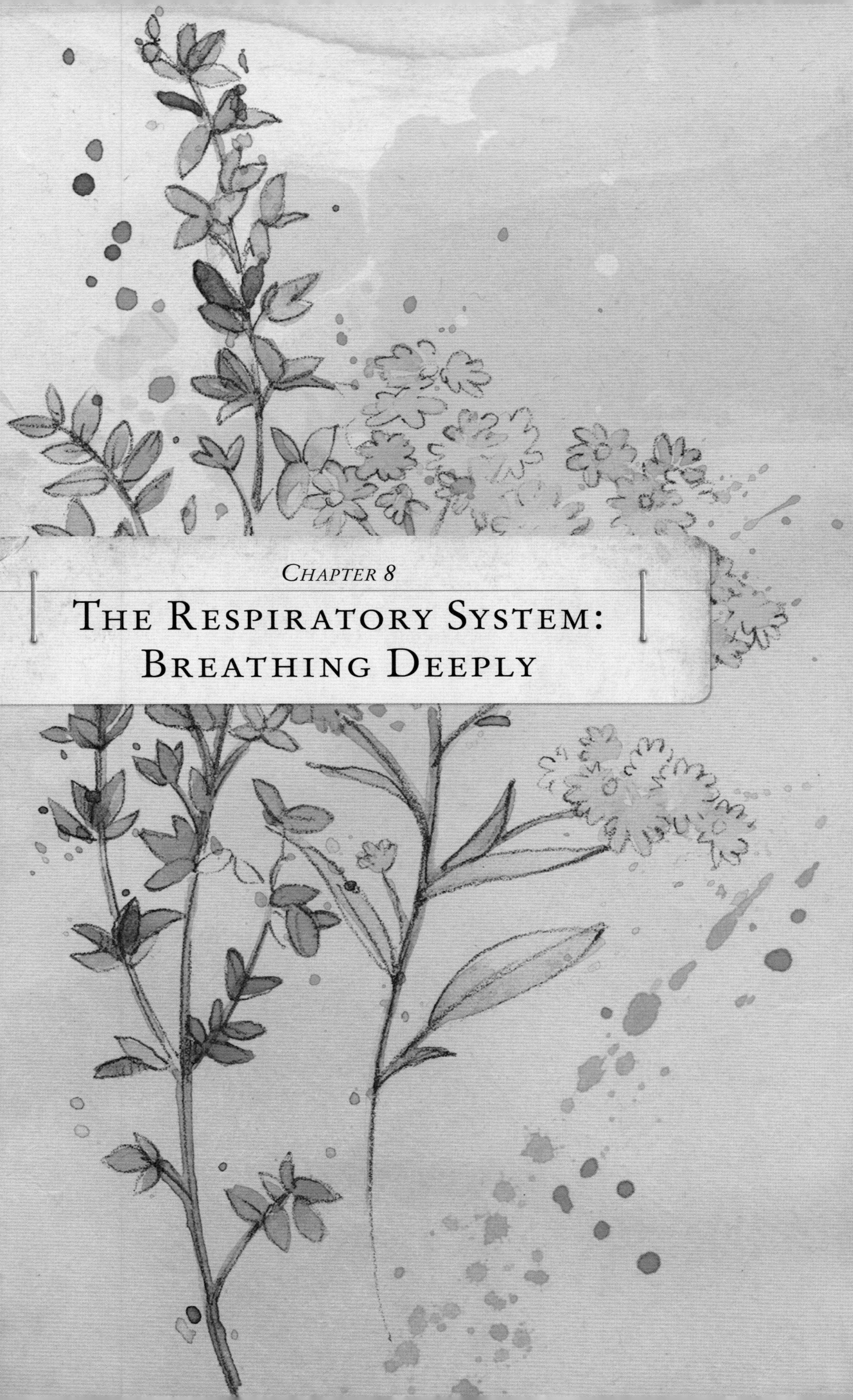

YOUR LUNGS COME second only to your heart as vital organs that symbolize life. Protected by the bars of your rib cage, these tender, spongy sacs rise and fall as they take in and expel air. With this action they filter contaminants from the outside air, release toxins from your body, and — most important of all — balance the levels of oxygen and carbon dioxide in your body. Fittingly, your bronchial tubes resemble an upside-down tree, and your respiratory system exists in symbiosis with the plant world, using and releasing the opposing gases that keep both alive. Your respiratory system branches around and cradles your heart. As oxygen comes into your lungs, it's transferred to your heart, where it's infused into the bloodstream to be delivered throughout your body. This elemental gas is essential for your ability to breathe, for your cells to make energy, and for your brain and immune system to function. If your oxygen levels begin to falter, your energy levels drop like a rock and everything else begins to fail.

The ability to take a deep breath is something most of us take for granted, but all of us, at one point or another, find ourselves congested and wheezy, whether due to a cold or something more serious. Potential respiratory issues range from infections (cold, flu, pneumonia) to inflammatory conditions (asthma, bronchitis) to physical damage (chronic obstructive pulmonary disease, silicosis). Fortunately, there's much you can do to support this important organ system and bring your whole body into better balance.

Treating *and* Managing Respiratory Issues

Herbs and natural therapies can be extremely helpful for everyday respiratory woes as well as more serious acute and chronic lung conditions; however, it's important to remember that any difficulty with breathing can be a serious matter. You may need to visit your doctor for assessment and diagnosis. A round of antibiotics or an emergency inhaler may be necessary, at least at the onset. However, even in cases where medical care is necessary, using herbs and lifestyle techniques alongside can be incredibly valuable to heal lung imbalances. They may minimize or eliminate the need for drugs or help pharmaceuticals work more effectively. Herbs do things no pharmaceutical can do. This is where herbalism shines: helping the body repair damage and bring the body back into balance. The ability of herbs to heal the lungs — even in serious conditions — can be nothing short of miraculous.

The basic strategies for treating and managing respiratory ailments center on the following principles:

- Open the airways (and improve oxygen utilization)
- Reduce histamine and mucus
- Soothe irritation and spasms
- Rebuild and repair lung tissue
- Fight infection
- Decrease inflammation
- Avoid respiratory irritants

Which tactics you take will depend, of course, on the particular respiratory problem you're having. We'll address each of these strategies in turn over the rest of this chapter.

As with many body systems, it's useful to double-dip when you choose a treatment plan for the respiratory system — that is, provide targeted herbs in at least two forms. It could be a tea and a tincture. A soup broth and a steam inhalation. Or a mushroom capsule and an herbal tea. The exact formulas will depend on your needs, personal preference, and the best methods of extraction and delivery for the herbs you want to use. You might have a few overlapping ingredients, but often the formula ingredients are a tad different and complement one another.

Open *the* Airways

Many lung issues, including asthma and bronchitis, involve a constriction or spasm of the lungs and bronchi. Though many herbs address this, mullein, elecampane, and yerba santa work so well and afford such a high degree of safety that they are my favorites. You will find at least one of them in almost every respiratory formula I create for my clients.

▸ Mullein

Verbascum thapsus

Availability: G+ W+ C

Key Properties: Mullein leaf is a go-to herb for respiratory ailments and lung issues, including asthma, bronchitis, impending respiratory infection, and lung irritation. Mullein relieves irritation in both infection and chronic cases, helping people take deeper breaths, and may even repair lung tissue. I've seen mullein allow singers to perform in spite of an oncoming infection and quickly clear up respiratory issues resulting from inhaling mold and other particles while cleaning water damage in a basement. It even has a reputation for helping to clear COPD, which is generally considered incurable. Mullein also cools and soothes harsh coughs, dryness, and seasonal allergies.

Additional Benefits: Mullein flowers can be added to formulas for their demulcent, soothing action. They're often infused in oil and applied for earaches.

Preparation: Harvest the soft, fuzzy leaves of this biennial weed whenever they look happy, from the earliest of spring into early winter. Use them fresh or dry as tea or tincture, being sure to strain out the irritating hairs through a tightly woven cloth, teabag, or coffee filter (metal strainers may not suffice). Standard herb doses (see page 298) apply. Inhaling mullein smoke can provide immediate results by targeting the tissues, but I prefer less smoky solutions.

Cautions and Considerations: Generally extremely safe, even for children and possibly during pregnancy (with supervision). Flowering mullein stalks are unmistakable, but you typically harvest mullein leaves before it blooms. Be sure to rule out potential look-alikes — foxglove being the most deadly potential mix-up. The hairs sometimes irritate sensitive skin and tissue on contact and should be well strained from formulas.

▸ Elecampane

Inula helenium

Availability: G C

Key Properties: This lovely sunflower relative produces pungent, balsam-y roots traditionally used to relieve bronchial spasms, fight infection, and move and clear congestion. The aromatic properties of this herb cause a slight irritation in the respiratory tract that is generally beneficial in that it stimulates better function. As your body attempts to release the aromatic essential oils via the lungs, this also helps to disinfect the air space. (Other aromatic respiratory herbs including bee balm, oregano, thyme, peppermint, and most evergreens have similar actions.) Though some may find elecampane too hot, dry, and irritating, others will find it amazing.

Additional Benefits: The bitter aromatics of elecampane root chug sluggish digestion back to life and may help expel parasitic worms. The roots are rich in inulin, a white fiber that feeds good bacteria.

Preparation: In the garden, elecampane prefers plentiful sunshine and good soil. It may take a few years to settle in, transitioning from scrappy rosettes (don't mistake them for weeds!) to robust, tall plants, but once it does, it should self-seed and produce large roots within just a few years. One autumn-harvested root can provide enough tincture for years; it's one of the most rewarding root medicines to grow. Most people prefer the tincture because of elecampane's strong flavor, but you can use it in tea blends and herbal honey. Don't be alarmed by a cloudy white substance at the bottom of your tincture or extract; it's just the inulin. Standard herb doses (see page 298) apply.

Cautions and Considerations: Generally safe in modest doses, but too strong (causing digestive complaints and more) in excessive doses. It's not recommended during pregnancy due to its emmenagogue effect.

▸ Yerba Santa

Eriodictyon spp.
Availability: W C-
Key Properties: This sticky shrub grows in California. Yerba santa leaf boasts a long history of use in both Native American and Eclectic circles for just about any lung issue, including emphysema, asthma, infection, bronchitis, common infections, and chronic cough, thanks to the aromatic resins and warming, drying nature of the leaves. It opens the bronchi, helps loosen mucus, fights germs, and acts as a carminative.
Additional Benefits: Its common name translates to "sacred herb," and it has a range of other uses, including improving digestion.
Preparation: It may be most convenient as a tincture (fresh or dry) but takes well to tea. The leaves taste sweet and aromatic, like a cross between cherry and eucalyptus. Don't be alarmed when the resins precipitate out in water and make your jars all sticky — that's normal. Standard herb doses (see page 298) apply.
Cautions and Considerations: No known side effects, including whether or not it's appropriate during pregnancy or nursing.

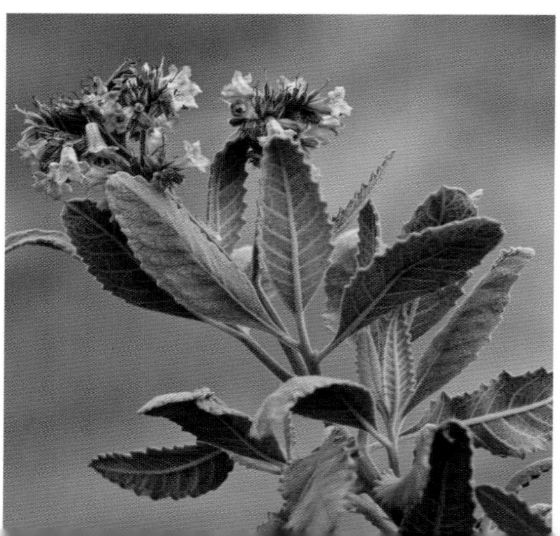

▸ Other Herbs for Opening the Airways

Two more controversial herbs are worth mentioning for opening the airways: **lobelia** and **ephedra.**

Lobelia tincture is not for the faint of heart — or sensitive of stomach — but those for whom it works love it and develop a sort of kinship with it. Tincture the fresh aerial parts as the flowers begin to go to seed. Taken in low doses — 1 to 5 drops as needed — lobelia provides *immediate* relief for spasms and allows deeper breaths. It's better to take more frequent rather than larger doses, and small amounts of lobelia will synergize a blend. Lobelia is especially effective for asthma and chronic spastic lung issues. It is rich in highly bioactive, acrid alkaloids that bind to similar receptor sites as nicotine. Because of this, it's sometimes smoked (and called Indian tobacco) or taken in more traditional herbal forms to help people quit smoking, both mellowing cravings and opening the airways to help get the crud out. In large doses, lobelia causes nausea and profound vomiting, earning it the nickname "puke weed." (The puke-'em-purge-'em Samuel Thomsonian herbal movement used lobelia as a core herb. Viewed within the context of Samuel Thomson's era, this seems safer than the bloodletting and mercury therapies that most nineteenth-century physicians were enamored of.) For respiratory ailments, we stay below the nausea threshold. Theoretically lobelia can be toxic in large doses, but the emetic effects prevent any real safety concerns.

Ephedra compounds resemble pseudoephedrine, and the herb acts as a bronchodilator. It can be used in small amounts for issues like asthma and allergies and in higher doses to avert an asthma attack. Ephedrine, the primary constituent in ephedra, works by stimulating the sympathetic fight-or-flight nervous system, which opens the airways and drains congestion in the sinuses and ears. However, because of its stimulating nature, it can be dangerous for sensitive people or if taken in high amounts. Death from stroke and

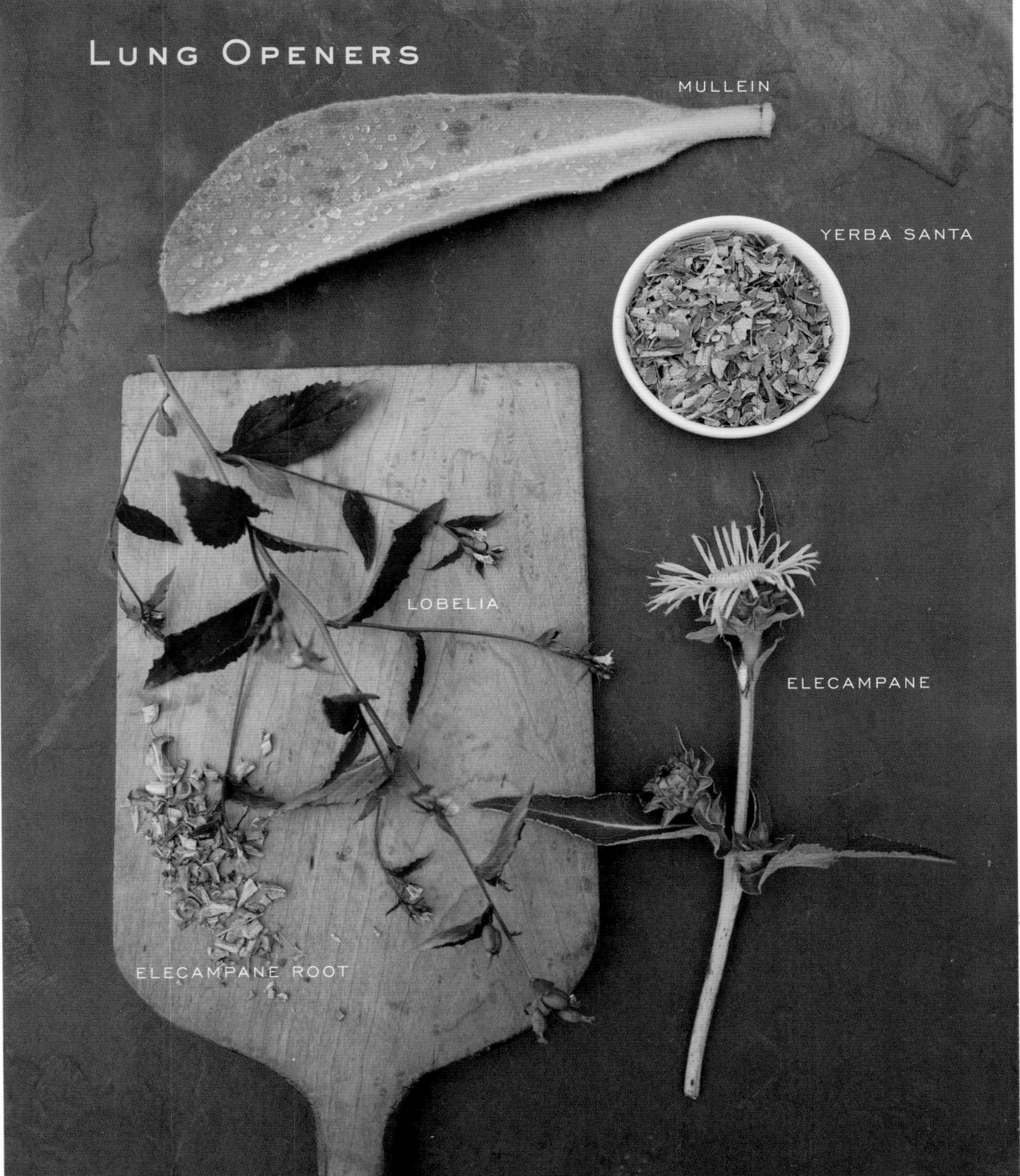
Lung Openers
MULLEIN
YERBA SANTA
LOBELIA
ELECAMPANE
ELECAMPANE ROOT

heart attack have been connected to the overuse of ephedra in diet and weight-loss products, forcing the U.S. Food and Drug Administration (FDA) to make it illegal to sell Chinese ephedra (*E. sinica*). (American species in the Southwest, like *E. viridis*, a.k.a. Mormon tea, tend to be less stimulating and are still available if you look hard enough.) The fact that ephedra and its over-the-counter equivalent can be used to make recreational drugs like methamphetamine have made access to this plant even more controversial in spite of its benefits for lung health. It's one of the few herbs that can avert an acute asthma attack, but it's probably safer (and more legal) to stick to your inhaler.

Reduce Histamine *and* Mucus

The healthy production of histamine occurs via cell signaling in your adaptive or acquired immune system. Histamine is a component of your immune system that stimulates inflammation and many of the symptoms we associate with colds and allergies. Once your body identifies a compound as an "invader," it marks it with antigen status and produces antibodies to it. Then whenever the body senses that antigen, immune cells amass on location, producing histamine with the goal of trapping and killing the pathogen. Unfortunately, histamine produces miserable symptoms, including thick, flowing mucus; watery eyes; and inflammation. The situation goes from bad to worse when your immune system gets sidetracked and begins reacting to otherwise harmless substances — like pollen and dander — as antigens.

Overreactive immune and histamine response is at the core of many respiratory ailments, including seasonal allergies, asthma, sinusitis, postnasal drip, congestion, and some cases of bronchitis. An immune-supportive lifestyle can reduce the severity and frequency of histamine response; this would include a healthy diet free from foods you're allergic or sensitive to, avoidance of respiratory irritants and toxins, stress reduction, adequate sleep, and immune-modulating remedies like astragalus, mushrooms, and probiotics. In addition, when symptoms kick up, try the following herbs, which shine for their ability to reduce histamine production and relieve symptoms.

WHAT IS AN EXPECTORANT?

Expectorants thin and move mucus so that it is easier to eliminate. They often relieve congestion and help make coughs more productive. Our most popular expectorant herbs also offer germ-killing (antimicrobial), slimy soothing (demulcent), airway-opening (bronchodilator), or cough-suppressant (antitussive) properties.

(In contrast, anticatarrhal herbs, like goldenseal and bitter berberines, eyebright, goldenrod, and garlic, clear mucus by drying it up and astringing tissues.)

General Uses: Cough, congestion, asthma, infections, cold, flu, bronchitis, allergies, sinusitis, pneumonia, et cetera

Examples: Elecampane, grindelia, lobelia, yerba santa, horehound, pungent mint-family herbs (bee balm, thyme, oregano, peppermint), and most evergreens (pine, fir, spruce, hemlock) are classic expectorants. Soothing expectorant-demulcents include marshmallow, slippery elm, licorice, violet, and plantain.

▸ Horehound

Marrubium vulgare

Availability: G W C

Key Properties: Horehound leaf thins mucus and helps clear it from the airways while quelling spasms. Though it's most famous for relieving wet coughs, I've found the herb incredibly useful in allergy-type issues with thick, damp mucus — postnasal drip, sinus congestion, bronchitis, chest congestion, seasonal allergies, and so on. It often works quickly and combines well with the herbal antihistamine goldenrod (see below).

Additional Benefits: Horehound also acts as a diaphoretic, helping to break a fever. Michael Moore found it incredibly effective for childhood asthma — he recommended horehound capsules with passionflower tea (calming) and echinacea tincture (immune boosting) — reducing the severity of symptoms and frequency of emergency room visits when used preventively.

Preparation: Try tincture of the fresh plant (my preference) or freshly dried herbs encapsulated. I use the aboveground parts of the plant, whether or not it's in flower. The herb's intense bitter flavor makes it less palatable for tea. Horehound candies, honey, and syrup work but tend to be less potent. Commercial horehound tends to be poor quality; use homegrown or buy from a reputable supplier. Standard herb doses (see page 298) apply.

Cautions and Considerations: It's so terribly bitter! Large doses can be nauseating. Don't use it during pregnancy due to its emmenagogue effects.

Similar Herbs: The budding aerial tops of the resinous **grindelia** also thin mucus so it can be expelled more easily and can be used similarly to horehound.

▸ Goldenrod

Solidago spp.

Availability: G+ W+ C-

Key Properties: Often (inaccurately) blamed for ragweed allergies, goldenrod actually contains anti-inflammatory, antihistamine properties and helps thin and drain mucus while toning the mucosal lining. It's fabulous for seasonal allergies, sinus congestion, and other scenarios involving thick, cold mucus buildup, often working quickly. It can also be taken as a tonic for the respiratory and kidney systems; in both places, thanks to its astringent-aromatic actions, it helps tonify the structure while improving the quality and production of secretions.

Additional Benefits: Goldenrod is better known as a diuretic kidney tonic, and it's a diaphoretic (inducing sweating, breaking a fever), so you can think of it as a very fluid-moving plant.

Preparation: Harvest the tops (leaves and flowers) just as the flowers are starting to open. I prefer tincture of the fresh plant for respiratory issues, but tea can also be used. Also consider goldenrod-infused vinegar. Standard herb doses (see page 298) apply.

Cautions and Considerations: Do not use it in cases of kidney disease without the supervision of a practitioner. The diuretic effects can be a nuisance — it's probably best not to take goldenrod before bedtime.

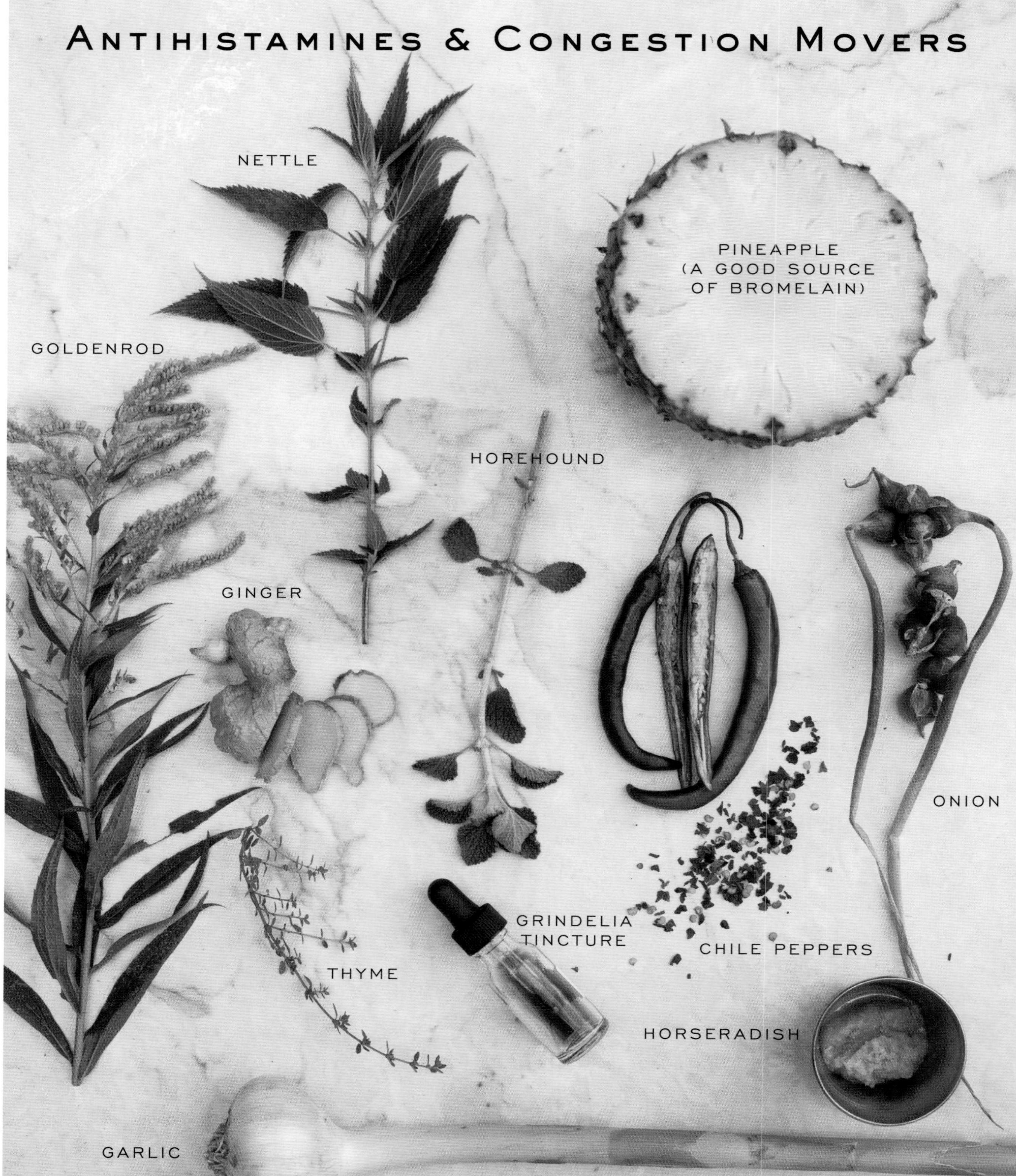
ANTIHISTAMINES & CONGESTION MOVERS
NETTLE
PINEAPPLE (A GOOD SOURCE OF BROMELAIN)
GOLDENROD
HOREHOUND
GINGER
ONION
GRINDELIA TINCTURE
CHILE PEPPERS
THYME
HORSERADISH
GARLIC

▸ Other Antihistamine Supports

Though best known for its nutritional benefits, **nettle** also offers mild antihistamine effects and helps keep the blood clear of compounds that irritate the immune system. Think of nettle for chronic, allergic, and respiratory ailments as well as mucus buildup. Consider it as a base for tea or in freeze-dried capsules, or just eat it as food. Maine herbalist Debbie Mercier combines tinctures of goldenrod and fresh spring nettles for fabulous, immediate allergy relief. For more on nettle, see page 33.

Quercetin and **bromelain** tend to work *better* than nettle for a broader range of people, and you'll often find the two supplements in combination, often with added nettle, vitamin C, or other allergy remedies. Quercetin (a bioflavonoid found in grapes, apples, and other substances, but typically extracted from corn for supplements) reduces histamine production, while bromelain (a protein-digesting enzyme from pineapple) helps break down histamine that's already been released. Start taking them a few weeks before allergy season to prevent or lessen symptoms; they take time to build up. Both compounds are generally safe and well tolerated. Quercetin has mild phytoestrogen effects, and bromelain thins the blood, which may be contraindicated with some drugs and conditions.

Aromatic, pungent, warming herbs can help loosen up and clear congestion and resolve infections. Consider fresh ginger (especially in honey-based syrups), onions lightly cooked with curry spices, fresh thyme, ample cayenne and hot peppers, and other pungent herbs. Harvest fresh evergreen needles of balsam fir, white pine, spruce, or hemlock tree to use as tea, tincture, or infused honey. Also consider any of the other aromatic herbs described on page 135.

DO YOU NETI?

For many, a neti pot is the number one answer for relief of sinus issues. If you have chronic nasal congestion, allergies, sinusitis, or sinus infections, consider using a neti pot or other nasal irrigation system regularly. Also consider it for episodes of congestion from colds and flu. Flushing your sinuses with warm salt water (¼ teaspoon of noniodized sea salt per cup of water) helps clear out bacteria and fungi (both of which tend to take hold when you're chronically congested) as well as pollen and dust, relieve mucus congestion, tone the mucosal lining, and make it easier to breathe. (If you're fighting an active infection, you can use herbal tea in place of the water, or add a squirt of tincture, in either case using antimicrobial herbs like goldenseal, yerba mansa, or yarrow. Still add about ¼ teaspoon salt per cup.) After using the neti pot, gently blow your nose using both nostrils to eliminate any remaining salt water and mucus; avoid forceful blowing. To avoid *introducing* microbes from your water supply (of particular concern in warm climates), boil the water in advance or use distilled bottled water. Thoroughly wash and dry equipment between uses. Follow the directions on the box.

Soothe Irritation *and* Spasms

Many of the same herbs we use to soothe and heal tissue in the throat and digestive tract are equally valuable for the whole respiratory system. These include herbs that slime/coat, soothe, and heal, as well as other herbs that directly relieve spasms.

Demulcent and Vulnerary Herbs

These herbs are generally slimy (demulcent) or wound healing (vulnerary) by nature, and they make a lovely supportive base for other herbs in teas and syrups. In the respiratory tract, they counteract dryness, irritation, heat, and inflammation while supporting the formation of healthy respiratory tissue and healthy levels of mucus.

- **Classic "slimers."** These include marshmallow root, almost any malva family leaf or flower (*Althaea* and *Malva* species), and slippery elm bark; all provide a soothing mucilage that coats, protects, soothes, and heals the mucosal tissues. They are best taken as tea.
- **Licorice root.** Licorice root is a demulcent with added immune-supportive and expectorant properties, and it lends a pleasant flavor to blends; however, it can aggravate blood pressure and kidney issues in some sensitive people.
- **Plantain.** Plantain leaf has anti-inflammatory, demulcent, and vulnerary properties that soften and support other herbs in a formula (taking the edge off warming herbs that stimulate better function by being mildly irritating, like oregano and elecampane).

For more on these herbs and other demulcents, see pages 77 and 220.

Antispasmodic Herbs

Antispasmodic herbs and remedies soothe in a different way, by relieving spasms and calming both the respiratory and nervous systems. Consider them for chest tightness, a spastic cough reflex, and general irritation in the bronchi. Some good ones to consider include the following:

- **Wild cherry bark.** Wild cherry bark specifically quells dry, irritated, hacking coughs and soothes lungs irritated by things like wood smoke. Think: tight, dry, spasm; overstimulation; anxiety. Cherry bark works well as a simple (on its own) or in blends for coughs and various respiratory issues. Compounds in the bark relax respiratory spasms while also calming the nerves. It blends very nicely — both in taste and action — with honey. Cherry bark should be dried before being made into a remedy and is best if you don't overheat it. If you make a tea, steep it in not-quite-boiling water rather than decocting it to retain the most strength. I prefer a tincture of the dried bark, sometimes combined 50/50 with honey. Cherry bark infuses nicely in honey (using the raw method; see page 309).
- **Horehound.** Horehound, mentioned previously (page 129), soothes wet coughs by making them more productive.
- **Honey.** Honey works well for any kind of cough; it even outperforms over-the-counter cough suppressants. Try slowly licking a spoonful of crystallized or creamed honey for immediate relief, or add it to teas and use it as a syrup base.
- **Aromatics.** Aromatic herbs — particularly peppermint and its primary constituent menthol, as well as evergreens like pine and balsam — relieve spasms while opening the lungs and expectorating mucus. Consider them as cough drops, syrups, steams, or infused honeys or as a synergist in tea and tincture blends.

Rebuild *and* Repair

We tend to think of damaged lung tissue — for example, in cases of COPD, emphysema, and silicosis — as irreparable. While it's *not easy* to undo damage, targeted herbs and mushrooms can often move things in the right direction. We're constantly learning more about how the human body works and discovering that, when given the nudge, the body has an amazing capacity for regeneration. Most of our respiratory remedies strengthen and support not only the respiratory system but also immune function. With this sort of support, the body has the tools it needs to live with — and sometimes even rebuild or repair — damaged lung tissue. Depending on the level of damage, it could take months or even years to see improvements. While nothing is guaranteed, why not try some potential remedies?

The following remedies are all excellent respiratory tonics with strong immune support — and the *potential* to help the body rebuild and repair damaged lung tissue.

- **Reishi and cordyceps.** All of our medicinal mushrooms have immune-supportive benefits, but reishi and cordyceps particularly strengthen respiratory function and structure. When used regularly, they make you less susceptible to repeat infections like bronchitis and pneumonia, boost oxygen utilization, decrease fatigue, improve red blood cells, and modulate the immune response. **Chaga** also seems to aid respiratory health. Some relief may be noted within a few days, but the effects build over a few weeks or months. They are generally quite safe, though cordyceps is a tad zippy. (For more on medicinal mushrooms, see page 115.)
- **Respiratory and immune adaptogens.** Several *Aralia* species, like spikenard, along with astragalus and schizandra (as well as the aforementioned reishi), have a reputation as adaptogenic herbs with an affinity for strengthening the lungs while lessening fatigue. They work well with mushrooms and in more complex herbal formulas.
- **Lung tonics and antihistamines.** Additional herbs that are also noteworthy for their exceptional ability to improve a range of respiratory conditions include mullein, yerba santa, and horehound, all described earlier in this chapter.

Fight Infection

Many of the respiratory herbs have some level of antimicrobial effect, either directly discouraging germs or enhancing the body's immune response. Aromatic, balsam-y, and pungent herbs can be particularly helpful; think: the evergreens, as much raw garlic as you can stand, and biting aromatic mint-family herbs like oregano, bee balm, hyssop, and thyme. Ample amounts from a diversity of plants are usually necessary in acute infections. We tend to excrete the aromatics of these herbs through our lungs — this is partly how they work to disinfect them — so don't be surprised if your breath smells like a pungent pizza for a few days. (If you're taking high doses or an essential oil product, you may even start to smell it on your skin.) Tea, tincture, food, soup, capsule — take them however you can!

Antimicrobial herbs target the microbes directly, but don't forget to support the immune system itself. In long-standing weak or autoimmune situations, consider immune-tonic herbs like astragalus (page 115) and medicinal mushrooms (page 115). For more acute situations (meaning sudden-onset or short-term infections), consider herbs like elderberry (an antiviral) and echinacea (to boost white blood cell activity and lymph movement). Lesser-known andrographis and umcka have performed very well in studies for acute respiratory infections like the common cold and bronchitis. Regional lung herbs like osha and balsam root have the ability to warm and to increase circulation, open the lungs, and fight infection . . . but they are slow-growing wild roots that only exist in limited ranges, so they can be difficult to find commercially or raise ethical concerns with overharvesting.

Rest, rest, rest is incredibly important in acute phases of chronic issues as well as during the *whole* recuperation from illness.

Decrease Inflammation

Inflammation is a key component of many types of lung issues, particularly those that are chronic. Asthma sufferers notoriously suffer from food sensitivities and allergies, often undiagnosed, with gluten/wheat and dairy leading the pack. Eliminate these foods while opting for a whole-foods diet rich in bioflavonoids and anti-inflammatory compounds: a rainbow of vegetables, dark leafy greens, berries, wild foods, herbs, spices and plants of all types as well as pastured or wild animal products in moderation. Vitamin D also decreases inflammation and improves immune function, especially if there is a deficiency. Omega-3 fatty acids from fish oil supplements or food sources decrease inflammation while helping cells throughout the body repair and function better. Goldenrod, a bioflavonoid-rich herb, decreases the histamine response, thins mucus, and drains congestion, especially when combined with other lung herbs. Petadolex, a special extract of butterbur, decreases inflammation and is especially helpful for allergies, migraines, and sinusitis.

Respiratory Irritants

When dealing with respiratory issues — especially conditions like asthma, bronchitis, COPD, and emphysema — do whatever you can to limit exposure to respiratory irritants. This includes avoiding smoking (cigarettes or otherwise), secondhand smoke, and indoor air with a lot of particles from woodstoves. Also be aware of mold, dust, animal dander, chemicals (including new paint, carpets, furniture, cars, and workplaces that use solvents, including salon products), pesticides and herbicides (such as lawns, ball fields, playgrounds, places near farms), and smog (especially on hot, humid days). Ensure good ventilation indoors and use a HEPA filter if necessary.

LUNGS AND EMOTIONS

EMOTIONAL TRAUMA OFTEN TRIGGERS chronic lung issues, and the inability to breathe immediately sets off panic alarms. Incorporating therapy, mindfulness, and other forms of mind-body balance can be incredibly helpful to your respiratory response. Consider adaptogenic and calming herbs as supportive players in your lung formula: holy basil, codonopsis, ashwagandha, astragalus, schizandra, reishi, roses, and hawthorn. More overt sedatives like passionflower and low-dose pulsatilla can be helpful in formulas where stress or anxiety worsen your symptoms. Some lung herbs, like wild cherry bark, also sedate the nerves. Also consider deep breathing exercises, which have a profound ability to reset your nervous system into a calmer "rest and repair" state (see page 28 for one such example, the 4-7-8 breathing exercise).

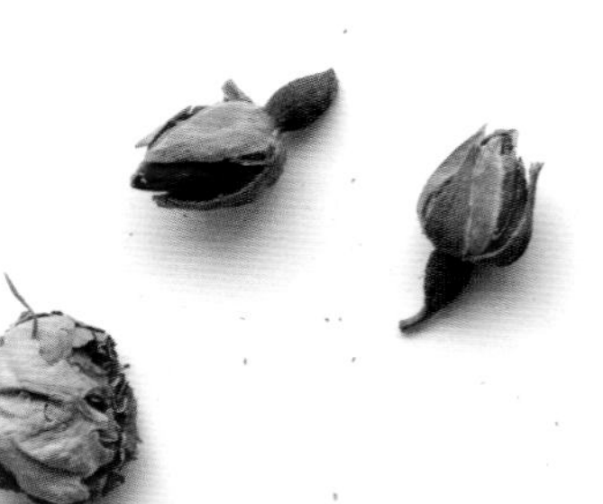

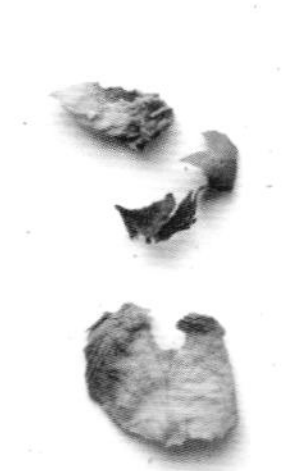

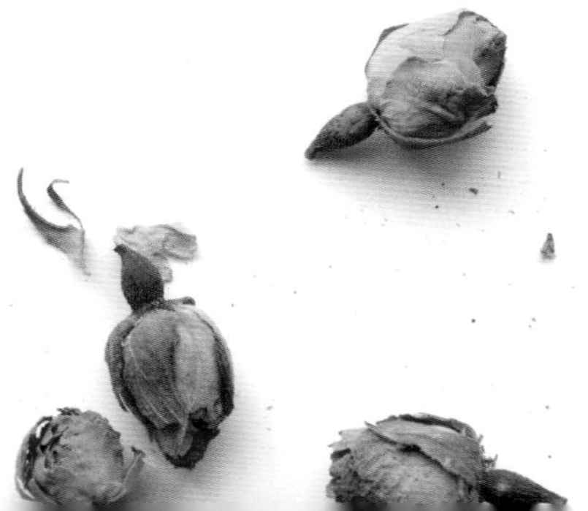

PROTOCOL POINTS

Asthma

In asthma, the airways become inflamed and constricted, making it difficult or impossible to breathe. There may also be an autoimmune connection, and asthma tends to coincide with dermatitis, eczema, allergies, sinus issues, and headaches or migraines. Although asthma is a serious respiratory condition that may require medical care or a practitioner's oversight, herbs can often reduce the severity of chronic symptoms, address the root of imbalance, and decrease the frequency of asthma attacks. Children who are not exposed to a variety of normal germs and everyday infections in their youth appear to have a greater risk of developing asthma. Overexposure to respiratory irritants is another underlying factor.

Diet: Identify and eliminate food sensitivities and allergies (such as dairy or gluten), and eat a balanced whole-foods diet, rich in anti-inflammatory foods, and limited in sugar and other pro-inflammatory foods. Consider eating more omega-3 fatty acids (try fatty fish and flaxseed oil) and adding fermented foods (like kimchi) to your routine.

Lifestyle: Limit exposure to respiratory irritants. Support mind-body-lung balance through mindfulness, stress reduction, and breathing exercises.

Herbs: Herbs for asthma vary quite a bit depending on the individual scenario, and *many* herbs can lend a hand. Consider nettle, astragalus, reishi, cordyceps, chaga, and other medicinal mushrooms for support. Lung tonics that open airways (e.g., mullein, yerba santa, elecampane, thyme) blend well with soothing herbs (e.g., marshmallow, plantain, horehound, cherry bark) for both acute and chronic formulas. If appropriate, incorporate calming herbs into your formula. Keep your inhaler nearby for emergencies, but hopefully they will be fewer and farther between.

Seasonal Allergies

Although some remedies can bring immediate allergy relief, your best bet is to start your routine a few weeks prior to your anticipated allergy season. Addressing food reactions and using a neti pot can produce amazing results for chronic sufferers.

Diet: Identify and eliminate sources of food sensitivities and allergies (such as dairy or gluten), and eat a balanced whole-foods diet limited in sugar and other less healthy foods.

Lifestyle: Get plenty of rest, and consider daily use of a neti pot or other nasal irrigation system. Limit exposure to respiratory irritants.

Herbs: Preventively, try nettle, quercetin, or bromelain. In cases of mucus stagnation and overproduction, consider horehound, goldenrod, nettle, and/or bee balm in a blend. Diffuse aromatic herbs into the air. Modulate your immune system function and strengthen your respiratory system with medicinal mushrooms or astragalus.

AROMATIC HERBS

AROMATIC HERBS LIKE PEPPERMINT, eucalyptus, evergreens (spruce, hemlock, fir, pine), oregano, rosemary, thyme, and bee balm do quite nicely as an herbal steam (using dried plants or essential oils), slowly sipped as tea, infused in honey, taken as a cough drop (think: Ricola), or diffused in the air — they simultaneously open the lungs, thin and loosen phlegm, relieve spasms, and fight germs. They make fabulous synergists for respiratory blends, too.

AT A GLANCE

Herbs for the Respiratory System and Sinuses

General Congestion

Astringent Antimicrobials

- Yerba mansa
- Bitter berberines (goldenseal,* coptis/goldthread, Oregon grape root, barberry)

Mucus Dryers

- Antihistamines (quercetin, nettle leaf, ragweed,* goldenrod, etc.)
- Bitter berberines (goldenseal,* coptis/goldthread, Oregon grape root, barberry)
- Eyebright
- Hyssop
- Sage
- Thyme

Mucus Drainers

- Horehound
- Goldenrod
- Expectorants (grindelia, osha, balsam root, evergreens, etc.)
- Sinus drainage herbs (horseradish, cayenne, ginger, onion, etc.)

Lungs

Lung Soothers

- Marshmallow
- Slippery elm
- Comfrey*
- Plantain leaf
- Mullein leaf
- Fenugreek
- Coltsfoot*

Lung Strengtheners and Tonics

- Cordyceps
- Reishi
- Chaga
- Aralia
- Andrographis
- Umcka
- Astragalus
- Ashwagandha

Lung Openers

- Elecampane
- Mullein leaf
- Yerba santa
- Horehound
- Thyme
- Pleurisy root
- Lobelia*
- Ephedra*

Aromatic Antimicrobials

- Bee balm
- Oregano
- Thyme
- Hyssop
- Evergreens (balsam fir, white pine, hemlock tree)
- Balsam root
- Elecampane
- Ginger
- Alliums (garlic, onion)
- Myrrh

Expectorants

- Grindelia
- Osha
- Balsam root
- Evergreens (balsam fir, white pine, hemlock tree)
- Ginger
- Pleurisy root
- Horehound

Antitussives

- Honey
- Horehound (wet cough)
- Cherry bark (dry cough)
- False Solomon's seal
- Aromatic antimicrobials (bee balm, oregano, thyme, hyssop, evergreens, etc.)

Sinuses

Antihistamines

- Quercetin
- Nettle leaf
- Ragweed*
- Goldenrod
- Asters
- Eyebright
- Butterbur (PA-free supplement)
- Ephedra*

Sinus Drainers

- Horseradish
- Cayenne
- Ginger
- Onion
- Turmeric and other curry spices
- Goldenrod
- Bee balm
- Nettle
- Horehound

Antimicrobials

- Bitter berberines (goldenseal,* coptis/goldthread, Oregon grape root, barberry), internally or in a nasal wash
- Bee balm
- Oregano
- Alder bark and twig (dry)
- Usnea lichen

Throat

Throat Soothers

- Licorice
- Slippery elm
- Marshmallow
- Hibiscus
- Honey
- Sage
- Salt (nasal rinse/neti)
- Comfrey*
- Ginger

Antimicrobials

- Bitter berberines (goldenseal,* coptis/goldthread, Oregon grape root, barberry)
- Aromatic antimicrobials (bee balm, oregano, thyme, hyssop, evergreens, etc.)
- Yerba mansa
- Sage (garden, white)
- Salt (gargle)
- Ginger
- Propolis
- Echinacea
- Spilanthes

Throat Numbing

- Echinacea
- Kava
- Cayenne
- Salt (gargle)
- Bitter berberines (goldenseal,* coptis/goldthread, Oregon grape root, barberry)

Ears

Pain Relievers and Infection Fighters

- St. John's wort oil (as ear drops)
- Mullein flower oil (as ear drops)
- Garlic oil (as ear drops)
- Calendula oil (as ear drops)
- Xylitol (internally)

**Be particularly aware of cautions and/or ecological status before using plants marked with an asterisk.*

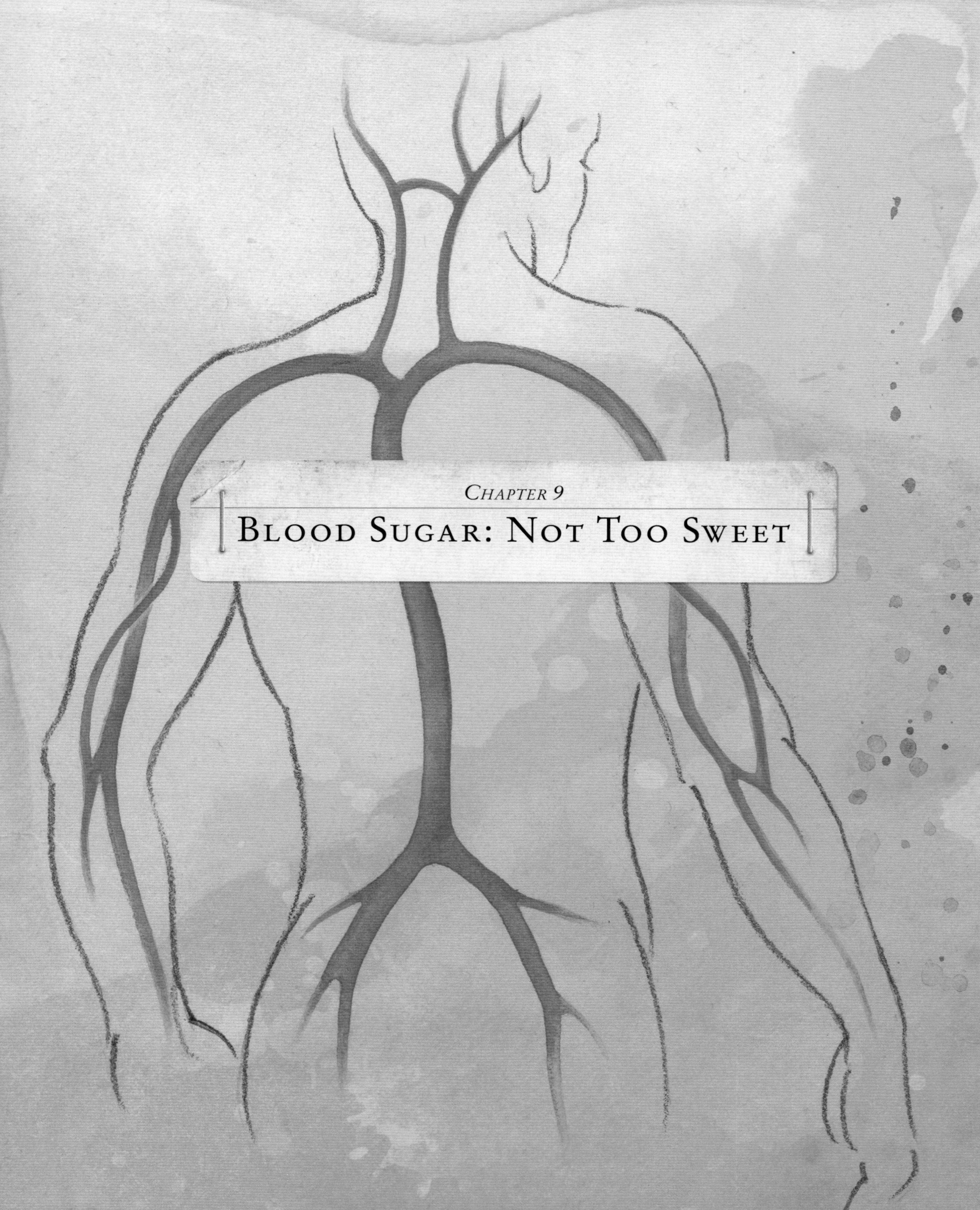

Chapter 9

Blood Sugar: Not Too Sweet

BLOOD SUGAR BALANCE has a profound effect on your overall health — including your cardiovascular system, mood, brain function, immune health, body weight, cancer risk, and, of course, diabetes risk. The most significant forces that influence blood sugar levels are what you eat and how you move. In ancient times, you wouldn't have had to pay much attention to such trivialities because humans generally ate smaller portions of whole foods and moved their bodies *constantly* in order to work and survive. Technological advancements have made life easier and food tastier — to the detriment of our health, unfortunately. While certain people are more susceptible to the ill effects of sugar excess (and movement deficiency), the modern lifestyle isn't good for *any* of us.

Sugar *in the* Body

Sugar isn't just the stuff of "sugar blues," roller-coaster moods, and deadly diseases. It's also *essential* for your body's proper functioning. Your body relies on the simplest forms of sugar to fuel almost every aspect of its function. Your brain prefers glucose over any other energy source, and when you exercise, you burn a lot of — you guessed it! — sugar.

Sugar comes in many forms. When you eat sweets and carbohydrate-rich foods, your digestive system breaks them down into simple forms, including glucose, fructose, and lactose. As you absorb these sugars through your intestines, they enter your bloodstream.

Sugar needs to get inside your cells for your body to be able to use it. And in order for that to happen, you need insulin.

The Importance of Insulin

Your pancreas (the same organ that makes digestive enzymes) has specialized cells, called beta cells, that produce insulin, a hormone that "unlocks" the doors of cells to let sugar in. When sugar levels rise, the beta cells flood your bloodstream with insulin, triggering cells to take in the sugar, which they use as fuel. However, the process doesn't always work the way it should.

Most of us consume far more sugar than we actually need, and after a while your cells become desensitized to insulin. Eventually your cells get sick of it, block the door, and say, "Forget about it, I'm not letting you in! I've seen too much of you lately, and I don't need any more sugar." At first your body panics and produces *more* insulin to bang down the doors of the cells. And because it's more insulin than you actually *need* for the amount of sugar at hand, you might notice a sharp blood sugar crash once the sugar does get into the cells — fuzzy brain, fatigue, and sugar cravings.

At this stage, blood sugar tests might not pick up any major issues. At a quick glance, you're still "normal." But if you were tested shortly after eating, your insulin levels would be higher than they should be. This all-too-common scenario is generally called insulin resistance, though it also goes by other names including metabolic syndrome, prediabetes, and syndrome X.

As the condition progresses and insulin resistance mounts, blood sugar levels will become notably higher than they should be, at which point you have officially developed type 2 diabetes. In later stages of type 2 diabetes, the beta cells often conk out and slow down or stop producing insulin altogether.

The Woes of Sugar Excess

Now your bloodstream is flooded with sugar, and your liver — the great metabolizer and detoxifier — must figure out what to do with it all. Some of it is packaged into triglycerides and very low density lipoproteins (a.k.a. *very* bad cholesterol), some is turned into stored sugar (glycogen) and placed in fat cells, and some of it gets excreted in the urine (the term "diabetes mellitus" translates as "honey urine," arising from early doctors noticing that bees were attracted to the sweet urine). So from this, we tend to see high cholesterol, abdominal weight gain (a major indicator), and increased risk of urinary tract infections. These symptoms often begin to develop during the early stages of insulin resistance.

Insulin wobbles and intense sugar highs and lows are incredibly damaging to your whole body. They go hand in hand with inflammation, obesity, high levels of cortisol (a hormone involved with stress and blood sugar metabolism) and oxidative stress, increased heart disease and cancer risk, and cranky mood. Ironically, they also *increase* your cravings for sugar and junk food. This all puts extra demands on your blood vessels, especially the capillaries (tiny blood vessels), as well as nerves, and over time these systems break down, resulting in poor eye health, poor circulation, neuropathy, increased risk of Alzheimer's and dementia, and poor wound healing. Insulin creates whole-body inflammation, including in the blood vessel lining. Your body tries to patch inflamed spots with cholesterol Band-Aids, which turn into plaque and ultimately harden the arteries and dramatically increase your risk of a life-threatening cardiovascular event.

Addressing the Epidemic

Imbalances of blood sugar, insulin, and metabolism set you on a dangerous road to travel. It becomes impossible for your body to function optimally, and your risk of premature death increases dramatically. Unfortunately, most of America has already begun the journey. According to the American Diabetes Association, an estimated 50 percent of adults and 75 percent of seniors have diabetes or prediabetes. The incidence in children has risen alarmingly as well. The earlier you can catch and address blood sugar issues, the better off you'll be. Even if you and your family don't experience overt blood sugar issues, integrating diet, lifestyle, and tonic sugar-balancing herbs can help keep you healthy. And if you or a loved one have already developed type 2 diabetes, take comfort in knowing that it's *always possible* to work your way back to better health and vitality.

FACTORS THAT INCREASE YOUR RISK OF DIABETES

Diet

- Excessive food
- Excessive fats (especially fried foods and trans fats)
- Excessive sugar/carbohydrates
- Excessive refined food
- Lack of fiber
- Lack of nutrients, especially chromium, omega-3s, magnesium, vitamin C, vitamin D
- Lack of bitter foods
- Food reactions (especially to dairy or gluten), which may trigger an autoimmune response and contribute to diabetes

Lifestyle

- Not enough movement/exercise
- Overexposure to pesticides
- Overexposure to plastics (especially BPA)
- Overexposure to environmental toxins and electromagnetic frequencies
- Viral exposure, which can trigger an immune response that contributes to diabetes

Other

- Obesity (your risk doubles for every 20 percent increase in body weight over "normal")
- Genetics
- Insufficient beneficial bacteria/probiotics
- Parents ate excessive junk food
- History of gestational diabetes
- History of autoimmune disease

Movement Matters

Exercise may be the least sexy answer to blood sugar balance, but it may exceed any other "remedy" in effectiveness. It's why Asians can eat all that white rice, the French can munch on their baguettes, and Italians can pack in the pasta and still remain trim and healthy. They move! Constantly! These cultures thrive on farming and manual labor and biking or walking everywhere they need to go. Forget a few hours of exercise — they often perform physically demanding tasks 20 hours or more a week. Here in the United States, on the other hand, we tend to sit most of the day, walking only to and from the car.

Regular cardiovascular exercise — walking, hiking, biking, gardening, dancing, paddling, et cetera — helps your body burn through sugar. Strength-training, weight-bearing exercise like lifting weights, boxes, or babies shifts your body to burn more fuel (sugar) at a resting state and also improves the cell's sensitivity to insulin. Staying sedentary for as little as half a day (!!) will begin to shift your blood sugar metabolism to your detriment. Do whatever you can to integrate more movement into your day. Hit the gym, take up a new hobby like kayaking, swing by a fitness class, bike to work, or take a walk during your lunch break.

Glycemic Index *and* Glycemic Load

The sugar and carbohydrates from your food hit your bloodstream at different speeds depending on, primarily, five factors:

1. How easily carbohydrates in a food break down into sugar in the bloodstream

2. How that food is broken down or prepared (boiled versus fried potato)

These two factors together make up the food's "glycemic index."

3. How many carbohydrates (sugar) are actually in the food

All of the above factors are incorporated into the "glycemic load" the body will have to shoulder.

4. How the sugar is packaged up in that particular food (with fiber, fat, protein, et cetera)

5. How the meal itself is balanced with other ingredients

AN IMMUNE CONNECTION

AT FIRST GLANCE, immune function and diabetes seem totally unrelated. However, type 1 diabetes is usually caused by autoimmune disease. The primary reason that someone with type 1 diabetes can't produce insulin is because the body has attacked the beta cells that produce insulin. Although they are less of a factor in type 2 diabetes, immune health and autoimmune disease may also play a role. The underlying reasons for the autoimmune response are poorly understood, but viral exposure, a cross-reaction to dairy, history of autoimmune disease, and poor overall health seem to be factors.

Scientists have tested various foods to give you a ballpark number that indicates foods that break down quickly (high glycemic) or slowly (low glycemic). Glycemic effect isn't the be-all and end-all for a healthy diet — it doesn't take into account *other* nutrients in the food. An 8-ounce glass of heavy cream is lower on the glycemic index than an 8-ounce glass of milk, but it definitely isn't healthier for you. However, glycemic index is a good piece of the puzzle of creating a healthy diet, and it's of particular importance for people with insulin resistance, diabetes, and an unhealthy diet and lifestyle. Chowing down on a lot of high-carbohydrate, high-glycemic foods sets you up for the blood sugar imbalances that we discussed on page 139. This puts you at greater risk for insulin resistance and diabetes (especially type 2), as well as related conditions, including high cholesterol, hardening of the arteries, obesity (especially abdominal weight gain), and an increased risk of cancer, heart attack, stroke, and Alzheimer's disease.

Balancing Your Plate

While noting a food's glycemic ranking is helpful, keep in mind that it doesn't take into account how the food combines with other ingredients in the meal. Be sure to balance your plate with some protein, some good carbs, plenty of produce, and a little bit of healthy fat — and keep your portions reasonable. For more on this topic, see page 21.

GLYCEMIC RANKINGS

You can find much more specific glycemic lists in books; the website of the University of Sydney (www.glycemicindex.com) offers a searchable database. Most of these rank foods from zero to 100; the higher the number, the greater the blood sugar effects. Although the minutiae of the glycemic index and load can be mind-boggling, emphasizing low-glycemic foods in your diet will make a major difference.

Low Glycemic

- High-protein or high-fat foods that are low in carbs
- Meat, poultry, fish, shellfish, and eggs (lean protein preferred)
- Fats, oils, cream, butter, avocado, coconut
- Soy, nuts, and seeds
- Most nonstarchy vegetables, especially leafy greens
- Nonsweet citrus
- Berries
- Herbs, spices, plain tea, black coffee, stevia

Medium Glycemic

- Foods with a high fiber content (like whole foods), which slows down the sugar breakdown
- Starchy vegetables like carrots, winter squash, sweet potatoes
- Whole grains (intact grains preferred over flour)
- Most beans and legumes
- Full-fat dairy
- Most fruit

High Glycemic

- Sugar, honey, maple syrup, et cetera
- Soda, juice, other sweet or sweetened drinks
- White flour (and to a lesser extent whole-grain flour)
- White starches like potatoes, processed corn, rice
- Puffed grains
- Nonfat dairy
- Most processed food, baked goods, candy, crackers, et cetera
- Super-sweet tropical fruits like bananas and dates

(Note: Artificial sweeteners trick the body into releasing sugar into the bloodstream, aggravate healthy sugar/insulin metabolism, and are not recommended, ever.)

A Tale *of* Two Diets

You can't ignore it: no matter what herbs or drugs you take, what and how you eat make the biggest difference in your disease risk, recovery, and overall health.

When it comes to blood sugar management, you'll find two dueling diet philosophies. Though they differ significantly, both have their merits, and you can combine the best aspects of each to find a plan that suits your individual constitution and taste buds. The best diet for *you* will be one that makes you feel better while keeping blood sugar in check *and* that you can maintain long term without feeling miserable and falling off the wagon.

High-Fiber, High-Carbohydrate (HFC) Diet

The name of this diet might raise your eyebrows. *High* carbohydrates? But the HFC diet isn't so much a high-carb approach as it is one that focuses on plant foods with carbs coming from whole grains (ideally intact, not flour), beans, vegetables, nuts, seeds, and some fruit. Essentially, it's a mostly vegan, whole-foods diet. Studies show that 60 percent of type 2 diabetics can discontinue medication once they follow the HFC diet, and the remaining 40 percent can reduce their medication doses. Studies also suggest that the HFC diet outperforms the diet recommended by the American Diabetes Association. At the forefront of this type of diet is Dr. Dean Ornish, who proved that it is possible to not only *slow* but also actually *reverse* heart disease using diet, exercise, and mindfulness (yoga, meditation). The diet features very little fat and animal products — mainly focusing on fish, nuts, and olive oil — which can be a challenge for some. Similar diets include Dr. Andrew Weil's anti-inflammatory diet, the Mediterranean diet, and the Okinawan diet. The star of all these diets is plants: rich in nutrients, rich in antioxidants, but most of all rich in *fiber*. Think of complex carbohydrates in the form of real, whole foods as "slow-burn carbs." Fiber slows down the release of the carbohydrates in the bloodstream like a time-release capsule and makes the body work harder to get all those nutrients and sugars out. Yet most Americans eat only half the fiber they need.

Low-Carb Diet

Thank Dr. Robert Atkins for helping us take a closer look at sugars and simple carbs and the role they play in disease and weight gain. His diet starts by completely eliminating sweets and classic carbs in favor of protein and fat, which forces your body into ketosis (because of the lack of sugar, your body uses fat and protein as fuel). This helps flip a switch that gets you out of fat-storage mode, insulin-resistance patterns, and the carb-craving cycle. People on a low-carb, high-protein diet tend to lose weight even if they're eating more calories. Fat- and protein-rich foods help you feel more satisfied for a longer period of time and make your taste buds happy. Usually, good-quality carbs are gradually added back in modest amounts.

Unfortunately, the low-carb diet can have pitfalls and doesn't have as much evidence for long-term vitality as HFC. First off, many people use a low-carb diet as an excuse to live on steak, cheese, and bacon — hardly healthy foods to binge on. Lean meats and plant protein accompanied by plenty of vegetables would be better, and newer low-carb diets (South Beach, Paleo, books by Dr. Mark Hyman) make this switch. Consider keeping the carb count to 6 to 24 grams (deduct any fiber grams) per meal. Low-carb diets — especially the less healthy versions — can put a tremendous amount of stress on your liver and gallbladder (which must deal with the dietary fats) and kidneys (which process the nitrogen from all that protein). Watch out for low-carb diets that rely on processed fake foods like margarine (full of trans fats) and artificial sweeteners — that junk's not really good for anyone. Steer clear, and stick to real ingredients.

Top Remedies *to* Balance Blood Sugar

The remedies we'll discuss here are generally considered to be hypoglycemics: they lower blood sugar, which is generally good but may cause hypoglycemia (too low blood sugar), which can be dangerous or even deadly. *Slowly* introduce these hypoglycemic remedies into your routine to gauge your body's response. Take them *with meals*, not on an empty stomach (when your blood sugar is already likely to be low). If you have diabetes, take medications, or are pregnant, work with your health-care practitioner to determine how best to incorporate these herbs into your routine.

▸ Chromium

Key Properties: You'll find this trace mineral in a wide range of whole foods; it's essential for the proper metabolism of glucose. Unfortunately, eating a processed diet can give you a double-whammy chromium deficiency: not only are you not getting any chromium from the food you eat, but eating excessive carbs causes your body to excrete chromium. If you suspect chromium deficiency or your doctor has diagnosed it with lab tests, taking a chromium supplement or adding chromium-rich foods (brewer's yeast, broccoli, whole foods) into your diet may improve glucose tolerance and insulin sensitivity and reduce blood sugar.

Additional Benefits: Some studies suggest that chromium also improves triglyceride and cholesterol levels, normalizes metabolism, and contributes to weight loss.

Preparation: Try a commercial supplement or brewer's yeast (*not* nutritional yeast), 200 to 400 mcg of chromium daily, taken with food. Or switch to a whole-foods diet. Eating more foods rich in vitamin C improves chromium absorption.

Cautions and Considerations: If you're not deficient in chromium, supplementing with it probably won't help. Chromium may worsen hypoglycemia. Some medications (e.g., antacids, proton pump inhibitors) reduce chromium absorption. Other medications can have a synergistic effect when taken with chromium.

WHAT IS A HYPOGLYCEMIC HERB?

A hypoglycemic herb, remedy, or food is one that decreases blood sugar levels, ideally bringing high blood sugar into a healthy range. Different remedies work in various ways: improving cells' insulin sensitivity, improving insulin output, decreasing the glycemic effect of food, improving the function of the beta cells that make insulin, altering the way your body absorbs, stores, and releases sugar, et cetera.

General Uses: These remedies are generally taken with meals to help prevent blood sugar spikes and crashes, thus keeping blood sugar in an overall healthier range. This can benefit both types of diabetes, insulin resistance, obesity, and high cholesterol in particular. Most remedies also offer antioxidant and anti-inflammatory properties, which indirectly improve blood sugar levels while also lessening the collateral damage of chronic hyperglycemia (high blood sugar).

Examples: Blueberry and bilberry leaf and fruit, cinnamon, gymnema, chromium and brewer's yeast, fenugreek (large doses), soluble fiber (including glucomannan, apple and citrus pectin, oat fiber, mushrooms, beans, pears), prickly pear pads (nopales), mulberry leaf, tea, coffee, yerba maté, bitters (artichoke, bitter melon), vinegar, holy basil, ginseng, garlic, onions

Blood Sugar Support

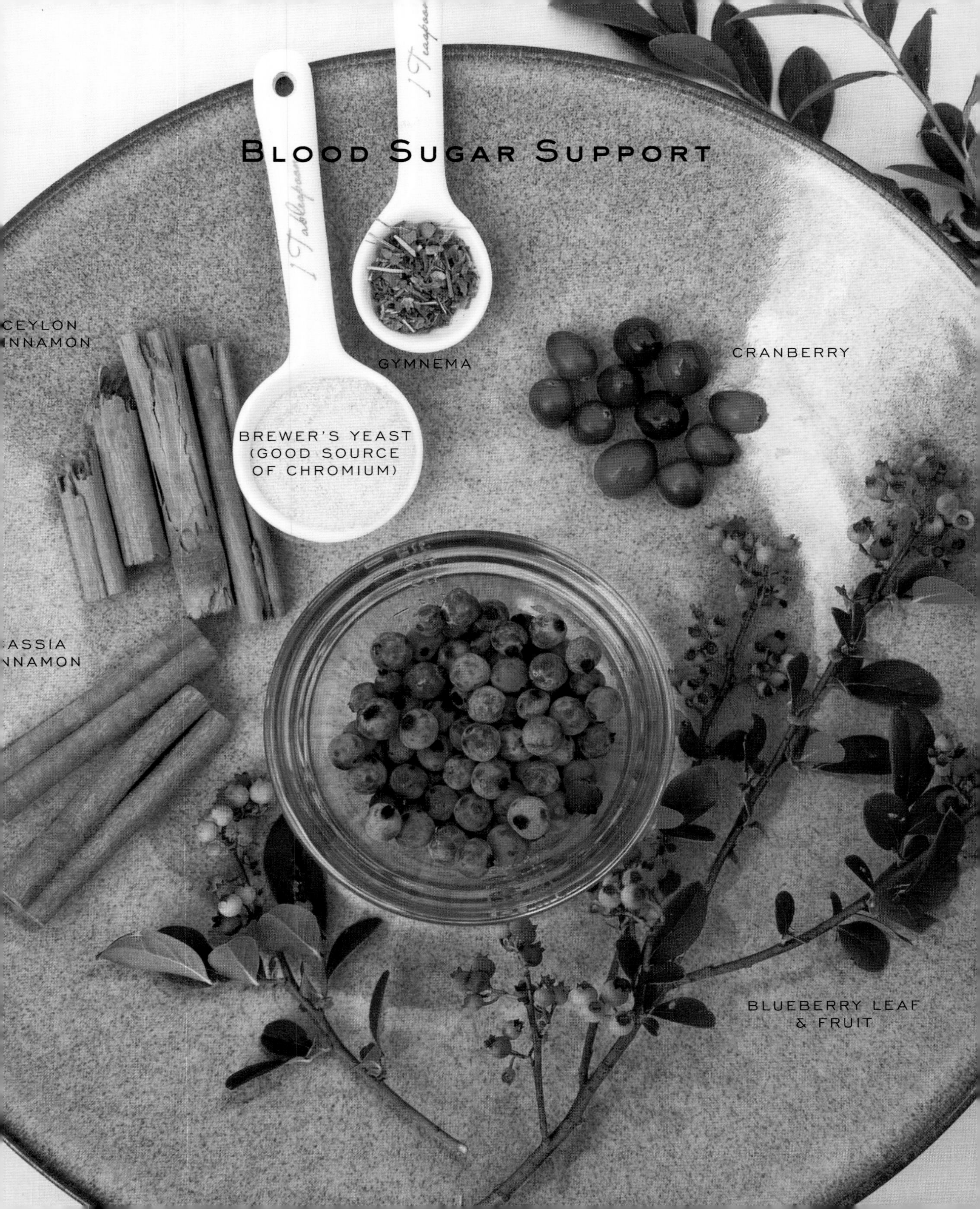

▸ Blueberry and Bilberry

Vaccinium spp.

Availability: G+ W+ C+

Key Properties: This is a whole-package plant for diabetes — it's amazing how many ways both the berries and the leaves balance blood sugar and reduce the side effects of diabetes. For the most specific hypoglycemic effect, drink the leaf tea. Folk herbalists have long used blueberry leaf tea to lower blood sugar and fight urinary tract infections (compared to its relatives, it's a tad stronger than blueberry and cranberry fruits and gentler than uva ursi leaves). New preliminary studies on *Vaccinium* spp. leaves support their ability to lower cholesterol and blood sugar, protect your body from sugar-related damage, and possibly even act like insulin and help regenerate damaged beta cells. They can be used, carefully, in cases of type 1 and type 2 diabetes as well as insulin resistance.

Additional Benefits: The low-glycemic berries can be enjoyed fresh, frozen, juiced, or as a supplement on a daily basis. Though they lower and modulate blood sugar (a little), they particularly excel at supporting the *other* areas of the body negatively affected by diabetes and blood sugar imbalance. They're loaded with antioxidants and deep blue-purple pigments that strengthen capillaries and blood vessels, discourage urinary tract infections, enhance circulation, improve beta cell proliferation, fight oxidative damage, and improve eye health, cardiovascular well-being, and brain function. Most research revolves around the European bilberry (*V. myrtillus*); however, our local blueberries offer similar benefits.

Preparation: Eat the berries (wild and frozen are most potent) or make tea with the leaves from wild or minimally cultivated plants. Dried leaves can be harder to find in commerce. Standard herb doses (see page 298) apply for the leaf tea; start on the low side to gauge your personal response. Eat one or two large bags of frozen blueberries weekly, or ½ cup daily.

Cautions and Considerations: The berries are incredibly safe and can be enjoyed as food. The leaves generally are safe; however, they contain tannins that may irritate the kidneys if used in high doses or long-term. Younger leaves boast fewer tannins; however, studies suggest that late-summer leaves may have a more profound anti-diabetes effect. When harvesting leaves, nibble a few first: leaves with a blueberry tang make better medicine, and the level of bitterness and astringency indicates tannin content.

Similar Herbs: The fruit of **cranberry**, a close relative, shares many of the same benefits.

A TOUCH OF BITTER

FOODS WITH BITTER OR SOUR FLAVORS improve your body's ability to deal with sugar and, surprisingly, help quell sugar cravings. Experiment with bitter greens, lettuce, arugula, dandelion, artichoke, endive, chicory, grapefruit, lemons, orange peel, and exotics like tamarind paste and bitter melon. Adding vinegar or pickled veggies to meals can also decrease the overall glycemic effect.

Blueberry-Vanilla Tea

Enjoy this tasty tea after meals or alongside a healthy dessert. If you don't have vanilla-infused rooibos, you can use plain rooibos plus one-quarter of a vanilla bean or a squirt of vanilla extract. It's also delicious iced, and it tastes mildly sweet even though it contains no sugar or honey.

- 1 teaspoon blueberry or bilberry leaf
- 1 teaspoon dried blueberries or bilberries
- 1 teaspoon vanilla-infused rooibos
- ½ teaspoon hibiscus
- Shake of powdered cinnamon
- Pinch of stevia

Combine the herbs. Pour 2 cups boiling water over the herbs and let steep, covered, for 15 minutes. Strain and enjoy.

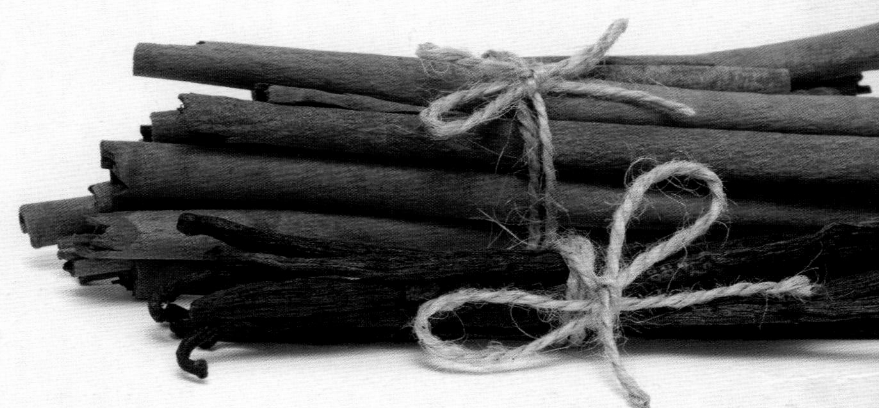

Sweet Cinnamon Tea, Two Ways

Easy and delicious, this tea could stand in for dessert. If your cinnamon doesn't taste sweet, it's probably too old or poor quality. The recipe takes time; let the cinnamon sticks steep or simmer while you're making and eating dinner.

- 2 sticks cinnamon

Infusion Method: Place the cinnamon sticks in a thermos, cover with 2 cups boiling water, and let steep, covered, for 1 hour or longer. Strain and enjoy.

Decoction Method: Place the cinnamon sticks and 2 cups water in a pot and simmer, covered, for approximately 20 minutes. Strain and enjoy.

▸ Cinnamon

Cinnamomum spp.

Availability: C+

Key Properties: Yet another hypoglycemic herb you already have in your kitchen! Cinnamon has been elevated to pop star status thanks to a surge of studies over the past 15 years that have focused on its ability to modestly lower blood sugar and improve insulin sensitivity. The results have been mostly good, though sometimes inconsistent.

Additional Benefits: Cinnamon may also help relieve diabetic neuropathy, promote weight loss, and lower triglyceride and cholesterol levels. The spice has classically been used as a treatment for digestion, diarrhea, and bleeding and as a potent antimicrobial, astringent, anti-inflammatory, and antioxidant herb. The sweet flavor can also stand in for sugar in some recipes.

Preparation: Most studies have used approximately 2 grams (½ teaspoon) of powdered cinnamon (*C. cassia*) per day, while a few preliminary studies used true or Ceylon cinnamon (*C. zeylanicum*). You can also take cinnamon as a tea, tincture, or capsule. Cinnamon gets gloppy in water and over time as a tincture. Use sticks or chips for tea and tinctures to avoid "cinnamon slime." When tincturing, add 10 percent glycerin to your alcohol, which delays the sludge effect. Standard herb doses apply (see page 298); for carbon dioxide extracts, follow label directions.

Cautions and Considerations: Cinnamon has a strong record of safety in clinical studies and thousands of years of traditional use; however, concerns have recently been raised regarding cassia cinnamon's levels of coumarin, a compound that can be liver toxic in excess. The real risk of toxicity from cinnamon seems low, but if you're concerned, you can opt for Ceylon cinnamon, which is very low in coumarins. The most likely issues you would have with cinnamon would be a little stomach upset or low blood sugar (especially if taken on an empty stomach) and constipation (it *is* a diarrhea remedy). Therapeutic doses of cinnamon are not appropriate in type 1 diabetes.

▸ Gymnema

Gymnema sylvestre

Availability: C

Key Properties: The traditional Ayurvedic name for this plant, *gurmar*, translates to "sugar destroyer," which indicates gymnema's history of use in India. (If you roll the herb around on your tongue, sip the tea, or take the tincture, your ability to taste sweet will be diminished for up to 3 hours. This *could* help you eat less sugar, but most people take gymnema in capsules to avoid the effect.) Gymnema research is preliminary but impressive. Compounds in the leaves appear to regenerate beta cells in the pancreas (this alone is amazing!), block glucose absorption in the intestines, encourage insulin production, and improve insulin uptake in the cells. It may even be beneficial in type 1 diabetes: one study found that taking just 400 mg of gymnema leaf allowed patients to reduce or eliminate their insulin medications. Another study used 800 mg of a standardized extract for type 1 and type 2 diabetics with good results.

Additional Benefits: Gymnema is primarily used as a hypoglycemic herb, but it also appears to reduce cholesterol levels and fight obesity, likely due to the blood-sugar-lowering effects.

Preparation: Most often taken as a capsule (400 to 800 mg of a standardized extract) or in standard herb doses (see page 298) of crude herb. Start on the low end to gauge your personal response. Take with meals.

Cautions and Considerations: Be careful: Gymnema may cause sudden drops in blood sugar and aggravate hypoglycemia. Work with your doctor, particularly in cases of type 1 diabetes. Gymnema is not a substitute for insulin, but it may lower the doses needed to maintain homeostasis.

PROTOCOL POINTS

Type 1 Diabetes

In this chapter, most of our discussion revolves around insulin resistance and type 2 diabetes, both of which are largely lifestyle related and are well managed, and often reversed, by diet, exercise, and herbs. Although there is quite a bit of overlap in beneficial diets, lifestyle changes, and herbs with type 1 diabetes, this condition is quite different and requires medical care. In type 1 diabetes, the beta cells are destroyed — often at a young age due to an autoimmune attack — and do not produce insulin. No amount of herbs will cure this condition, and some herbs can be dangerous. The goal, holistically, in type 1 diabetes is to maintain optimal health, minimize blood sugar spikes and crashes, and reduce the risk for secondary complications with TLC for blood vessels and plenty of antioxidants. Blood sugar must be carefully monitored, and insulin will need to be adjusted accordingly. When in doubt, work with your doctor *and* a qualified holistic practitioner such as a naturopath, herbalist, nutritionist, or dietitian.

Conventional Care: Insulin therapy and careful blood sugar monitoring are *required*.

Diet: The diet and lifestyle therapies discussed in this chapter for type 2 diabetes also benefit type 1 diabetes by keeping blood sugar levels more stable.

Lifestyle: General good lifestyle, including regular fitness, sleep, and mind-body balance. Interestingly, toxin and electromagnetic frequency (EMF) exposure seem to negatively affect the way your body deals with sugar.

Herbs: Type 1 diabetics must be *extremely* careful when adding herbs into their routine as the herbs are likely to affect blood sugar quickly. Herbs that increase insulin absorption — like cinnamon — are less beneficial because cell sensitivity is not generally the issue. Gymnema and blueberry may be beneficial but should be taken under the guidance of a practitioner and with careful blood sugar monitoring. The herbs are not a replacement for insulin, though they may reduce the doses needed. Increase antioxidants and nutrients to support your body against the common side effects of diabetes.

Type 2 Diabetes and Insulin Resistance

Essentially, this *whole* chapter has been about type 2 diabetes and insulin resistance. Here are the key points:

Diet: Eat a high-fiber carbohydrate (HFC) or low-carbohydrate diet, or a mix of both. Key components include avoiding refined foods, sugar, and flour in favor of whole foods. Get plenty of fiber and plant foods alongside quality protein, and balance your plate. Eat berries, especially blueberries, daily. Consider a chromium supplement (or brewer's yeast) if you are deficient.

Lifestyle: Daily exercise and activity is ideal, including a strength-training workout a few times a week. Adequate sleep, stress management, mind-body balance, and toxin avoidance will also support your body's ability to function optimally.

Herbs: Take hypoglycemic herbs — cinnamon, blueberry leaf, gymnema, et cetera — with or just before meals. Antioxidant, bitter, nutrient-dense, and adaptogenic herbs will help support you. Slowly introduce remedies and work with your doctor if you're on medications, as they will likely need to be adjusted to keep your blood sugar levels in a good range.

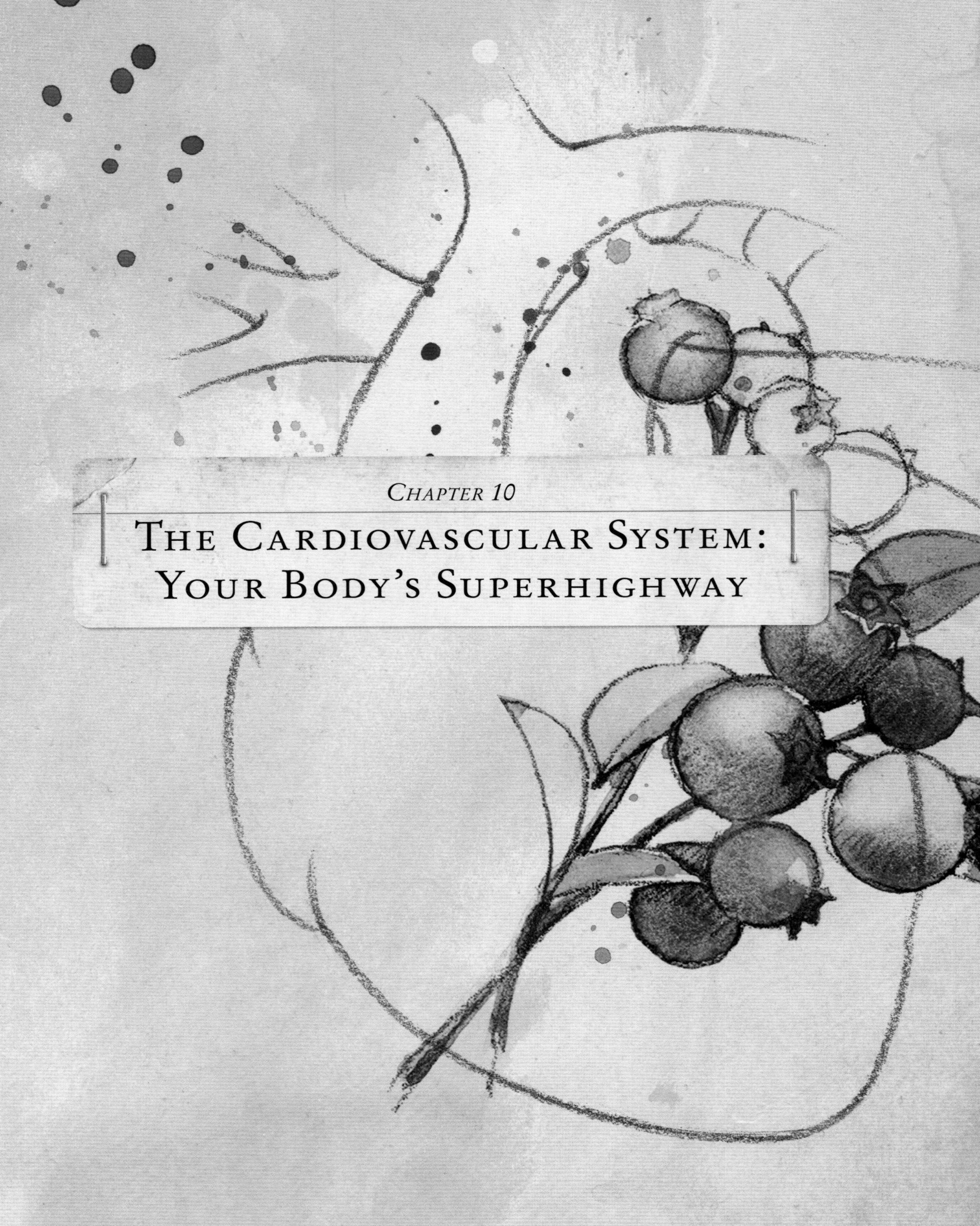

Chapter 10

The Cardiovascular System: Your Body's Superhighway

IN THE UNIVERSE of your body, your heart serves as the capital city, pumping lifeblood in, out, and around your body via a complex system of highways (arteries), back roads (capillaries), and superhighways (major arteries). Neatly packaged cells and compounds are transported rapidly through this system — it only takes about a minute for the same pint of blood to cycle through and return to your heart.

In collaboration with the lungs, your heart infuses oxygen into your blood, which is necessary for each of your cells to produce ATP, the primary source of energy for the body. The blood also delivers nutrients, hormones, immune cells, and other special packages, picks up waste, dumps the waste while passing through the liver, and then continues back to the heart (via veins), where, in conjunction with the lungs, new oxygen is infused into the blood and it's pumped back out again.

Your heart needs to be strong to pump all that blood, and its contractions are stimulated primarily by electrical impulses. This contract-relax action gives you your heartbeat, which sounds and feels like a drumbeat to which the rest of your body dances. Its tempo and strength will affect your vitality or lack thereof. Each day, your heart beats approximately 100,000 times, moving approximately 2,000 gallons of blood.

The health of your heart affects all other aspects of your health and vice versa. Heart disease is the leading cause of death in America, and stroke (cardiovascular attack in the brain) is not far behind. High cholesterol, hypertension, and elevated inflammatory markers like C-reactive protein (CRP) and homocysteine serve as early warning signals for cardiovascular distress. However, sometimes symptoms are barely perceptible, and cardiovascular well-being is also closely linked to energy levels, brain health, sexual function, and risk or progression of diabetes, obesity, and more. Therefore, the more you can do to take care of your ticker and keep the roadways running smoothly, the better off you will be and the longer you're likely to live.

Heart-Healthy Basics

The work of Dr. Dean Ornish and scientists researching, among other things, the Mediterranean diet has helped shed light on how to prevent, treat, and even reverse the effects of heart disease. As with so many aspects of human health, the basic approach to both prevention and management of cardiovascular disease is undertaking appropriate exercise, mind-body balance, and diet — with herbs to support more specific aspects of heart health, as needed.

Exercise

Regular cardio workouts strengthen the function of the heart and help burn through excess sugar in the bloodstream, which keeps your heart healthy, blood pressure steady, and cholesterol levels in range. Add in some strength-training exercises a few times a week to improve your body's resting metabolism to burn more and improve how your body deals with sugar and cholesterol throughout the day. If you're in poor health, talk to your doctor before starting a routine. If you already have heart disease, you may need to start a routine slowly.

Mind-Body Balance

Meditation, breathwork, and exercises with a mind-body component like yoga and tai chi have been shown to reduce heart-damaging stress and slow and even *reverse* heart disease.

Heart-Healthy Diet

The general diet recommendations detailed in chapter 1 also work nicely for a healthy heart, but there are some key things to pay attention to:

- **Primarily plants:** Veggies, fruits, plant-based protein (beans, nuts, seeds), and whole plant foods in general (including whole grains) feed a healthy heart. That's because they're loaded with fiber, anti-inflammatory compounds, antioxidants, and phytonutrients, including magnesium. Aim for five to nine servings of fruits and vegetables daily (heavy on veggies, leafy greens, and berries), which helps improve heart health and blood pressure in particular. If you have high blood pressure, note that leafy greens, other green veggies, parsley, burdock, celery, and dandelion have potent anti-hypertension effects via their diuretic effects.

- **Soluble fiber:** Found in whole plant foods (particularly beans, apples, pears, citrus, blueberries, oats, flaxseeds, psyllium), soluble fiber slows the release of sugar and other compounds from food into the bloodstream — which helps lower triglycerides and cholesterol — and also helps the body eliminate cholesterol and fats more efficiently through the colon. Try to eat foods in the most whole form possible, such as intact seeds, or eating a fruit skin and all, to get the most benefit.
- **Fish, seafood, avocados, and olive oil:** These are key components of the heart-healthy diet of the Mediterranean and other areas of the world, and they provide your body with good fats (including omega-3s and monounsaturated fats) that reduce inflammation and boost good cholesterol. Aim for 2 teaspoons of extra-virgin olive oil per day and at least two or three servings of fish and seafood per week. Also consider other sources of good fats and omega-3s, like nuts and seeds.
- **Red-blue-purple foods:** Berries, red wine, purple grapes, and other plant foods in the red-blue-purple family are loaded with heart-happy antioxidant and anti-inflammatory pigments (anthocyanins and related compounds) that fight heart disease and keep your blood vessels flexible and smooth. See page 157 for more on these "red tonics."
- **Pungent herbs, spices, and tea:** Garlic, onions, turmeric, hot peppers, and other herbs and seasonings, as well as green tea and cacao, decrease inflammation and tone the cardiovascular system. Herbs and spices work in synergy with the other ingredients in your meal, providing even more antioxidant activity together than they would alone.
- **Low sodium:** Salt gives your body important electrolytes for homeostasis, but excess sodium increases blood pressure in some people. Major sodium-saturating culprits include restaurant fare and highly processed foods, which usually include several sodium-based compounds for flavor and food preservation, while the minerals like potassium that would help balance sodium in the body are lost in the processing. The Dietary Approaches to Stop Hypertension (DASH) diet recommends limiting sodium to 1,500 to 2,300 mg (⅔ to 1 teaspoon of salt) daily. It's easy to stay under this limit if you eat home-cooked food made from scratch with whole foods and just a sprinkle of salt to taste.
- **Bitters:** Bitter greens like lettuce, radicchio, chicory, dandelion, endive, and artichoke — or an herbal bitters formula — not only improve digestion and liver function but also help lower blood sugar and cholesterol and keep heart disease at bay.
- **High-quality animal foods:** Worldwide, the most promising heart-healthy diets feature fish and seafood but otherwise very little (if any) meat and dairy, treating them more as seasonings than a main course. Though delicious, the latter are often high in saturated fat and tend to increase inflammation. If/when you eat meat, dairy, and eggs, keep them in moderation and opt for organic, wild, or pasture-raised sources. The food we get from animals that eat good food and move outdoors has a healthier fat profile, including more omega-3s, and more nutrients than the food we get from their factory-farmed counterparts. We aren't just what *we* eat but what *the animals we eat* eat!

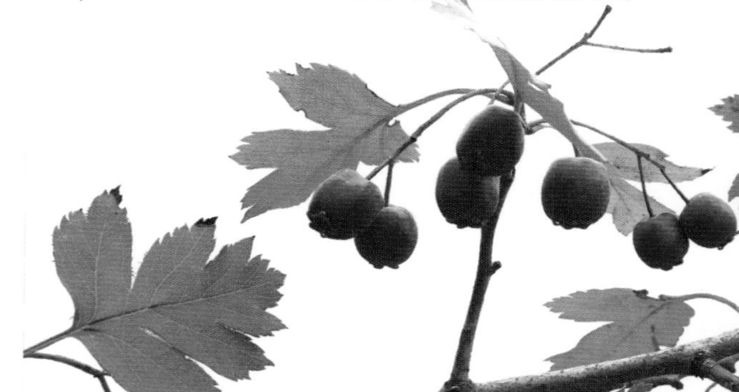

Heart Tonics

Red blood, red tonics: most of our key cardiovascular tonics follow the Doctrine of Signatures — which suggests that the plant looks like the part of the body it helps — with a deep red hue like the blood. Specifically, that deep red color indicates that the plants contain anthocyanins and related red-blue-purple pigments that act as potent antioxidants, protecting your heart from oxidative damage and helping to maintain good endothelial (blood vessel lining) health.

▸ Hawthorn

Crataegus spp.

Availability: G W C+

Key Properties: Hawthorn's affinity for the human heart never ceases to amaze me. This thorny shrub-tree improves *every* aspect of cardiovascular health, working from various angles to fight oxidative stress, decrease inflammation, prevent and reverse blood vessel damage, relax and tone the blood vessel lining, reduce high blood pressure, improve circulation, and strengthen the heart muscle itself. Hawthorn helps modulate and improve blood pressure, working as a slow, gentle ACE inhibitor (ACE, or angiotensin-converting enzyme, raises blood pressure by causing blood vessels to constrict). It may modestly lower bad cholesterol levels. However, hawthorn's ability to prevent, treat, and potentially reverse congestive heart failure remains the most impressive and best-researched benefit. In congestive heart failure, the heart gets weak and sometimes thick and enlarged and blood begins to pool; hawthorn seems to gradually normalize and restore vitality to the heart in these cases. Hawthorn also slowly lessens angina (chest pain) and atherosclerosis (hardening of the arteries). It may prevent heart attack and improve the body's ability to heal after an attack. It does all this while being totally nontoxic and safe enough to eat as a food. Isn't that remarkable? If you have heart issues or a family history of heart disease, it's worth considering adding hawthorn to your daily routine.

Additional Benefits: The herb also "gladdens" the heart and calms the nerves, and when you put all of these uses together, you can expect to notice better mood, strength, and energy levels with regular use. It can be used in formula with other herbs for grief, broken heart, hyperactivity, memory problems, and brain injury.

Preparation: Traditionally people have used the autumn-harvested berries; however, the spring-flowering twigs (leaves and buds or newly opened flowers in particular) can also be used. Many herbalists combine these parts for a full-spectrum remedy in tincture, elixir, tea, or capsule. Standard herb doses (see page 298) apply, and larger quantities may be even more beneficial. A few companies make delicious and potent solid extract pastes that you take by the quarter teaspoon — a favorite form! You'll see the *monogyna* and *laevigata* species most often used (*C. oxyacantha* ambiguously refers to either); hawthorn is one of the most difficult plants in the world to identify definitively to the species, partly because it hybridizes like crazy. Fortunately almost all species can be used interchangeably. It blends well with other heart herbs, as well as nervines, adaptogens, berry antioxidants, and anti-inflammatories.

Cautions and Considerations: Although hawthorn is incredibly safe, it can interact with a handful of medications — especially digoxin and blood pressure meds — acting synergistically to increase their activity. Some doctors purposely prescribe them together, getting equal results and fewer side effects with a lower drug dose. However, you'll need to work with a qualified practitioner to safely find this balance point. Also keep in mind that hawthorn itself is a tonic herb and not a drug. In acute situations, it's not likely to be fast or strong enough. It works slowly and needs to be taken in substantial doses over months before you gradually begin to see the effects. But because of this tonic effect and high degree of safety, it can be taken on an ongoing basis for years to attain or maintain a healthy heart.

Antioxidant-Rich Heart Tonics

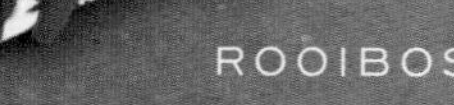

▸ Rooibos and Hibiscus

Aspalathus linearis and *Hibiscus sabdariffa*

Availability: C+ (rooibos)/G- C+ (hibiscus)

Key Properties: The tasty red-hued, caffeine-free herbal teas made from rooibos leaves and stems and hibiscus flowers (technically the calyx of the flower) are loaded with antioxidants including polyphenols, rutin, and anthocyanins. Scientists have just begun to confirm their heart benefits. In one study, about 3 cups of hibiscus tea daily for 6 weeks reduced systolic blood pressure — the higher the blood pressure, the better it worked. In other studies, hibiscus worked liked an ACE inhibitor (not quite as strong as the drug counterpart lisinopril but equal to captopril) and reduced sodium levels without affecting potassium, with a high degree of safety and tolerability. Hibiscus also has a positive effect on cholesterol and triglycerides and protective effects for the capillaries, helps normalize blood sugar and insulin response, and protects the liver.

Much like hibiscus, early research is showing that rooibos protects the liver and reduces cholesterol and blood pressure. In one study, participants who drank 6 cups of rooibos tea daily for 6 weeks (as opposed to just water) showed increased blood levels of polyphenols and nutrients, decreased cholesterol oxidation (when fats and cholesterol oxidize in the blood, which increases the risk for blood vessel damage), increased function of the body's natural antioxidant systems, decreased low-density lipoprotein (LDL) cholesterol and triglycerides, and increased high-density lipoprotein (HDL) cholesterol. Other studies suggest that it reduces hypertension by inhibiting ACE and improving nitric oxide.

Additional Benefits: Rooibos remains a popular daily naturally caffeine-free tea for enjoyment and overall health in its native South Africa. Central Americans drink hibiscus (a.k.a. roselle and rosa de Jamaica) as a tasty tea — especially iced and sweetened — to cool down on a hot day. Most fruity and red teas and antioxidant drinks include hibiscus for flavor and color.

Preparation: Drink 3 to 6 cups a day of a standard infusion. If 3 to 6 cups of tea a day seems ridiculous, keep in mind that each 1-cup serving is 8 ounces, yet most of our travel mugs and coffee cups hold 16 ounces or more. (Just one of Starbucks' supersized "Trenta" equals about *4* cups.) Bottoms up!

Cautions and Considerations: Both appear to be quite safe and are drunk widely in large quantities in their native lands by people of all ages. Extreme doses of hibiscus may mildly reduce the rate of conception (though it seems fine *during* pregnancy). Tart acids in hibiscus can wear away at tooth enamel, as would drinking fruit tea, juice, or lemon in your water — rinse or brush afterward. They may interact with some medications, clearing them out of the system a little quickly. They are somewhat diuretic.

▸ Cacao and Dark Chocolate

Theobroma cacao

Availability: C+

Key Properties: Cacao may be our most delicious heart tonic — and it has some good competition! Native people who consume cocoa beverages have a reduced incidence of hypertension, and researchers back that up with clinical studies on more than 66,000 people showing that cacao/cocoa consumption reduces the risk of death due to heart disease. Beneficial compounds in the beans — including antioxidant flavonols and magnesium — seem to work together to have broad-reaching cardiovascular benefits. Preliminary studies show that chocolate reduces the oxidative stress that aggravates atherosclerosis and plaque formation, decreases the inflammation known to aggravate cardiovascular disease, increases circulation, decreases blood pressure, improves the integrity of the endothelium, and may also improve cholesterol levels. However, the sugar and milk used in making chocolate from cacao can dilute the benefits. The higher the

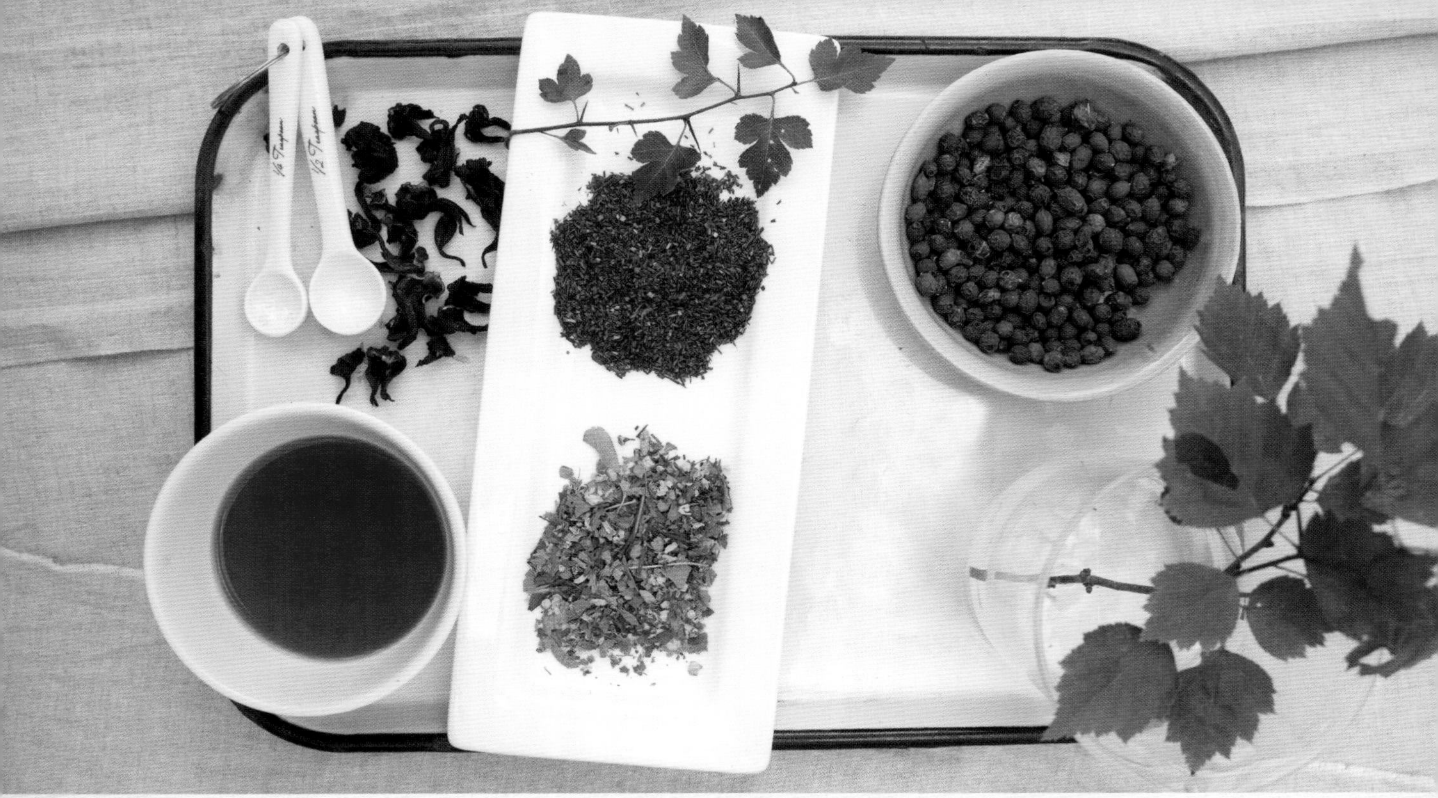

Red Heart Tea

A lovely and gentle tonic blend! Drink approximately 3 cups daily.

- 1 teaspoon hawthorn berry
- 1 teaspoon hawthorn leaf/flower
- 1 teaspoon rooibos
- 1 teaspoon hibiscus
- 1 teaspoon linden
- 1 teaspoon rose hips
- Honey (optional)

Combine all the herbs. Pour 2 cups boiling water over the mixture and let steep, covered, for at least 20 minutes. Strain, sweeten with honey, if desired, and enjoy.

Choco-Vanilla Rooibos Tea

I love this posh blend, which I got from a NATURAL HEALTH *magazine article years ago, and it just happens to include nice heart-tonic herbs! It definitely has the flavor of chocolate but is subtler, not like hot cocoa at all. If you don't have a vanilla bean, you can use a squirt of vanilla extract instead, or vanilla-infused rooibos, but the bean is best.*

- 1 teaspoon rooibos
- 1 teaspoon cocoa nibs
- ¼ vanilla bean, snipped into pieces

Combine the rooibos, cocoa, and vanilla bean. Pour 1 to 2 cups boiling water over the mixture and let steep, covered, for 15 to 30 minutes. Strain and enjoy. It will get less tasty and more bitter (from the cocoa) if it steeps too long — there's a careful balance to get nice cocoa undertones.

cacao content, the better the effects. Dark chocolate has 120 to 150 mg of beneficial polyphenols, while pure cocoa has almost five times that amount and milk chocolate has almost none.

Additional Benefits: Cocoa (without all the cream and sugar) also appears to reduce glucose levels and promote weight loss. And it boosts your mood! The modest dose of caffeine and mood-boosting properties make it a nice synergist for energy blends.

Preparation: Enjoy a few squares of dark chocolate as a treat, and incorporate a spoonful or two of cocoa nibs or cocoa powder into smoothies, teas, and other recipes. You can also tincture cacao to add to herbal blends.

Cautions and Considerations: Cocoa is generally safe; however, it may aggravate anxiety, irritability, and insomnia in caffeine-sensitive folks, and some people just don't tolerate chocolate and xanthine compounds well. Most xanthines (a category of purines), such as caffeine, theobromine, and theophylline, have a stimulating effect, and they are present not just in chocolate but also in coffee, tea, and yerba maté. In sensitive people, xanthines may aggravate pain and migraines, fibroids, gout, and kidney stones.

Similar Herbs: **Tea** (*Camellia sinensis*), whether green, white, or black, also shows promise in studies for lowering cholesterol and improving overall heart health.

▸ Red-Blue-Purple Heart Tonics

Pomegranates, cherries, berries, purple grapes, red wine — if you have a dark red, purple, or blue fruit in front of you, there's a good chance it will improve your heart health! A range of antioxidant and anti-inflammatory compounds are associated with the pigments that yield these colors, including resveratrol, anthocyanins, and the pigment precursors oligomeric proanthocyanins (OPCs) and proanthocyanidin oligomers (PCOs). They are part of broad classes of compounds called flavonols and flavonoids, which are themselves part of an even broader class of compounds called polyphenols. These are some of the sciencey buzzwords you'll hear associated with these fruits and their health benefits. (Hawthorn can also thank many of these compounds for its heart benefits.) Although alcohol, consumed in moderation, has its own potential heart tonic effects, red wine provides a double whammy of goodness with its deep red hue. And because alcohol can also have ill health effects, daily consumption of the fruits fresh, frozen, or juiced (read the ingredients label to ensure you have the real deal) provides benefits without the pitfalls. Powders, capsules, and dried berries may also work well. Studies suggest that high-antioxidant berry consumption improves the health of blood vessels, improves blood pressure and cholesterol levels, and reduces inflammatory markers.

The Center *of* Emotion

Your heart isn't just a blood-pumping, oxygen-infusing machine. It's also a primary seat of emotion (as are the lungs and belly). When you experience immense grief, your heart breaks. Anxiety feels like a heart attack. And when you're snuggled up in peace and love, those feelings radiate from your heart. Just laughing improves blood flow by approximately 20 percent.

Stress is one of our greatest triggers of heart disease. In Japan, where long work hours and intense stress remain the norm, stress-induced heart attack and stroke in the working class are so common that "death by overwork" has a name: *karoshi*. In the United States, scientists have noted that you're more likely to have a heart attack on Monday morning than any other time of the week. (Personally, I think the jolt of the alarm plus out-of-routine sleep deprivation are at least partly at fault.) It's important to remember this heart-mood connection when using herbs for your cardiovascular system. While your core protocol for the heart may involve heart tonics and herbs to lower blood pressure and cholesterol levels, don't forget to tend to your mental state and stress levels.

Blood Pressure Balance

Your blood pressure is affected by the volume and viscosity of your blood, as well as the level of tension in the blood vessel lining itself. Hypertension — both the low-grade chronic form and acute spikes — can be incredibly dangerous because the pressure can damage blood vessels, which increases the risk of heart disease, stroke, and other issues. Thick blood, plaque-filled arteries, excessive sodium, excessive insulin and blood sugar levels, and stress all raise blood pressure. Hypotension also poses problems, including dizziness and fainting as the body tries to cope with less-than-adequate blood flow.

Your kidneys help regulate blood pressure and the general homeostasis of body fluids. In your bloodstream, sodium and potassium help increase and decrease blood pressure, respectively. The kidneys work with the liver to release angiotensin, a compound that encourages sodium to increase blood pressure. Many antihypertensive drugs work by inhibiting angiotensin-converting enzyme (ACE) and are called ACE inhibitors. Nitric oxide also reduces blood pressure by relaxing the lining of the blood vessels. Diuretics — as drugs, diet, or herbs — lower blood pressure by making you pee more and releasing fluid (and, thus, pressure) from the system. Many of our heart tonic herbs have mild effects on blood pressure compared to medications, though they can encourage modest drops.

To bring mild to moderate hypertension into balance, it is (once again!) best to start with a heart-healthy diet and exercise. Key in on eating more vegetables and less sodium, complemented by blood-pressure-lowering herbs and diuretics (see below). Seek the advice of a professional to slowly and safely begin a good exercise routine. When stress is a factor, mind-body balance techniques including yoga, tai chi, meditation, and breathwork help.

▸ Celery

Apium graveolens

Availability: G C+

Key Properties: Celery shows promise for lowering blood pressure by approximately 15 percent due to the diuretic effect as well as specific blood-pressure-lowering compounds that — unlike drugs — also improve blood flow to the brain. The seeds are the most potent (and researched) part of celery; however, the celery stalks are also effective, and safer.

Additional Benefits: Celery helps dissolve uric acid crystals to clear them from the body, reducing symptoms of gout. It also boosts general detoxification via the kidneys and is a good source of potassium and B vitamins.

Preparation: Start off with four fresh stalks of celery daily, raw or juiced. Or try celery seed capsules, following the dosage instructions on the product label.

Cautions and Considerations: Choose organic; celery bioaccumulates sodium nitrate and pesticides from conventionally farmed soil. Fresh celery juice, applied or splashed on the skin, can burn when exposed to sun (as can other parsley family juices), appearing almost like poison ivy or an acid burn. Phototoxicity — though rare — has also occurred with ingestion of large quantities of celery root (no reports for juice or seed ingestion). The seeds can irritate and inflame the kidneys and should not be taken during pregnancy or if you have a history of kidney disease or inflammation.

▸ Other Herbs for Blood Pressure

Several of the heart tonics profiled earlier in this chapter also have blood-pressure-lowering effects, including **hawthorn**, **hibiscus**, and **rooibos. Garlic** is effective for lowering blood pressure, too. Diuretic herbs may be useful, as both food and medicine, in reducing the body's overall pressure. Ones to try include **dandelion** (leaf and root), **burdock root**, **chicory root**, and **parsley** (leaf or seed). These and other vegetables are high in calcium, potassium, and magnesium, which balance sodium's blood pressure effects.

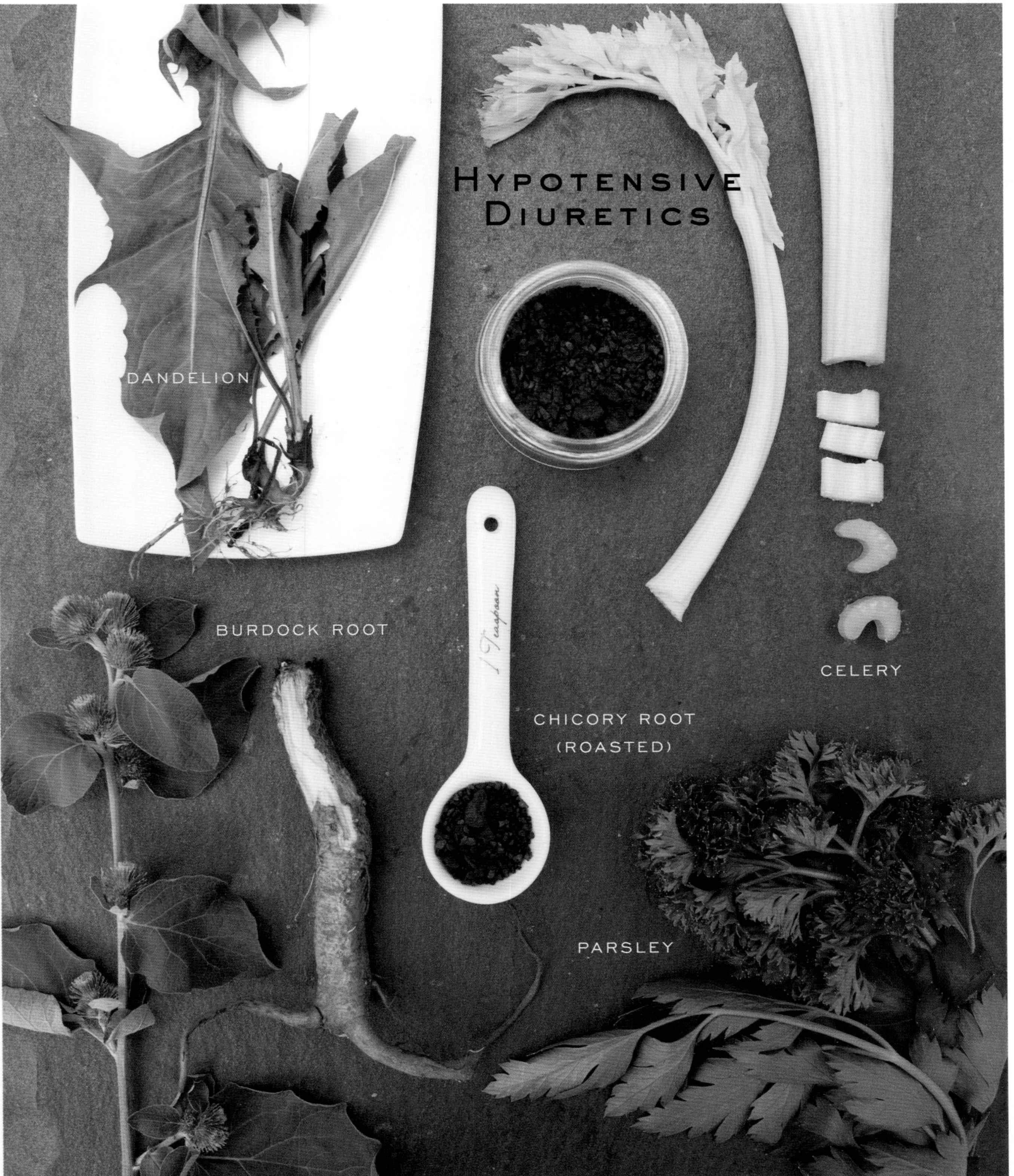
HYPOTENSIVE
DIURETICS
DANDELION
BURDOCK ROOT
CELERY
CHICORY ROOT
(ROASTED)
PARSLEY
1 Teaspoon

PROTOCOL POINTS

High Cholesterol and Triglycerides

In heart disease, high cholesterol and triglyceride levels function more as warning signs and risk factors than diseases in and of themselves. Don't simply look to suppress them — try to incorporate changes and herbs that will correct the imbalance at its root — and also pay attention to your other risk factors for heart disease, including stress, family history, blood pressure, blood sugar instability, abdominal obesity, and inflammation.

Diet: Enjoy a low-glycemic, plant-based diet (such as the vegan or Mediterranean diet) featuring plenty of vegetables, fruit (especially berries, apples, pears, citrus), beans, whole grains, nuts and seeds, olive oil and avocados, some fish and seafood, and eggs, and plenty of garlic, onions, ginger, and other herbs and seasonings. Such a diet will be rich in soluble fiber, which improves cholesterol elimination. Limit sugar, bad fats, excessive meat and dairy, and refined, fried, and processed food. Try to include bitter-tasting foods and herbs with your meals. Berries, tea, dark purple grape juice, and red wine may also help offset some of the damage of fatty foods as you eat.

Lifestyle: Move daily, including cardiovascular exercise and strength training. Also address stress, and adopt activities that support mind-body balance. Maintain a healthy body weight, in particular a good hip-to-waist ratio.

Herbs: Bitters hold promise, and artichoke leaf extract has been shown to help lower cholesterol. Also consider turmeric powder or extract, garlic pills, guggul, or cinnamon. Medicinal mushrooms including oyster and maitake — eaten amply in the diet — have cholesterol-lowering fiber and some natural statin activity. If you really need to drop numbers and don't find the previously mentioned tips sufficient, red yeast rice and beta-sitosterol (marketed as Benecol, Basikol, and Basichol) work well. Red yeast rice acts as a natural low-dose "fuzz" of various statins (though less common, they also have similar side effects), and beta-sitosterol blocks cholesterol absorption in the gut. Both appear effective and safer than statin drugs; however, like statins, they don't get to the root of the problem.

Hypertension

Hypertension should always be taken seriously. Both chronic low-grade hypertension or more extreme spikes can be life threatening. Mild to moderate hypertension often responds favorably to diet, lifestyle, and herbal therapies. Severe or unresponsive hypertension may require medication, although you may be able to combine herbs with lower doses of medications with your doctor's supervision.

Diet: Focus on a healthy whole-foods diet, and especially key in on plenty of veggies (ideally 9 or 10 servings of produce daily) and reduced sodium intake. Enjoy diuretic, high-mineral veggies daily: celery, parsley, dandelion, burdock, chicory, and nettle. Note that alcohol intake raises blood pressure for some; you may need to avoid it. Adequate intake of minerals, including calcium, magnesium, and potassium — from food, nutrient-dense herbs (e.g., nettle super infusion), or mineral supplements — may balance blood pressure, too.

Lifestyle: Regular cardiovascular exercise (you may need to start slowly to allow a weak/diseased cardiovascular system to adjust) and mind-body balance

Herbs: Alongside the diuretic veggies, consider garlic, hawthorn, rooibos, or hibiscus. Linden and passionflower may help for mild stress-related hypertension. Dandelion leaf-root tincture works wonders for some, more often for those of Central American ancestry. Also try tea or tincture made with dandelion, burdock, and chicory roots, which have a sodium-leaching diuretic effect. See the recipes for Bitter Brew (page 95) and Red Heart Tea (page 156). Herbs generally work slowly and reduce blood pressure by only 10 to 15 percent. Medication may be necessary for severe or nonresponsive hypertension.

PROTOCOL POINTS

Varicose Veins, Hemorrhoids, and Spider Veins

Although our standard heart tonics also benefit vascular health, really key in on approaches that relieve pressure on the valves and strengthen the lining of the veins.

Diet: Focus on the general heart-healthy diet (see page 151). Pay particular attention to foods that improve and tighten the endothelial tissues. These include foods high in bioflavonoids, including rutin (in buckwheat as well as hawthorn, tea, citrus fruit and rinds, mulberries, cranberries, aronia berries), as well as the red-blue-purple anthocyanin pigments (in blueberries, bilberries, cranberries, blackberries, dark purple grapes, mulberries, hibiscus, hawthorn, black rice, purple potatoes, purple corn, red cabbage . . .). Aim for at least ½ cup of berries daily, fresh, frozen, or 100 percent juice. For hemorrhoids, insoluble fiber (seeds, fruit skin, root veggies, whole grains) and adequate water intake help ease constipation and pressure.

Lifestyle: Regular movement is crucial. Try not to stand or sit too much. Support hose and elevating your legs help with varicose veins.

Herbs: Alongside those mentioned in the diet section, consider herbs that improve circulation while tightening and toning the endothelium. Horse chestnut standardized extract capsules can be extremely beneficial and are well researched. (Crude herbal formulas may be mildly toxic.) Also consider yarrow, hawthorn, dry alder, or gotu kola in any form. Topically, apply creams made with the infused oil, hydrosol, or tincture of horse chestnut, gotu kola, yarrow, witch hazel, or (to a lesser extent) calendula. Caffeine and tea, applied in a cream, may also help with varicose veins; however, they can also be stimulating.

Vein Health: Ensuring *a* Smooth Return Trip

Blood flows through your arteries as it's pumped away from the heart, and it travels more slowly as it takes the return trip through the veins. Because the veins lie farther from the pumping action, blood flows more slowly. Your veins have a system of valves that ideally only allow the blood to flow in one direction, but sometimes they get weak from poor vascular health, poor circulation, gravity (including too much sitting or standing, excessive body weight, pregnancy), and lack of exercise and movement. Valves may give out, allowing blood to pool and blow out the vein. This can cause cardiovascular insufficiency, varicose veins, spider veins, and hemorrhoids (which are also aggravated by constipation and lack of fiber because of the pressure hard feces put on the blood vessels near the rectum).

Promote better vascular health in a variety of ways. Exercise and regular movement help maintain circulation and avoid undue pressure on the valves in your veins. Foods rich in blue-purple pigments and rutin help to tone the endothelial lining of the blood vessels to improve its strength and flexibility. For more suggestions, see the protocol points above.

AT A GLANCE

Herbs for the Heart

The herbs listed here are grouped by their beneficial action for the heart, with my favorite, most effective, safest, and most common herbs listed first. Because blood sugar imbalance often coincides with and causes cardiovascular disease, herbs that help balance blood sugar levels are also important for heart

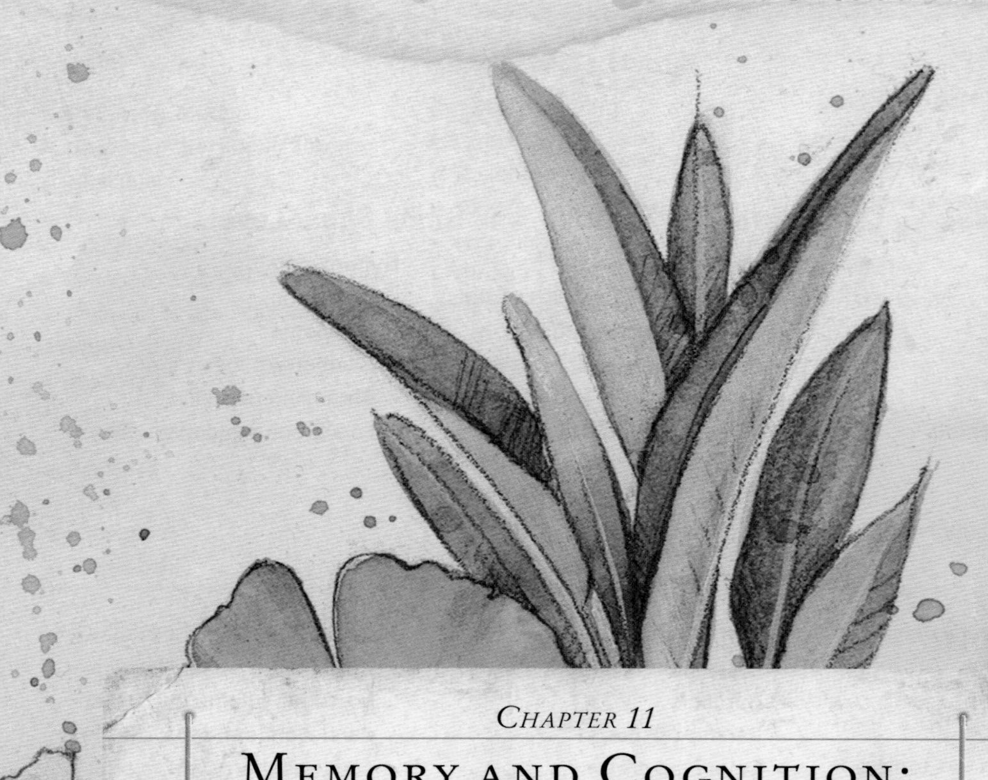

Chapter 11

Memory and Cognition: Sharpening Your Mind

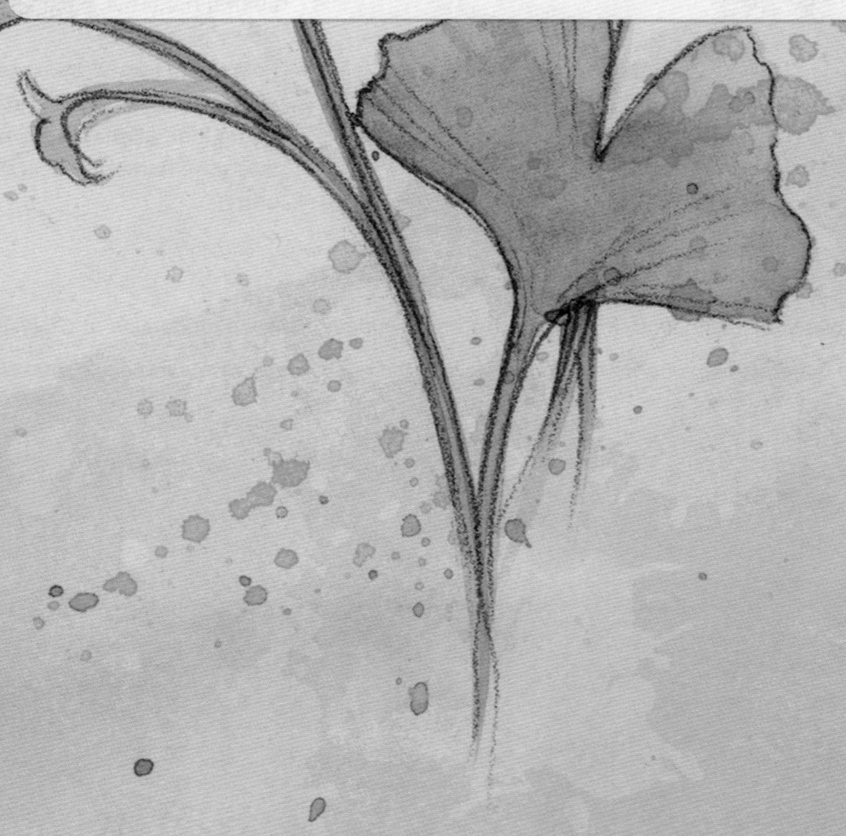

YOUR BRAIN SERVES as the primary control center for your body. It's the original portable computer: weighing in at just a few pounds (a small percentage of your total body weight), it contains 100,000 miles of blood vessels and 1 quadrillion neurons, and it consumes 25 percent of your body's oxygen and nutrients and 70 percent of its glucose (the brain's preferred fuel). But what's really amazing about your brain is that it's what makes you human. Alongside all the complex calculations and overview of all body functions, your brain is an electric neural forest rich with memories, emotions, dreams, and desires. It controls how you see the world, taste your food, hear music, smell aromas, and absorb the wonders of the world around you. So much of your identity stems from your brain and how it works.

It's easy to take your brain for granted, until it starts to falter: flighty attention, difficulty remembering names and where you left the keys, or the inability to perform cognitive tasks for work and play. Your neural forest ecosystem begins to degrade into a jumble of tangles that interfere with data transmission. Problems with memory and cognition come in many forms and for many reasons, from chronic or acute stress to brain trauma or aging. As you age, the health of your brain becomes a greater priority, especially if dementia or Alzheimer's runs in the family. But whether you're 20 or 90, it's never too early or too late to start tending your neural forest.

Jumping *from* Synapse *to* Synapse

Memory and cognition are functions of the neural network, the web of neurons (nerve cells) that make up the brain and innervate the body. Like Tarzan swinging across the jungle from tree to tree, neural signals fly through your brain and body via electrical impulses that jump across gaps (synapses) between one neuron and another. They're lightning fast! One nerve impulse can travel at a rate of up to 100 yards a second.

As their name would imply, neurotransmitters are the substances responsible for transmitting these electrical impulses across the neural synapses. When their job is done, enzymes (their names often end in *-ase*) or neurotransmitter transporters (a type of protein) break down the neurotransmitters. Reuptake inhibitors — including the well-known antidepressant selective serotonin reuptake inhibitors (SSRIs) — inhibit the breakdown of specific neurotransmitters so that more of those neurotransmitters will be present in the body.

Neurotransmitters do a wide range of things, and an excess or deficiency of them plays a role in many different diseases. Acetylcholine (ACh) is a major transmitter for basic body functions, including contraction and control of muscles and involuntary actions. Low ACh levels are assocated with Alzheimer's, and many of our mint-family brain-boosting herbs (sage, rosemary, lemon balm, mint) boost ACh levels by inhibiting the enzyme that breaks it down. Other cognition- and mood-related neurotransmitters include adrenaline, norepinephrine, dopamine, GABA, serotonin, glutamate, and endorphins. In this chapter, we'll key on the neurotransmitters that contribute to cognition and memory, and the things that you can do to naturally improve and protect these functions of the brain.

Diet, Lifestyle, Mind-Body Balance

In chapter 1 we talked about diet, lifestyle, and mind-body balance as the foundations of health, vitality, and well-being, and these topics have come up repeatedly in terms of their importance for each of the body's major systems. Well, here they are again. These three factors play a *major* role in the overall health of the brain, and in particular memory and cognition. There are, of course, herbs, remedies, and pharmaceuticals you can take that combat oxidation, enhance circulation, reduce inflammation, and boost mood, all of which will support good memory and cognition, but without a healthy diet, lifestyle, and mind, these remedies will tend to address symptoms, not the core problems. So begin your journey toward a better-functioning brain here, with the following guidelines.

Diet

Remember that the food you eat provides your body with the raw materials it needs to make cell and nerve linings, neurotransmitters, enzymes, fuel, and more. Therefore, what you eat plays a significant role in brain function. A poor diet gums up the works, while a healthy diet gives your brain and nervous system exactly what they need to thrive.

High-Quality Fats

As much as 60 percent of your brain is made of fat, and the myelin sheath that protects nerve endings is also primarily fat. Add this to the fact that the lining of *all* your cells includes fatty acids, and you see that being a "fathead" isn't an insult, it's a reality!

The types of fat available for use by the body to construct and cushion all of this come primarily from your diet. Quality counts! Load up on omega-3 and monounsaturated fat-rich foods, including cold-water wild fatty fish, olive oil, avocados, nuts, and seeds. A diet rich in these fats is associated with a 40 percent reduced risk of Alzheimer's and dementia, better brain volume, improved performance on memory and reasoning tests, and reduced levels of beta-amyloid plaque (which hinders nerves and brain function). Low levels of omega-3 fatty acids are associated with brain shrinkage, memory loss, declines in cognitive function, and a greater risk of Alzheimer's disease and dementia. Fatty fish (salmon, sardines, herring, mackerel, trout) is the *most* important source of omega-3s. Studies show that in countries with the greatest fish consumption, people have better moods and fewer cognition issues.

Too many "bad fats" gum up the works, so keep fried food, packaged food, and trans fats to a minimum. Saturated fats (animal products, coconut oil, palm oil) and polyunsaturated fats (soy, corn, and most vegetable oils) have positive and negative effects, so enjoy them in moderation.

Complete Protein

Neurotransmitters (among many things in your body) are made with amino acids, the building blocks or protein. You don't necessarily need megadoses of protein, just steady, adequate amounts of *complete* protein. Aim for 0.8 gram of protein per 2.2 pounds of body weight, which comes to 60 grams daily for a 150-pound person. Animal products contain complete protein, but it may be even better to get it by combining sources of vegetarian protein — beans and grains, nuts, seeds, et cetera. Eggs are amazing brain food; besides offering easily digested complete protein, they contain omega-3s (if raised on pasture or given omega-rich feed), choline in the yolks (which helps you make acetylcholine), and vitamin D.

GETTING YOUR OMEGA-3S

WILD FATTY FISH (sardines, black cod, salmon, herring, mackerel, trout) are the most potent sources of omega-3s; eat at least two or three servings weekly. Plant sources — though less effective — include flax, hemp, and chia seeds (and the oils made from them), walnuts, purslane, and pasture-raised eggs. Omega-3 supplements can serve as backup and work best when taken daily, 1.5 to 5 grams of total EPA (eicosapentaenoic acid) and DHA (docosahexaenoic acid), which are the most efficiently utilized forms of omega-3s; taking them with some fatty food will help your body absorb them more efficiently and limit fishy burps. Most omega-3 supplements are some form of fish oil. Get a freshly made product from a quality manufacturer, store it in the fridge, and use it quickly. A strong fishy flavor or odor indicates rancidity. (Note that fish oil may interact with blood thinners.)

In one study, Swiss researchers found that eating eggs for breakfast improved overall cognitive performance (and promoted healthy body weight).

Low Sugar

Even though glucose is the brain's primary fuel, most of us eat too much sugar, which increases blood sugar levels, aggravates inflammation, and can worsen mood and brain health. Stick to low-glycemic foods and "slow burn" carbs from whole foods. See chapter 9 for more details.

Organic

Pesticide and herbicide residues are associated not just with poor memory and cognition but also with low acetylcholine levels, Alzheimer's disease, reduced brain processing speed, and lower IQ. They pose the greatest risk for children and the elderly. Key in on organic grains, dairy, and meat, and avoid the "dirty dozen" fruits and veggies (identified by the Environmental Working Group as the foods with the highest levels of pesticide and herbicide residues; see the EWG website for rankings).

Plenty of Antioxidants

Found in berries, veggies, beans, herbs, and spices — especially those with a vivid hue or flavorful aromatics — these compounds fight oxidative damage that can worsen brain function.

Pungent, Spicy Foods

Garlic, onions, hot peppers, and other pungent, spicy foods and herbs improve blood flow throughout the body, including the brain.

Lifestyle

When you exercise your body, you exercise your brain. No matter what your age or mental capacity, getting your body moving improves your brain function and adds years to your life span. Exercise stimulates your brain to produce more neurons, provides a positive challenge, and protects your neurons from damage. Going from couch potato to cardio king increases brain volume and nervous system well-being in just 6 months. Exercise also balances neurotransmitters such as serotonin, norepinephrine, and dopamine that play a role in mood as well as overall function. Numerous studies find a correlation between activity level and brain function in older adults. But you don't have to be old to reap the rewards—high schools that encouraged students to take morning fitness classes found that test scores also improved.

Exercise helps your brain produce more brain-derived neurotoxin factor (BDNF), which is like Miracle-Gro for your brain. BDNF boosts structural growth, creates new neurons, improves signal strength, and prevents damage, all of which can help with day-to-day function and reduce your risk of Alzheimer's. The more you change up your fitness routine, learn something new, or introduce more complicated exercises, the better the results.

Exercise is essential for a healthy brain (and body!), but here's another axiom to keep in mind: Use it or lose it. Using your brain — challenging it, testing it, learning with it — has been shown to prevent losses in memory and cognition. There are many, many ways to keep your brain actively engaged:

- Meditate
- Learn a new language
- Play an instrument
- Read
- Take up an art or craft
- Get some sun
- Spend time in nature
- Play
- Get some culture
- Improve your social connections
- Volunteer
- Spend time with animals
- Do crosswords, games, puzzles — mix it up!

Mind-Body Balance

The importance of mind-body balance in attaining and maintaining healthy memory and cognition becomes obvious when you realize that meditation is one of the best-researched brain-boosting "remedies" around. Likewise, while some of our brain tonics improve "hardware functioning" by averting damage (oxidation, inflammation) and allowing delivery of adequate nutrients and removal of waste (circulation), others work on a higher level to improve brain function. Nootropic, nervine, and adaptogenic herbs help revitalize neurotransmitter and nerve function, promoting a better state of mind.

Mint-Family Memory Tonics

Several common mint-family garden herbs help keep your brain young and improve memory and cognition. They notably inhibit acetylcholinesterase (AChE) — enemy number one in aging and Alzheimer's — and they also have circulation-enhancing, antioxidant, anti-inflammatory, mood-boosting properties. Work them into your daily routine as tea, tincture, or food.

- **Lemon balm.** Best known for its antianxiety and uplifting properties, lemon balm also improves the ability of acetylcholine — an important neurotransmitter that often declines as we age — to do its job. In one study, lemon balm improved cognitive performance and lengthened attention span. Improvements were seen in as little as one dose in 1 hour! And the higher the dose, the better the response. Use the fresh or recently dried herb for tea, or take a tincture. It blends well with holy basil, skullcap, bacopa, and milky oat seed, especially for improving attention while decreasing hyperactivity in children and adults. (For more on lemon balm, see page 59.)

CLEARING THE COBWEBS: WHAT DRAINS YOUR BRAIN

NO MATTER WHAT HERBS you take, also address the underlying cause of your brain fog. Here are some common cognitive pitfalls to sleuth out and address.

- Sleep deprivation (during sleep, your body cleans up metabolic wastes and toxins in the brain that would otherwise contribute to Alzheimer's disease and neurological disorders)
- Poor diet: dehydration, excessive sugar, food allergies/sensitivities, bad fats, lack of key nutrients such as vitamin B_{12}, omega-3s, or iron
- Lifestyle: sedentary behavior, smoking, heavy metal or toxin exposure
- Obesity
- Stress
- Menopause (stress and insomnia)
- Poor circulation to the brain
- Inflammation and oxidative damage
- Pharmaceutical drug side effects
- Diseases: attention deficit hyperactivity disorder, Alzheimer's and dementia, diabetes and insulin resistance, heart disease, arteriosclerosis, hypertension, hypo- or hyperthyroid, anemia, Lyme disease and coinfections

You may also support some of these underlying issues with herbs. For example, you can use adaptogens or nervines for stress, sedatives for insomnia, digestive herbs to support dietary changes, circulatory herbs, anti-inflammatory or antioxidant herbs, and so on.

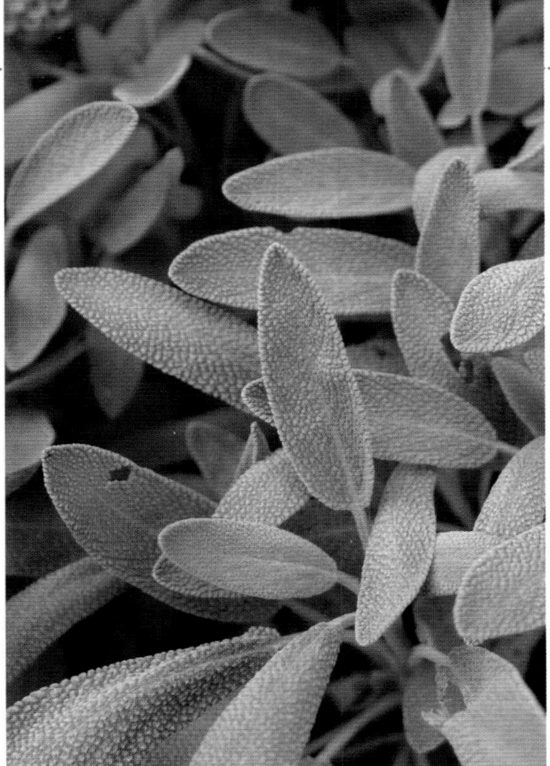

- **Sage.** Though perhaps better known as a seasoning for stuffing, sage potently inhibits AChE and has been shown to improve scores on word recall tests. Inhaling the aroma of Spanish or garden sage improves mood and cognition. Due to sage's thujone content, this herb is best used sparingly.
- **Rosemary.** In "seasoning" doses of around 750 mg, rosemary has been shown to improve memory recall speed in elderly patients. Simply inhaling the aroma of the herb or essential oil perks up the senses and significantly improves memory. High doses (around 6,000 mg) aren't necessary and may even dampen memory.
- **Spearmint.** Spearmint extract was shown in one study to boost memory and scores in cognitive tests designed to measure reasoning, attention, and planning, with some benefit seen within just 1 day. Attention and concentration scores more than doubled after 30 days, and reasoning scores improved dramatically, too.
- **Peppermint.** Peppermint essential oil, as aromatherapy, has been shown to improve many aspects of alertness and memory, including recall and reaction time.

Mint Memory Medley

Enjoy the invigorating internal and aromatherapeutic benefits of these herbs as you sip! Also play with chocolate mint, apple mint, holy basil, culinary basil, sage, and lemon balm.

- 1 teaspoon peppermint
- 1 teaspoon spearmint
- 1 sprig fresh rosemary, or ½ teaspoon dry
- 1 teaspoon honey (optional)

Combine the herbs. Pour 2 cups boiling water over the herbs and let steep, covered, for at least 10 minutes. Strain, sweeten with honey, if desired, and enjoy.

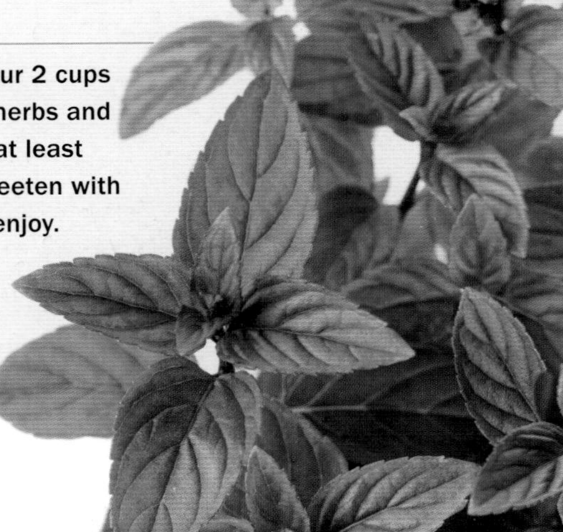

Circulation, Oxidation, *and* Inflammation

Your brain requires voluminous blood flow to function properly. Blood delivers essential nutrients, including oxygen and glucose; shuffles out waste; and transports hormones. Tiny blood vessels network throughout your brain, so microcirculation and the health and strength of those capillaries is crucial. Our cardiovascular tonics (see chapter 10), therefore, play a major role in preserving brain health.

Likewise, oxidation and inflammation really gum up the works, inhibiting blood flow and creating roadblocks in your neural roadways. Some damage may become obvious immediately, but long-term signs — including Alzheimer's and dementia — take decades to accumulate and are revealed only in your elder years, when it's more difficult to reverse the pattern. Scientists are just beginning to analyze inflammatory markers in the blood as early warning signs of cognitive damage and the risk of developing dementia. Most scientific research keys in on the use of nonsteroidal anti-inflammatory drugs (NSAIDs), but herbalism offers us promising, safer natural solutions. Diet, stress, sleep, and exercise have the most profound effects on inflammation and oxidation in your body; however, several herbs — like the nootropic gotu kola and ginkgo, profiled below — may also provide targeted care.

▸ Gotu Kola

Centella asiatica

Availability: G C

Key Properties: This Ayurvedic herb remains one of my favorites due to its impressive history of use in addition to a multitude of "side benefits" that apply to many. Indians have revered it as a memory and brain tonic for at least 2,500 years. Sanskrit texts claim that gotu kola juice will improve memory and intellect in just 1 week, and with long-term use, photographic memory and longer life span. Studies support gotu kola's ability to improve mood and cognitive function while decreasing anxiety in the elderly, and it also improves circulation and blood vessel integrity, as well as the body's ability to use glucose (the primary brain fuel) for energy when blood sugar levels are low. Indian children eat it when they go back to school.

Additional Benefits: Gotu kola also acts as a calm-energy adaptogen to relieve stress. It decreases anxiety without making you sleepy. It supports the health of connective tissues and the repair of tissue damage.

Preparation: Tea, tincture, capsule, juiced, powdered in smoothies, or as food. Standard herb doses (see page 298) apply. The leaves have a peppery flavor that easily blends with other herbs. Asian pennywort drink is made with this herb. Gotu kola and bacopa both go by the name *brahmi*, so when you're buying, check the Latin name to ensure you have the right herb.

Cautions and Considerations: Generally safe for all ages, but it shouldn't be used during pregnancy or nursing without supervision, may thin blood, and interacts with a few medications. Seek organic sources or grow your own; it naturally grows in sewage-sludgy conditions and can be contaminated with bacteria, including *E. coli.*

WHAT IS A NOOTROPIC?

Nootropics are "smart herbs" (or drugs) that improve memory, brain function, and intelligence.

General Uses: As brain tonics, these remedies help maintain and attain memory and cognitive ability while improving levels and function of neurotransmitters. Nootropics are typically reserved for brain concerns; however, they may also aid mental health and any condition that has a neural component.

Examples: Many Ayurvedic herbs work as nootropics, in particular bacopa, gotu kola, and holy basil, as well as rosemary, lavender, ginkgo, rhodiola, and, from the fungal world, reishi, lion's mane, and cordyceps. Nervines and stimulants may also have value.

Brain & Memory Support

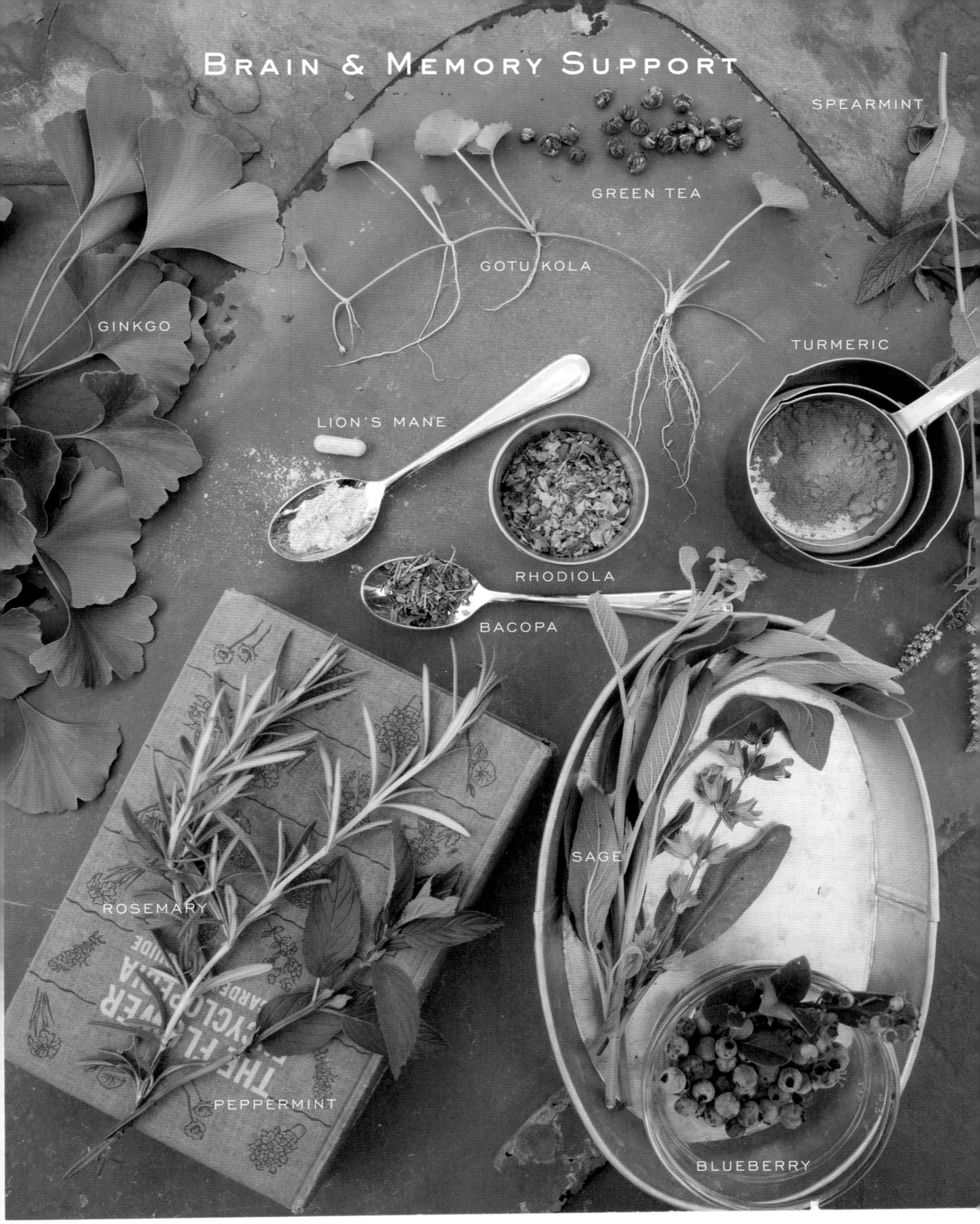

SPEARMINT

GREEN TEA

GOTU KOLA

GINKGO

TURMERIC

LION'S MANE

RHODIOLA

BACOPA

SAGE

ROSEMARY

PEPPERMINT

BLUEBERRY

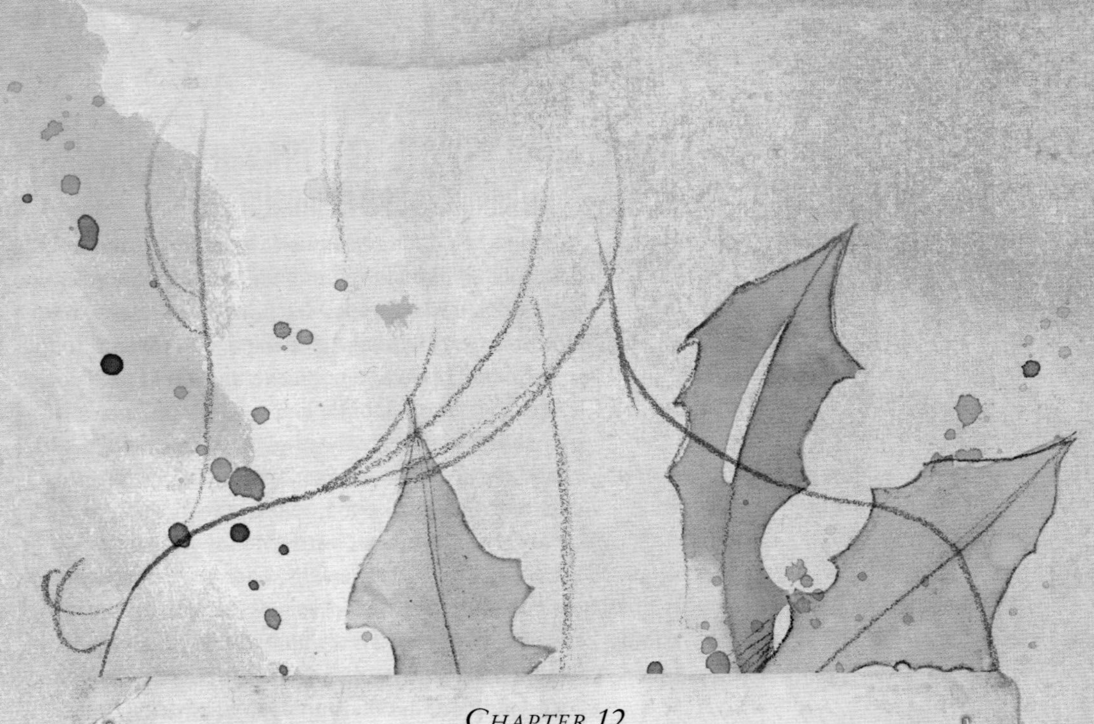

Chapter 12

Managing Pain: Listening to Your Taskmaster

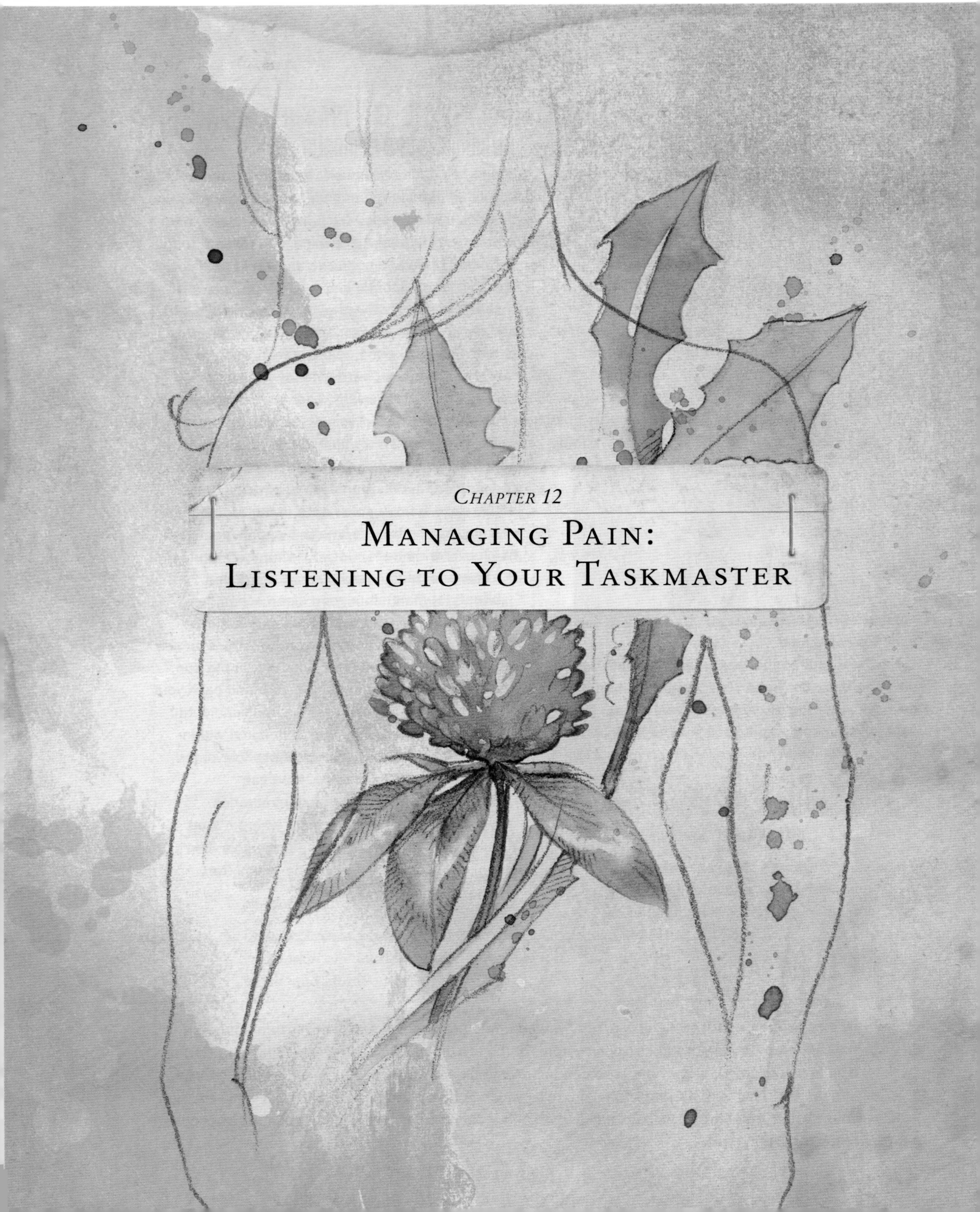

WHAT YOU PERCEIVE as "pain" is largely caused by inflammation. In your body, inflammation is a lot like fire. Short bursts of inflammation play an important role in your body's healthy functioning: drawing attention to a problem area, and telling you to give it a rest until the situation improves. In this way inflammation works to speed healing. Unfortunately, many factors common in the American lifestyle feed the fire, causing inflammation to flare up out of control, with potentially devastating effects. Excessive or long-term inflammation can ultimately damage tissue, impair function, and put you in a chronic state of pain. Many different compounds and signaling pathways elicit inflammation, including prostaglandins, cytokines, eicosanoids, and certain enzymes, including lipooxygenase (LOX), cyclooxygenase-1 (COX-1), and cyclooxygenase-2 (COX-2). When inflammation begins to get out of control, it can set off an inflammatory cascade, with each aspect of irritation initiating a new round of inflammatory response and unpleasant symptoms for you — not only pain but also, for example, an increased risk of heart disease and cancer and susceptibility to infections.

Conventional medicine is relatively good at turning down pain volume. NSAIDs (including ibuprofen, aspirin, and naproxen) decrease pain by inhibiting compounds that cause inflammation, such as COX-1, COX-2, and prostaglandins. This widespread action makes NSAIDs useful for almost any kind of pain — at least for a while. The body adapts quickly, however, producing more prostaglandins and causing an inflammatory rebound effect. Chronic users of NSAIDs often end up with worse and lingering pain compared to people who never used anything. NSAIDs also paradoxically increase inflammation in the gut, increasing the risk of reflux and ulcers. Prescription pain medications, including steroids and morphine-related drugs, work harder to stop the pain response; however, they come with a host of dangerous side effects and a risk of addiction.

Take a step back and ask — as we do with any health concern — *why* is this happening? Pain isn't really your enemy. It's a signal. Your body uses pain to tell you something is wrong. An injury or imbalance creates inflammation in your body, and your nerves communicate the pain to you, saying, "Stop. Rest. Let it heal, and change whatever you've done to create this issue in the first place."

Think of pain as a helpful taskmaster: it lets you know that work needs to be done to correct an imbalance. If you address the underlying cause holistically, you can often eliminate or drastically reduce pain with very little likelihood of side effects. In fact, you'll probably improve *other* areas of health as well, because that's how holistic medicine works!

Proper Diagnosis

When you're dealing with severe or chronic pain, it's always helpful to visit a practitioner to get a proper diagnosis. Knowing *why* you have pain will help you develop a targeted, more effective approach to dealing with it. You will also want to rule out more serious conditions like cancer or Lyme disease that may require additional medical care.

Conventional medications have such broad anti-inflammatory action that it may not really matter exactly what the underlying pattern or cause is in order for the medications to work. Herbs are a different story. We don't have *any* herbal analog for ibuprofen. Pain-relieving herbs are highly specific to the type of pain and the individual. Cramp bark might wipe out your menstrual cramps in minutes but do zip for your sister — or your headache.

The general anti-inflammatory lifestyle approach applies to almost anyone: eat an anti-inflammatory diet, avoid foods that irritate you, move regularly, sleep well, and reduce stress. Simply maintaining these core aspects of health will minimize or eliminate most chronic pain. However, the herbal approach will be much more specific to the person, and some trial and error may be needed to find what works. Knowing whether you have rheumatoid arthritis or osteoarthritis, cramps from a tilted uterus or from endometriosis, and the specific kind of headache you're experiencing matters. Sometimes, frustratingly, you never know the cause. But the more you do know, the easier it will be to find an herbal approach that helps.

Herbal Aspirins

Herbal "aspirins" are herbs that contain a variety of NSAID-like salicylate compounds that have an energetic cooling effect on hot, acute inflammation and are most appropriate for short-term use. They include the following:

- **Willow and meadowsweet.** The salicylic acid in willow bark and meadowsweet inspired the creation of pharmaceutical aspirin, and both herbs continue to be used as natural, weaker analgesic anti-inflammatories. Willow might upset the stomach, but meadowsweet is gentler, particularly the flowers. They're most often taken as tea or capsules. Meadowsweet has a pleasant wintergreen-cherry flavor, whereas willow tastes bitter, like chewing aspirin.
- **Wintergreen and birch.** Wintergreen leaves and birch bark contain methyl salicylate, which gives them their wintergreen scent and flavor. They are helpful as analgesics; however, methyl salicylate can be toxic in high doses, so reserve them for occasional use in low-modest doses, as just 5 to 10 percent of a pain formula, or topical applications.
- **Peony.** Certain species of peony root contain lesser amounts of methyl salicylate than wintergreen and birch and are more appropriate for regular use.
- **Poplar.** Poplar bud, a willow relative that contains salicin and populin, is often applied topically.

Note: If you're asthmatic or allergic to aspirin, avoid herbal aspirins to be safe. They may also interact with blood thinners and other medications.

KNOW YOUR TRIGGERS, AVOID INFLAMMATION

INFLAMMATION IS AN OVERRIDING theme in pain, but the underlying causes vary widely. When you stack up a variety of inflammatory factors, your risk of pain increases. The following unhealthy habits and conditions encourage inflammation in the body and can worsen pain. See if one or more of them is a trigger for you. By keeping them to a minimum, you can often achieve a dramatic reduction in pain and inflammatory disease symptoms.

- Injury and overwork
- Sleep deprivation
- Stress
- Lack of movement
- Inflammatory diet: high sugar, bad fats, food sensitivities, processed foods
- Foods from the nightshade family: potatoes, tomatoes, peppers, eggplant, et cetera (but only for some people)
- Blood sugar imbalance (too high or low)
- Caffeine withdrawal/fluctuations
- Nutrient deficiency (for example, magnesium, vitamin D, B vitamins, calcium)
- Bad posture or wrong pillow or mattress
- Autoimmune response
- Overloaded detox system
- Infection (from a simple cold to Lyme disease and lupus)

Topical Remedies

Consider slathering on these great herbs for both acute and chronic pain woes. They often work quickly.

- **Arnica.** Arnica can be applied topically (as an herbal or homeopathic preparation) and taken internally (in a 30C homeopathic potency or one drop of tincture) to prevent and resolve bumps, bruises, aches, and pains, particularly those resulting from trauma. It should not be applied to broken skin and is toxic internally in greater-than-homeopathic doses. If you want to make your own, arnica is possible (but tricky) to cultivate. You can make an infused oil or liniment with the local substitute **elder** leaves for topical use only; **comfrey** and **plantain** infused oils sometimes help, too.

- **St. John's wort oil.** This herbal oil, made by infusing the fresh buds and flowers in olive oil until it turns a deep red hue, is traditionally used for gentle yet fast relief for nerve pain and may even heal nerve damage when applied regularly over the long term. As a gentle yet profound wound-healing herb, it's fine for use on broken skin. Studies suggest it quickens repair and reduces scarring, though it may not be sufficient to treat infections. St. John's wort interacts with many medications, but this is unlikely when it is used topically. Learn more about St. John's wort on page 57.

- **Cayenne or capsaicin cream.** The cream, which you can obtain commercially or make yourself, relieves pain by depleting substance P, which transmits pain signals through the nervous system. Cayenne may also improve circulation and stimulate the body's natural anti-inflammatory response to the area, though it may sting or burn the first few times you apply it. Research supports its use for a range of pain, particularly osteoarthritis, nerve pain, and neuralgia. Don't apply it on broken skin, and keep it away from your eyes and genitals.

- **Peppermint.** Peppermint, along with menthol and camphor, has counterirritant, pain-relieving properties. Peppermint quickly relaxes tight muscle spasms, including headaches and gut pain. Use the essential oil, diluted in a carrier oil to avoid burning your skin.

- **Wintergreen and birch.** Being good sources of methyl salicylate, these two have fast-acting aspirin-like pain-relieving properties for headaches, muscle pain, and so on. Use the essential oil, making sure you dilute it well in a carrier oil because you can absorb methyl salicylate through the skin and large doses are toxic to the liver. Internal use of the essential oil is not recommended.

Acute Pain

Acute pain results from, say, accidentally hammering your thumb, or strenuous exercise that gives you sore muscles. Think of it as heat. Your body immediately responds to the trauma with localized swelling, inflammation, redness, and heat as it attempts to contain and repair the damage. Rest and a healthy body's innate ability to heal will usually get you up and running in a short amount of time. For more serious injuries like a sprained ankle, the traditional sports-medicine approach of compression and elevation, followed by a good balance of rest with gentle movement, encourages healing. Consider hot or cold packs, depending on what feels best — cold reduces inflammation but can also create stagnation and slow healing, while heat improves blood flow to the area, relaxes muscles, and speeds the healing response. For herbal and dietary support, consider simple anti-inflammatory herbs and foods, including herbal aspirins, turmeric, tart cherry juice, or bromelain (an enzyme found in pineapple).

If you're anticipating a long day of yard work or activity, taking a few preventive measures can prevent or lessen the risk of injury and acute pain. As you increase your level of activity, try to do it incrementally. Warm up and stretch first — this cuts your risk of injury in half. Be sure to stay hydrated and take electrolytes if you expect to sweat a lot. Rest when you need to. Ensure adequate calcium and magnesium intake before and afterward — powder packets that can be added to water work great, and nettle super infusions (naturally rich in calcium and magnesim) can also help. This gives your muscles the nutrients they need to contract and relax and can help prevent or treat post-exercise pain, aches, and spasms. Also consider taking turmeric or drinking tart cherry or pineapple juice before and afterward — both have documented anti-inflammatory effects.

Chronic Pain

In contrast to the swift, hot, localized action of acute pain, chronic pain tends to be cold and stagnant, with effects that wreak havoc throughout your body. Treating chronic pain generally takes time: months, maybe even years, to reverse the effects. It usually begins with general anti-inflammatory measures, followed by more targeted approaches based on the type of pain you're dealing with: muscle pain, nerve pain, joint pain, and so on. Often, it involves warming anti-inflammatory remedies, such as ginger, turmeric, cayenne, and cinnamon, which help break up congestion and bring blood flow and nourishment to repair stagnant, stiff areas.

Anyone who has successfully managed chronic pain will tell you their secret is hardly sexy: eat good food, avoid food irritants, keep moving, get enough sleep, rest when needed, and manage stress. Sure, almost *anyone* would benefit from such a routine, but the pain taskmaster is one of the best to keep people in line. People who successfully manage chronic pain become in tune with their bodies; once they bring things back into a good place, they are more aware and vigilant about maintaining a good lifestyle than perhaps anyone else.

FLOWER ESSENCES FOR PAIN

THESE HEAVILY DILUTED REMEDIES offer a gentle approach to healing and are believed to encourage the body to heal itself via energetic or vibrational (not biochemical) means. You can add a few drops of flower essences to your tincture blend or take them solo for pain patterns. Unlike some pain-relieving herbs, flower essences have no risk of herb-drug interactions and can easily be integrated into anyone's health plan. Here are a few of my faves:

- **Comfrey:** Deep healing; particularly when there has been serious or long-standing trauma, including brain injury or a car accident
- **Lavender:** Deep peace and calm spirit; for anxiety, stress, tight nerves, nerve pain, spiritual quandary, and related or concomitant pain; think of it for headaches, too
- **Valerian:** Deep calm; it's the energetic equivalent of the root medicine, for when people need to feel more grounded, be at peace, and sleep better in order to experience less pain
- **Blueberry:** Resilience; to help the body and mind bounce back from physical or emotional trauma more easily
- **Blue vervain:** Relax control; the energetic analogue to the tincture, useful for type A folks with tense necks, shoulders up to their ears, and headaches
- **Lilac:** Unburdened; for spine and back issues, to strengthen, straighten, and relieve the physical and emotional burden; especially think of it for the person with back pain that feels overwhelmed and overly depended on
- **Rescue Remedy or Five Flower Formula:** For trauma, shock, anxiety, panic, recent injury; think of them as the flower essence equivalent to homeopathic arnica

General Anti-inflammatory Support

When you're ready to undertake the journey back to a pain-free (or tolerable) life, take time to overhaul, focusing on your overall inflammatory state — again, as with most things, beginning with diet, lifestyle, and mind-body balance. Take huge strides or baby steps — whatever works best for you. Listen to your body as you go; it will educate and motivate you to do what's best for *you*. Start with simple steps that reduce your proclivity to inflammation, like eating whole foods, avoiding processed foods and sugar, figuring out whether you have food sensitivities and avoiding them, meditating, and going for regular walks or to yoga classes. Herbs and other natural remedies that combat inflammation in the body will make the transformation easier.

As you reduce your body's level of inflammation, you should start to notice improvements in your pain level and overall health over the following weeks and months. You might notice an overall reduction in pain or that acute episodes happen less frequently and pass more easily. It may come in waves — two steps forward, one step back — but should continue to improve over time.

The Anti-inflammatory Diet

This may be the single most effective tool you have to manage or eliminate chronic pain. You may notice some benefits immediately, but they will likely build over the course of a few months so that you feel dramatically better. Start with a balanced, whole-foods diet, keying in on these major areas:

- **Limit or avoid inflammatory foods.** They benefit no one. Sugar, white flour and simple carbs, trans fats and fried foods, excess alcohol, artificial and processed food. MSG (also look for "hydrolyzed" and "yeast extract" on labels) and artificial sweeteners often trigger the pain response. Excessive salt may also aggravate inflammation.
- **Avoid food allergens and sensitivities.** Though highly individualized, this makes a profound difference for many. Regularly consuming foods that don't agree with you can aggravate inflammation as well as autoimmune disease. Common culprits include wheat/gluten, dairy, soy, nightshade plants, corn, eggs, and coffee. Depending on your level of sensitivity, you may need to completely avoid them or simply stick to small, infrequent amounts. You don't need to avoid these foods unless they specifically bother you. Get an IgG food intolerance test (not always 100 percent accurate but handy) or try an elimination/rechallenge diet to sleuth out which foods, if any, you may not tolerate well. See page 84 for more details.
- **Balance meals.** Chronic blood sugar imbalance will catalyze inflammation. Keep blood sugar (and, hence, inflammation) in check by including protein, fats, and carbohydrates from whole foods whenever you eat. This also provides an array of amino acids, vitamins, minerals, and good fats so that your body can manufacture its own anti-inflammatory compounds and repair damage more efficiently. For more blood-sugar-balancing tips, see chapter 9.
- **Load up on veggies and fruit.** These plant foods contain potent anti-inflammatory compounds and important nutrients that decrease inflammation and help repair damage. Focus on a rainbow of veggies, berries, dark leafy greens, herbs, and spices. Look to whole-foods vegan, vegetarian, raw, Indian, Mediterranean, and Asian cuisine for anti-inflammatory recipe inspiration. Fill half your plate, or more!
- **Stay hydrated.** Water keeps the body functioning properly and makes it easier to eliminate waste and deliver nutrients. Dehydration can trigger a flare-up of many different kinds of pain issues.
- **Boost omega-3s.** Omega-3 fatty acids may be one of the most potent natural anti-inflammatories,

increasing your body's own anti-inflammatory compounds while inhibiting inflammatory compounds including 5-lipoxygenase (5-LOX), COX-2, cytokines, and certain prostaglandins. They also decrease the inflammation in and degradation of cartilage in osteoarthritis. See page 170 for a discussion of good omega-3 sources.

Mind-Body Approaches for Pain Relief

Relaxation techniques have a profound ability to reduce systemic inflammation, decrease pain, and improve overall vitality. They're also accessible to anyone, have great side *benefits*, and won't interact with medications.

- Deep breathing
- Meditation
- Sleep
- Yoga
- Tai chi
- Qigong
- Art therapy and music
- Regular, gentle exercise
- Time in nature

Anti-inflammatory Herbs and Remedies

Diet and lifestyle come first, of course, but herbs help along the way. Here are some of our most potent general anti-inflammatories that will jump-start the process and are safe to take long term, if needed. You might see some improvement within a week, but be patient: it often takes several weeks or months for the effects to build and become noticeable.

▸ Turmeric

Curcuma longa

Availability: G- C+

Key Properties: This traditional curry spice and its key constituent curcumin (a vivid yellow carotenoid) get a lot of attention for their superstar anti-inflammatory and antioxidant activity. Turmeric inhibits many inflammatory compounds, including COX-2, without the side effects associated with NSAID pain relievers. And it can relieve chronic pain, including rheumatoid arthritis and osteoarthritis.

Additional Benefits: It also thins the blood, improves circulation, prevents heart disease, fights cancer, alleviates depression, and improves digestion and liver detoxification. These effects build over time; give it at least a few months of regular use at a steady dose. Cultures that consume a lot of

ANTI-INFLAMMATORY FOODS

A WHOLE-FOODS DIET rich in vibrant plants and a rainbow of colors in general is ideal. Here are some anti-inflammatory superstars.

- Fish and seafood rich in omega-3s (see the list on page 170)
- Plants rich in omega-3s (see the list on page 170)
- Green and white teas
- Pineapple
- Cherries, especially tart
- Pomegranate
- Blueberries and bilberries
- Cranberries
- Other berries
- Turmeric and other spices
- Rosemary and other culinary herbs
- Ginger
- Garlic
- Mushrooms (cooked, or as broth or tea), especially reishi and chaga

turmeric in the diet — like those of India and Okinawa — have low rates of cancer and Alzheimer's.
Preparation: Capsules (standardized extracts or crude herb), following the dosage instructions on the product label. Aim for ¼ to ½ teaspoon of the ground root daily in food or smoothies. To tincture, high-proof alcohol works best: 95 percent for fresh root or 70 percent for dry. Though turmeric is not well absorbed in the gut, adding 1 to 2 percent black pepper in your formula boosts absorption 2,000 times. Heat also improves bioavailability. Rule of thumb: the brighter the color and stronger the stain, the more potent the medicine.
Cautions and Considerations: Turmeric (and, more often, black pepper) may aggravate reflux and acute ulcers and interact with blood thinners. Therapeutic doses aren't recommended during pregnancy without supervision. Turmeric's oxalic acid content may make regular use inappropriate if you have a tendency to develop kidney stones.

▸ Boswellia

Boswellia carteri, B. serrata
Availability: C
Key Properties: Also known as frankincense, this aromatic incense resin delivers potent and varied anti-inflammatory actions. Recent research lauds it as a safer alternative to NSAIDs for various types of chronic pain including rheumatoid arthritis and osteoarthritis, cluster headaches, and inflammation-based autoimmune diseases including inflammatory bowel disease. It specifically inhibits the inflammatory compound 5-LOX. One study found it effective for osteoarthritis pain in combination with ashwagandha and turmeric, and another found it as effective as an anti-inflammatory medication for osteoarthritis in the knee — taking slightly longer to have an effect but providing longer-lasting results.
Additional Benefits: Boswellia is primarily used as an anti-inflammatory aid in herbal medicine; however, like most plant resins, it also has antimicrobial and aromatic properties that have made it a popular incense. It's sticky and smells like a Catholic church (where it is burned as incense to create sacred space, bring prayers to heaven, and dispel negative energy).
Preparation: Most often taken as a capsule (follow the dosage instructions on the product label), though some people just swallow small resin nuggets. You can also tincture it, but you will need to use 95 percent alcohol (or as close to it as you can get) to effectively extract and stabilize it because resins repel water.
Cautions and Considerations: Generally safe. Boswellia may upset your stomach, so take it with food. Not recommended for use during pregnancy without supervision. Unfortunately, this biblical tree suffers from overharvesting due to incense and medicinal trade.

▸ Pineapple and Bromelain

Ananas comosus
Availability: C+
Key Properties: Bromelain, a protein-digesting enzyme from fresh pineapple, helps decrease inflammation thanks to its enzyme action. Enzymes break apart compounds, and in this case bromelain or pineapple taken on an empty stomach breaks down protein-based inflammatory compounds. They can be used for various types of inflammatory conditions including sprains, strains, tendonitis, rheumatoid arthritis and osteoarthritis, knee pain, and ulcerative colitis.
Additional Benefits: When taken on an empty stomach, bromelain also helps relieve sinus inflammation and seasonal allergy symptoms and is most often combined with the bioflavonoid quercetin. When taken with food, bromelain and pineapple help you digest protein-rich foods.
Preparation: Bromelain pills tend to be most helpful — follow the dosage instructions on the product label — but regular consumption of freshly juiced pineapple (include the core, where bromelain is concentrated) may also help.

Natural Anti-inflammatories

TART CHERRY JUICE

TURMERIC TINCTURE

PINEAPPLE (GOOD SOURCE OF BROMELAIN)

CINNAMON

HOLY BASIL

GINGER

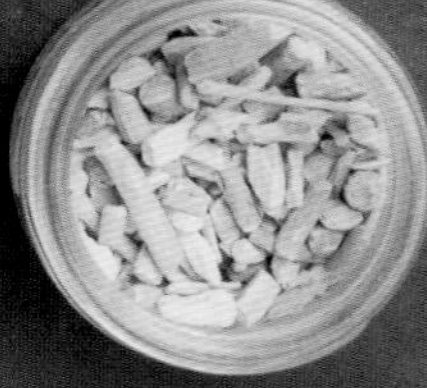

POMEGRANATE

ASHWAGANDHA

BOSWELLIA

Cautions and Considerations: Generally safe. They may interact with medications, particularly blood-thinning pharmaceuticals.

▸ Tart Cherry

Prunus cerasus

Availability: G C

Key Properties: All cherries and berries are antioxidant and anti-inflammatory powerhouses. The darker cherries — and particularly tart cherries — tend to be most beneficial. Tart cherries significantly decrease inflammation and have been shown to decrease the pain associated with working out and running races as well as gout, rheumatoid arthritis, and osteoarthritis.

Additional Benefits: They may decrease cancer risk, stroke risk, and age-related bone loss. Drinking cherry juice regularly also improves sleep and allays insomnia, possibly due to tart cherries' melatonin (sleep hormone) content.

Preparation: Drink two glasses of 100 percent tart cherry juice or two 1-ounce servings of cherry juice concentrate daily. Be sure to read the fine print on the ingredients list to ensure it hasn't been diluted with less beneficial juices. Tart cherry is also available in pill form; follow the dosage instructions on the product label.

Cautions and Considerations: Generally safe. Seek out organic sources when you can (they can be pricey); conventional cherries are often contaminated by pesticide residue.

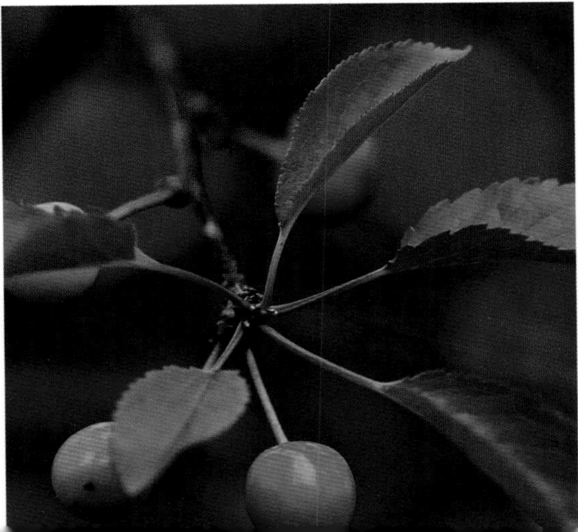

▸ Other Potent Anti-inflammatories

Ginger, turmeric's close relative and fellow COX-2 inhibitor, blends nicely with it and lends a warmer energy for cold, stagnant pain like arthritis. Though it may not be as potent an anti-inflammatory as turmeric, consider ginger if you have "cold signs" like poor, sluggish digestion and cold hands and feet. Drink it hot to amplify the effects (see a recipe on page 120) or take it in capsule form. Ginger makes a great synergist for "cold" folks in more complex formulas, though it may aggravate heartburn.

Fellow warm spice **cinnamon** sweetens the pot and also offers anti-inflammatory action (alongside digestive, astringent, antidiarrheal, and hypoglycemic effects). Steep a stick or two in a thermos for an hour — delicious!

Ashwagandha and **holy basil** (also called tulsi) are stress-relieving adaptogens with specific anti-inflammatory and calm-energy actions that can be particularly useful solo or in formulas for pain. Ashwagandha improves strength and vigor while nourishing the nerves and addressing autoimmune disease. It also gently supports and increases thyroid function. Studies show it works well for both types of arthritis, especially in combination with turmeric and boswellia. Holy basil inhibits COX-2, balances cortisol, and also gently modulates blood sugar, reduces sugar cravings, improves digestion, and helps protect your body from infection and other woes. It's often combined with fellow COX-2 inhibitors turmeric, ginger, rosemary, or green tea for pain. Both herbs are particularly helpful if you're stuck in the Bermuda triangle of mood-pain-stress. They can be taken in any form, but favorites include ashwagandha infused in milk (for a real treat, also add honey, cinnamon, cardamom, and nutmeg) and tulsi green tea. These herbs appear in almost every chapter of this book because they are so well tolerated and offer many benefits. Learn more about them on pages 50 and 53.

Muscle Pain: Muscle Relaxers *and* Antispasmodics

Many different pain issues stem from or include some kind of muscle pain, including sore and tender muscles, aches, and spasms. In some cases the muscles afflicted are skeletal; these are the muscles you generally have conscious control over, and tension, inflammation, and spasms here can lead to issues such as headaches and back pain. In other cases pain arises in smooth muscles, which are found in the digestive tract and reproductive organs, leading to various types of gastrointestinal pain (irritable bowel syndrome, inflammatory bowel disease) and menstrual cramps. Although certain herbs seem to work best for particular muscle types or pain conditions, you will also find many herbs and remedies that overlap a range of muscle pain issues. Antispasmodics and muscle relaxers really shine here.

Underlying causes and triggers for muscle pain include nutrient deficiency (especially magnesium, B vitamins, and calcium, which play a role in muscle contraction and relaxation, either due to a lack of intake or to poor absorption), injury, poor posture, the wrong mattress/pillow/chair, and lack of regular movement. Sleep issues — deprivation and a lack of deep sleep — are a significant trigger or cause of pain because muscles stay tense all night when they should be relaxed. Stress may also aggravate muscle tension and pain.

As we discussed earlier in this chapter, figuring out the root cause of pain is essential to breaking out of a pain pattern. Once you know what the problem is, you can address it directly and prevent future pain. In the meantime, to address muscle pain itself, there are a few herbs and remedies to try.

Magnesium Supplementation

Magnesium deficiency is common among people with muscle tension and related pain, including headaches, migraines, menstrual cramps, and muscle spasms. This important mineral performs hundreds of important roles in the body, one of which is helping muscles relax (calcium, the yang to its yin, helps muscles contract). You need B vitamins to properly absorb and utilize magnesium and vice versa. (Consider adding calcium if you anticipate physical exertion or notice bone aches, pain, or spasms after exercise or physical labor.) Generally powdered (to be mixed in water) or liquid magnesium supplements are most effective for preventing and treating muscle pain. Follow the dosage instructions on the product label. Our best food sources of magnesium include cacao, seeds, nuts, leafy greens, fish, beans, lentils, and whole grains. Poor nutrient absorption may also be a factor in magnesium, calcium, and B vitamin deficiency. Taking your supplements or food with bitters or a splash of vinegar can boost absorption, as will healing the gut in conditions like inflammatory bowel disorder and leaky gut. See chapter 5 for more on supporting digestive health.

Heat

Heat, in the form of hot water bottles, warm baths, and warm compresses, helps relax tight muscles and may improve the effects of massage, chiropractic adjustment, or pain-relieving herbs. Heat can aggravate acute inflammation, including inflamed nerves (cold would be better for this), so its appropriateness depends on the situation. Make a microwavable hot pack by filling a cloth (which could be as simple as a sock that you tie off at the end) with dry rice, buckwheat hulls, cherry pits, or similar material. Adding dry herbs or a few drops of essential oil makes it smell nice and may enhance its action. Microwave the pack in 30-second intervals to the desired temperature (beware of scalding). Apply to the area until the pack cools, approximately 20 to 30 minutes. The "hot" pack can also easily become a cold pack; just store it in the freezer.

Herbs

Although many herbs act as antispasmodics or muscle relaxers, I find the following plants most universally useful for various types of muscle pain.

▸ Blue Vervain and Wood Betony

Verbena hastata and *Stachys officinalis* (syn. *Betonica officinalis*)

Availability: G+ W C-

Key Properties: These beautiful yet bitter-tasting garden herbs provide relaxing, antispasmodic actions for tense muscles. They're not too sedating to take during the day yet also improve sleep and sleep-related pain. Both calm and nourish the nervous system. Blue vervain targets overly controlling, driven, type A personalities who have a lot of neck tension and headaches — just a few drops on the tongue may produce immediate results. Wood betony tends to be more general in its targets. Interestingly, most headache and muscle-relaxing herbs are bitter, which may be part of the therapy — grounding you, stimulating liver detoxification and digestion, and balancing blood sugar.

Additional Benefits: Both herbs boast a history of use as panaceas for almost any health condition even though they've not seen much use in recent years.

Preparation: Use aerial parts in flower. Most often taken as tinctures, these herbs are hard to find in stores but easy to grow. With good blending, wood betony makes a decent tea. Both of these herbs may work in low doses, just a few drops of tincture on the tongue, but can also be taken in standard doses (see page 298).

Cautions and Considerations: Generally safe but not appropriate during pregnancy. High doses (especially of blue vervain) can cause nausea. "Betony" may refer to wood betony or pedicularis, so check the Latin name — though they both help with pain, they're quite different and unrelated plants.

▸ Pedicularis

Pedicularis spp.

Availability: G- W- C-

Key Properties: It's among our best, safest herbs to relax skeletal muscles, highly effective for backaches, muscle twitches, and whole-body pain resulting from impact injury, like a car accident. It's usually not too sedating for daytime use and works quickly. Consider it as an adjunct to improve the effectiveness of bodywork, including massage and chiropractic care.

Additional Benefits: Pedicularis also relieves tension headaches, joint and muscle pain, sharp muscle spasms, sprains, and insomnia related to exhaustion and overexcitement.

Preparation: Use aerial parts. Most often taken as a fresh plant tincture, in standard herb doses (see page 298). Common names include betony, lousewort, and elephant's head. Unfortunately, you're unlikely to find it in any store because the big brands don't sell it. Pedicularis grows most abundantly along the Rockies and on the West Coast. Look to small-scale, skilled product makers if you don't have a stand to ethically wildcraft.

Cautions and Considerations: Pedicularis itself is quite safe, though little safety data is available. Be aware of what it grows near (and if those plants are safe) because this semiparasitic plant can take on compounds from its host plant (including toxic aconite and senecio). It is an endangered or at-risk herb in some areas. Consider cultivating it among yarrow in the garden.

▸ Other Herbs to Relieve Muscle Pain

Pain-relieving, muscle-relaxing herbs that also have a sedative action include **valerian, skullcap, passionflower, hops, California poppy, kava,** and **holy basil.** Depending on the herb and your sensitivity level, their sedative action can make you groggy if you take them during the day. They're superb for sleep-pain formulas. Other beneficial antispasmodic herbs include peppermint, cramp bark or black haw, and ginger.

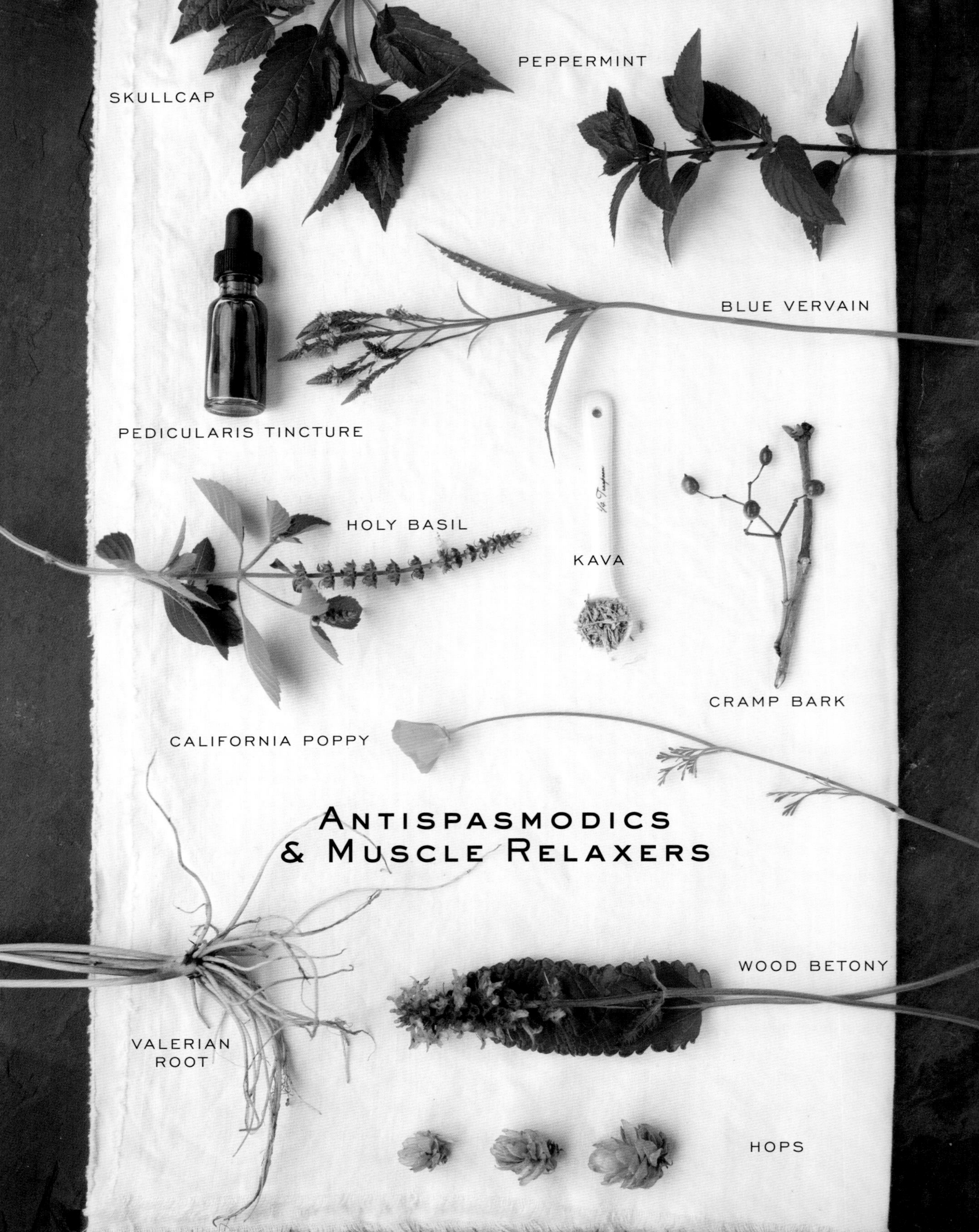

Antispasmodics & Muscle Relaxers

PROTOCOL POINTS

Headaches and Migraines

When it comes to the triggers and best remedies for headaches and migraines, the answers vary widely depending on the exact type of headache as well as the individual person. You may need some detective skills and trial and error to find the solution to your particular headache problem, but it's worth the effort.

Diet: When a headache comes on, do you feel like you've been suddenly hit by a Mack truck? Have you noticed that your headaches come in cycles? These are possible signs that your headaches are related to a food sensitivity. Sleuth out any dietary triggers, which vary widely from person to person but can include shellfish, red wine, chocolate, gluten, dairy, and blood sugar highs or lows. Dehydration, magnesium/B vitamin deficiency (common for headaches and migraines), and caffeine withdrawal or fluctuation (which can take a few days to kick in) can also be triggers.

Lifestyle: Nonfood triggers can include stress, poor posture, poor sleep habits, ill-fitting pillow or mattress (tension headaches and neck/back pain), mold, dust, animals (sinus headaches), the need for glasses, drug side effects, and NSAID rebound. Make sure to get enough good-quality sleep and consider meditation or breathwork for stress reduction. Bodywork, regular exercise, stretching, physical therapy, and chiropractic care can work wonders for headaches related to tight muscles and structural imbalances.

Herbs and Supplements: Magnesium, with B vitamins, should be the first thing you try. These nutrients can prevent, treat, and even allay oncoming migraines and other forms of muscle tension and pain.

All the muscle-relaxing herbs can help, particularly blue vervain (for the control-freak headache with neck pain), wood betony, and pedicularis. Butterbur root contains compounds that relax blood vessels and smooth muscles while zapping inflammation. Use Petadolex or a similar butterbur extract specially processed to remove liver-toxic pyrrolizidine alkaloids (PAs). Clinical studies support Petadolex for migraines, asthma, and seasonal allergies, even for children as young as 6. This herb can be phenomenally effective for preventing and treating migraines in particular, sometimes better than pharmaceuticals. PA-free butterbur is quite safe and unlikely to interact with medications; however, it makes some folks (myself included) feel sick to their stomach.

Feverfew, the best-known migraine prevention herb, reduces inflammation by inhibiting eicosanoids, leukocytes, and platelet aggregation and also decreases blood vessel constriction that can trigger migraines. In the 1970s, an ad in a British newspaper sought people who had successfully used the herb for headaches; they received more than 25,000 positive responses! Feverfew slowly shows its full benefit over weeks and months, so be patient. Take it as a tincture or capsule, or eat two to four fresh leaves a day; however, some people get mouth ulcers when they take it as a liquid or chew the leaves. It's not an issue with capsules.

Clematis is specific for cluster headaches. And just 250 mg of encapsulated ginger, taken at the onset of a headache or migraine, works as well as triptan drugs for reducing the severity of the headache, without the side effects.

Nerve Pain

Nerve pain can be a component of many types of pain patterns, including sciatica, carpal tunnel syndrome, injury, or more complex issues, including Lyme disease and multiple sclerosis. The approach you take will depend on your particular situation.

Triggers include inflammation, stress, misalignment of joints or bones so that they pinch or damage nerves, injury, repetitive use, poor posture/ergonomics, and lack of proper nervous system nourishment — particularly good fats and B vitamins. Caffeine, especially in coffee, aggravates sensitive nerves and can increase pain and overall symptoms, including anxiety, insomnia, and tremors.

Holistically, look to healing nerve damage and soothing nervous system malfunction more than simply numbing the pain response. The following herbs and supplements can help.

- **Omega-3s and good fats.** Omega-3 fatty acids and healthy fats slowly relieve nerve pain via a two-pronged approach. First, they have widespread anti-inflammatory action in the body. Second, they are a critical component of the lining of all the cells in your body, including the myelin sheath that protects the nerves. Having enough good fats in your diet improves nervous system function and nerve transmission. Be sure the diet limits or avoids bad fats. See the discussion of the anti-inflammatory diet (page 187) for more information about good fats and other tips to reduce chronic inflammation through your food choices.

- **St. John's wort.** It might surprise you to know that St. John's wort is historically better known as a nerve tonic and pain remedy than an antidepressant. It's one of the safest and most effective topical pain remedies — as an oil, salve, or liniment. Consider it for any kind of nerve pain that you can pinpoint, including postinjury care (use once the wound has closed; it also improves wound healing and prevents scarring), sciatica, and shingles. Long-term use may heal and regenerate the nerves. It sometimes helps other types of pain, too. The internal use is less common for pain; however, herbalist David Winston uses it in formula with bacopa, ginkgo, and holy basil for brain injuries. The serotonin-boosting, neurotransmitter-balancing effect of St. John's wort may also relieve pain that has a mood connection, including fibromyalgia. It's the same reason that doctors prescribe antidepressants for pain. Internal use of St. John's wort is contraindicated with most medications (and in rare cases it causes photosensitivity), but topical use should be fine. For more on St. John's wort, see page 57.

- **Lion's mane.** This mushroom (*Hericium erinaceus*) stimulates nerve growth, potentially heals nerve damage, improves cognition, and fights dementia, Alzheimer's, and other types of cognitive diseases. In traditional Chinese medicine, the mushroom is used for weak nerves and general debility and fatigue. Studies show that lion's mane stimulates nerve growth factor, helps generate myelin, and has an affinity for the brain. The mushroom may be best taken long term. Herbalists currently use this mushroom as a tincture or capsule for clients with nerve damage with impressive results, and they have seen similar results with related species (*H. coralloides* and *H. americanum*), although they have not been studied. Learn more about lion's mane on page 178.

- **Calm-energy adaptogens.** Some of the calming adaptogens have a particular affinity for soothing nerve pain while supporting overall well-being. They include gotu kola, bacopa, ashwagandha, and holy basil. Consider them for your pain formula and daily tea. See chapter 3 for more on these adaptogens.

- **Topical cayenne.** Topical cayenne or capsaicin cream specifically relieves nerve pain by depleting the neurotransmitter substance P, which transmits pain signals through the nervous system. Research supports its use for a range of pain, including nerve pain and neuralgia. Learn more on page 185.

PROTOCOL POINTS

Fibromyalgia

This complex and debilitating condition generally requires a whole-body approach to wellness.

Diet: Focus on an anti-inflammatory diet (see page 187), and sleuth out any potential food sensitivities. Gut dysbiosis may also be a factor (see page 89). If you're overweight, do your best to maintain a healthier weight.

Lifestyle: Make sufficient deep sleep and regular movement your top priorities! Use herbal sleep aids if you need to, and slowly work your way into mild to moderate exercise that suits you. Consider walking, swimming, yoga, or tai chi. Also consider bodywork, both for direct pain relief and the healing benefits of touch.

Herbs: Diet and lifestyle play the biggest roles in fibromyalgia, but specific herbs include those with a stress-mood component (gotu kola, ashwagandha, holy basil), as well as nutmeg and general anti-inflammatory herbs (turmeric, ginger, tart cherry).

Sciatica

Sciatica is one of the most common types of nerve pain. Structural damage or pinching causes inflammation of the sciatic nerve and pain radiating down the back of the buttocks, hip, and leg.

Diet: Focus on an anti-inflammatory diet (see page 187), including omega-3s and anti-inflammatory superfoods like turmeric, tart cherry, and pineapple. Mineral deficiencies — especially lack of magnesium, B vitamins, calcium, and vitamin D — may worsen the pain during exertion. Try supplements or high-nutrient foods like nettle super infusion, leafy greens, nuts, seeds, and high-quality dairy.

Lifestyle: Figure out whether specific activities aggravate your sciatica, such as awkward sitting positions and activities that involve bending over, like cleaning, gardening, and performing certain job-related tasks. There may be a herniated disc in the back or bone spurs along the spine. Rest, physical therapy, ergonomics, regular exercise and stretching, and bodywork like chiropractic would be the primary holistic therapies.

Herbs: Combine anti-inflammatory herbs (turmeric, tart cherry, boswellia, ashwagandha, holy basil) with nerve-pain tonics (skullcap, blue vervain). Try St. John's wort oil or liniment, which often provides immediate relief and lasting effects with long-term use.

Carpal Tunnel Syndrome

Carpal tunnel syndrome occurs when the median nerve running into your hand gets pinched or squeezed, which can cause numbness, tingling, and pain. It can be caused or aggravated by a congenital predisposition, injury, poor ergonomics, or other conditions that aggravate inflammation. Of all remedies, start with vitamin B_6, which sometimes completely alleviates the issue. In extreme and nonresponsive situations, surgery may be warranted.

Diet: Consider a general anti-inflammatory diet; see page 187 for details.

Lifestyle: Much like sciatica, carpal tunnel is a common form of nerve pain and inflammation due to a pinched nerve. The approach would be similar to that for sciatica (see above), but targeted to the wrist.

Supplements: Vitamin B_6 supplementation tends to be surprisingly helpful for relieving symptoms. You can also try the herbs and foods recommended for sciatica.

Painful Joints *and* Cartilage Degradation

Joint inflammation and structural damage to the cartilage that cushions the joints are key components of many types of pain, most notably osteoarthritis. Underlying causes include past injury, repetitive use, structural misalignment, systemic inflammation, family history, and other factors, and the usual inflammatory triggers are often at play. As cartilage breaks down, bones begin to rub against each other, causing inflammation, swelling, pain, and sometimes deformation of the joints. Circulation to the cartilage is poor. Once cartilage is damaged, it's slow and difficult (but not necessarily impossible) to repair.

Diet and Lifestyle

If you're suffering from joint pain, one of the best things you can do — as early as possible — is to regularly practice some form of gentle, low-impact movement such as walking, yoga, tai chi, or swimming. This stimulates your body to produce joint-lubricating compounds, relieves stiffness, and improves circulation to the area. This makes it easier for your body to remove inflammatory waste products and bring in the nutrients and compounds needed to gradually repair damage. You may need to rest during a flare-up, but chronic inactivity quickly accelerates the progression of disease and debility.

An anti-inflammatory diet and lifestyle are also important components of a holistic therapy plan; see page 187. Consider also the general anti-inflammatory herbs and remedies previously mentioned.

Supplements

Although anti-inflammatory herbs are certainly helpful, many of the remedies that best target cartilage-related pain are animal-based cartilage-like compounds.

- **Glucosamine and chondroitin.** These supplements are components in cartilage that decrease inflammation over the course of a few months and may slowly — over years — encourage cartilage repair. They first became popular as holistic veterinary remedies for pets and horses. Owners were impressed by how well their animals improved and began taking the supplements themselves. Research is promising, though conflicting, and anecdotal evidence suggests they work well for many people. Give them 2 or 3 months at the recommended dose (1,500 mg glucosamine and 1,200 mg chondroitin, divided into doses throughout the day) to see if they work for you. Bone broth made with cartilage-rich bones like beef knuckles and chicken feet tends to contain glucosamine and chondroitin as well as gelatin and collagen; consider taking 1 to 3 cups daily plain or in recipes. (For instructions on making bone broth, see page 42.)

- **MSM.** This sulfur compound, more properly known as methylsulfonylmethane, offers widespread anti-inflammatory action that may help with rheumatoid arthritis and osteoarthritis, as well as other types of pain and inflammation, by decreasing pain and improving range of movement. Research is somewhat limited, but many people report good results, sometimes more quickly than with glucosamine and chondroitin.

- **Hyaluronic acid.** Often touted as an antiaging miracle, hyaluronic acid is found throughout the body (in synovial fluid around joints, skin, brain) and has a lubricating, toning property, keeping your body supple, cushioned, stretchy, and functioning smoothly. As a supplement, it's extracted from rooster combs or made in a lab. It works quickly to relieve pain, decrease inflammation, and repair joint damage. Hyaluronic acid drew attention when researchers studied the people of Yuzari Hara for their antiaging secrets. This Japanese community's unique lifestyle and reliance on potato-like crops rich in hyaluronic acid seemed to help them live longer and with a much lower incidence of Alzheimer's, pain, and disease, while staying limber and looking young. The FDA has approved hyaluronic acid injections for targeted osteoarthritis relief. For self-treatment, take it as a dietary supplement.

PROTOCOL POINTS

Rheumatoid Arthritis and Osteoarthritis

Both of these common forms of arthritis are characterized by painful, stiff joints and chronic inflammation, which worsens over time and can become debilitating. However, they have different underlying causes and patterns, and the treatment approach — especially with conventional medications — varies. Osteoarthritis is caused by the physical wear and tear on joints and joint tissue, including cartilage. In rheumatoid arthritis, an autoimmune response causes the body to attack the tissue in the joints. In rheumatoid arthritis, we're more apt to see a sudden onset, possibly at an earlier age, with more swelling, and similar pain on both sides of the body. Stiffness often lasts longer, and you're more apt to feel fatigued throughout the day. Osteoarthritis often starts on one side of the body and may eventually migrate to both sides. Weight gain is a common aggravating factor, and you'll see more issues with weight-bearing joints like the knees, hip, and spine.

General Holistic Approach: Even though the pharmaceutical approach is very different for the two conditions, there's a lot of overlap among holistic and herbal remedies. Diet, lifestyle, omega-3s, and anti-inflammatory herbs like turmeric, boswellia, ashwagandha, and cherry juice tend to be equally beneficial for both types of arthritis.

Targeted Approaches: With osteoarthritis, use tissue/cartilage-supportive remedies like glucosamine and chondroitin, and address issues like weight gain and structural misalignments. For rheumatoid arthritis, it's important to address the underlying autoimmune issue alongside the anti-inflammatory support. The diet piece can be dramatic, particularly if you can avoid gluten, sugar, nightshade plants, and other common causes of food sensitivities and allergies, which are often at play in haywire immune responses. Enhancing the detoxification channels with diet and herbs also helps relieve rheumatoid arthritis and chronic pain associated with an autoimmune response or low-level infection, like Lyme disease.

GIN RAISINS

THIS OLD-TIME HOME REMEDY for arthritis pain and stiffness boasts next to no research, but it's worth a shot! Fill a jar approximately halfway with golden raisins, cover amply with gin, and drape a cloth over the top of the jar. Let sit for 2 weeks on the kitchen counter. You'll see some bubbles. If the alcohol evaporates below the raisins, add a bit more. After 2 weeks, seal the jar with a lid. Store at room temperature; so long as the gin covers the raisins, they'll last almost indefinitely. Eat 1 teaspoon of gin-soaked raisins daily, for example in cereal or on salad.

The benefits may be related to the healing properties of the juniper (an anti-inflammatory detox herb) in gin, the antioxidants in grapes, or the anti-inflammatory effects of the sulfur dioxide used to keep golden Thompson raisins pretty (although I get good results with organic unsulfured raisins, too). It may also be the complex polysaccharides in the grapes; polysaccharides are complex sugar compounds that may have pain-relieving, anti-inflammatory properties that help cushion and repair the joints. Whatever it is, people usually see improved mobility and decreased pain within a few weeks, so (as long as you tolerate raisins and gin) why not try it? We make gin raisins in my chronic pain classes, and students report back that it helps both rheumatoid arthritis and osteoarthritis, as well as frozen shoulder and other issues.

Other Chronic Pain Patterns

Although inflammation, muscle tension and spasms, nerve pain, and joint/cartilage degradation form the basis of most Americans' chronic pain issues, other patterns may also be at play.

The Detox Connection

Low-level toxicity often coincides with Lyme disease, rheumatoid arthritis, and other autoimmune- and infection-based forms of chronic pain. The body becomes overburdened with day-to-day toxins and the accumulation of metabolic waste increases inflammation and immune problems. In the ancient healing art of Ayurveda, arthritis and a variety of other inflammation-based conditions (eczema, psoriasis, cysts, cholesterol, heart disease, et cetera) are caused by a buildup of *ama* or metabolic waste. Herbs that support more efficient removal of waste — including turmeric, burdock, dandelion, and schizandra — may be helpful as part of your formula. See chapter 6 for more about these detox herbs.

Diet is also a phenomenal asset to boost detoxification and eliminate *ama*. Studies suggest that periodic short fasts (water only or vegetable and fruit juice fasts) offset or reduce the likelihood of a rheumatoid arthritis flare-up. Fasting is not appropriate for everyone; work with your health practitioner to determine if it's safe for you. Eating a whole-foods vegetarian or vegan diet also reduces inflammatory markers and flare-ups, at least in part because these diets reduce metabolic waste and provide ample antioxidant and anti-inflammatory compounds while boosting the body's natural detoxification response. Raw diets can also help, though they may be too cold for some individuals, are difficult to digest, and may increase the likelihood of developing select nutrient deficiencies (B_{12}, iron, vitamin D, omega-3s) over the long haul; the nutrients in some foods are better absorbed after they are cooked.

Tendon and Ligament Support

Tendons and ligaments are fibrous connective tissue that hold the skeletal and muscular systems together, connecting bone to muscle (tendon) or bone to bone (ligament). Injuries of these tissues — in the form of sprains, strains, and tears — can be acute or chronic because they heal slowly and are easily reinjured once they've weakened. New research suggests that the conventional RICE protocol (rest, ice, compression, elevation) may actually delay the body's natural healing response, and its proponents advocate for heat, movement, elevation, and traction instead. While the experts debate, I recommend listening to your body to see what feels right for you. But you can support either approach with massage, bodywork, physical therapy, and a diet rich in the nutrients and herbs that enhance connective tissue repair and health (see page 187). Natural anti-inflammatories like turmeric, tart cherry, and bromelain may better support the healing response than NSAIDs because they work with — rather than against — the body's healing response.

Certain herbs specifically target and tone tendons and ligaments while decreasing pain and improving healing. Thank modern herbalists Matthew Wood, Jim McDonald, and Kiva Rose for reigniting interest in these lesser-known plants. True Solomon's seal root, just a few drops or a squirt of tincture a few times a day, keeps connective tissues supple and aids those that are too tight, too loose, or damaged; chronic tendonitis slowly disappears, sprains heal more quickly, et cetera. It's quite remarkable and can also be used topically. There are no known side effects. Mullein root encourages proper joint alignment, helps heal sprains, relieves tendon and ligament pain, and improves muscle tone. Horsetail tincture may improve the healing of broken bones. And pleurisy root helps warm frozen shoulder and other joints, allowing them to move more freely and regain function.

The Immune Connection

Many of our most difficult-to-treat forms of chronic pain involve the immune system. For instance, the pain associated with autoimmune conditions, such as rheumatoid arthritis, lupus, inflammatory bowel disease, celiac disease, multiple sclerosis, and myasthenia gravis, may be caused by the inflammation and tissue damage that occurs when the immune system attacks a specific area of the body. Sometimes the pain is associated with a specific, complex infection — such as chronic fatigue syndrome, lupus, or Lyme disease and its coinfections — that aggravate inflammation and confound and derange your immune system. Start with the general approach to chronic pain: diet, lifestyle, anti-inflammatory herbs. Mind-body balance, adequate rest and relaxation, and the elimination of aggravating foods are also essential. Improving detoxification channels can help prevent metabolic waste buildup that increases inflammation, pain, and disease. You'll also want to include components that specifically modulate and strengthen the immune system without making it overreactive and causing a flare-up. This may not cure the condition, but it should significantly improve pain and disease management.

Medicinal mushrooms shine as food and medicine to encourage a healthy immune response. Some like chaga and reishi also have specific anti-inflammatory actions and may also fight infections directly. Include edible medicinals in your cooking repertoire — shiitake, maitake, enoki, lion's mane, oyster, et cetera. The medicinals (even those that are too tough to eat, like chaga and reishi) can be simmered into soup broth, tea, or double-extraction tinctures. Certain herbs also support and modulate the immune system in similar ways, especially astragalus, ashwagandha, and schizandra, all of which you can take in any form. Turmeric, ginger, and holy basil will play a supportive role.

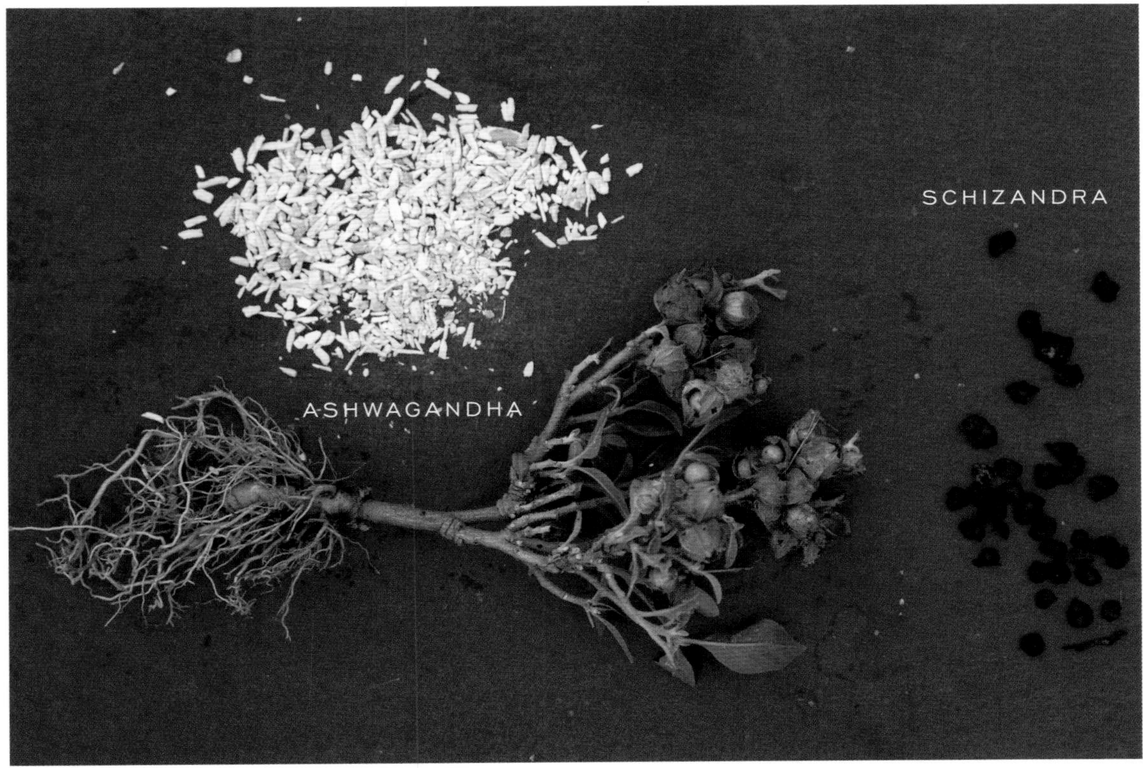

AT A GLANCE

Herbs for Pain Management

The herbs listed here are grouped by their beneficial action for chronic and acute pain, with my favorite, most effective, safest, and most common herbs listed first.

Natural COX-2 Inhibitors

- Turmeric
- Ginger
- Hops
- Baikal skullcap
- Holy basil
- Green/white tea
- Rosemary

Natural Aspirins and Opiates

- Willow bark*
- Meadowsweet
- Black birch/wintergreen*
- Peony root
- California poppy

Other Natural Anti-inflammatories

- Boswellia
- Bromelain and protein enzymes
- Anti-inflammatory diet
- Omega-3s and GLA
- Ashwaghanda
- Cherry fruit (especially tart)
- Yucca
- Bunchberry leaf

Antispasmodics

- Wild yam
- Peppermint
- Cramp bark

Muscle Relaxers and CNS Sedatives

- Magnesium (with B vitamins)
- Hops
- Valerian
- Jamaican dogwood*
- Pedicularis
- Kava*
- Passionflower
- Wood betony
- Blue vervain
- Skullcap

Warming and "Juicy" Herbs**

- Ginger
- Pleurisy root
- Prickly ash
- Cayenne

Remedies to Repair Joints/Tendons/Ligaments

- Bone broth
- Gelatin
- Collagen
- Glucosamine
- Chondroitin
- Hyaluronic acid
- MSM
- Vitamin C
- B vitamins (especially B_6)
- Gotu kola
- Gin raisins
- Solomon's seal root
- Mullein root
- Horsetail

Herbs to Relieve Nerve Pain

- St. John's wort (topically and internally*)
- Skullcap
- Blue vervain
- Wood betony
- Lion's mane mushroom

Topical Counterirritants

- Cayenne (capsaicin)
- Peppermint (menthol)
- Camphor
- Essential oils of peppermint, juniper, wintergreen, rosemary, eucalyptus

Other Topical Remedies

- St. John's wort oil
- Arnica oil/cream
- Dandelion flower oil
- Elder leaf oil

Natural Antihistamines

- Butterbur
- Quercetin
- Citrus bioflavonoids
- Grape seed and skin extract (OPCs/PCOs)
- Pycnogenol
- Bromelain

Herbs to Improve Circulation (Lymph and Vascular)

- Feverfew
- Clematis
- Cayenne
- Horse chestnut*
- Gotu kola
- Red root

Serotonin Boosters

- St. John's wort*
- 5-HTP
- Tryptophan

Energy Connection: Adaptogens

- Asian and American ginseng
- Eleuthero
- Rhodiola
- Gotu kola
- Schizandra
- Reishi, cordyceps, other medicinal mushrooms
- Holy basil
- Ashwagandha

Autoimmune Connection: Immune Supports

- Medicinal mushrooms
- Astragalus
- Schizandra
- Ashwagandha
- Detoxification/fasting

Detoxification Connection: Detox Support

- Diuretics (dandelion, parsley, nettle, celery, cornsilk)
- Turmeric
- Guggul
- Triphala
- Magnesium (high doses)
- Milk thistle
- Schizandra
- Ginger
- Lemon
- Fermented foods
- Raw foods, broths, juicing
- Vegetarian/vegan diet
- Fasting
- Low-glycemic/low-carb diet

**Be particularly aware of cautions before using plants marked with an asterisk.*

***Consider for cold, stagnant, frozen pain issues or as a formula synergist.*

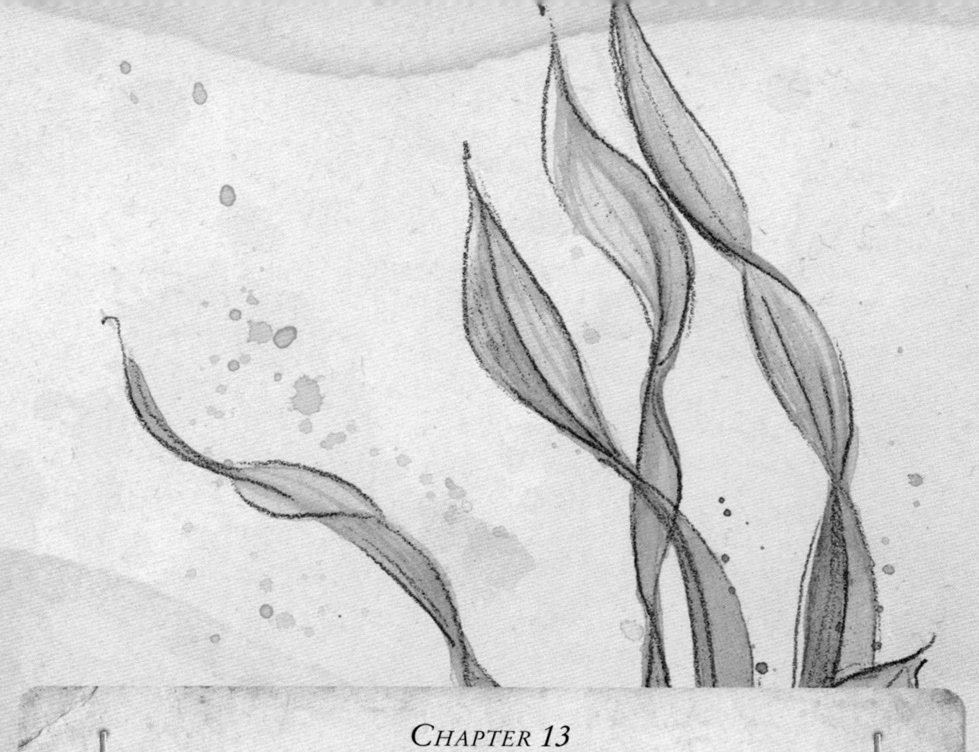

Chapter 13

The Thyroid: Butterfly in Balance

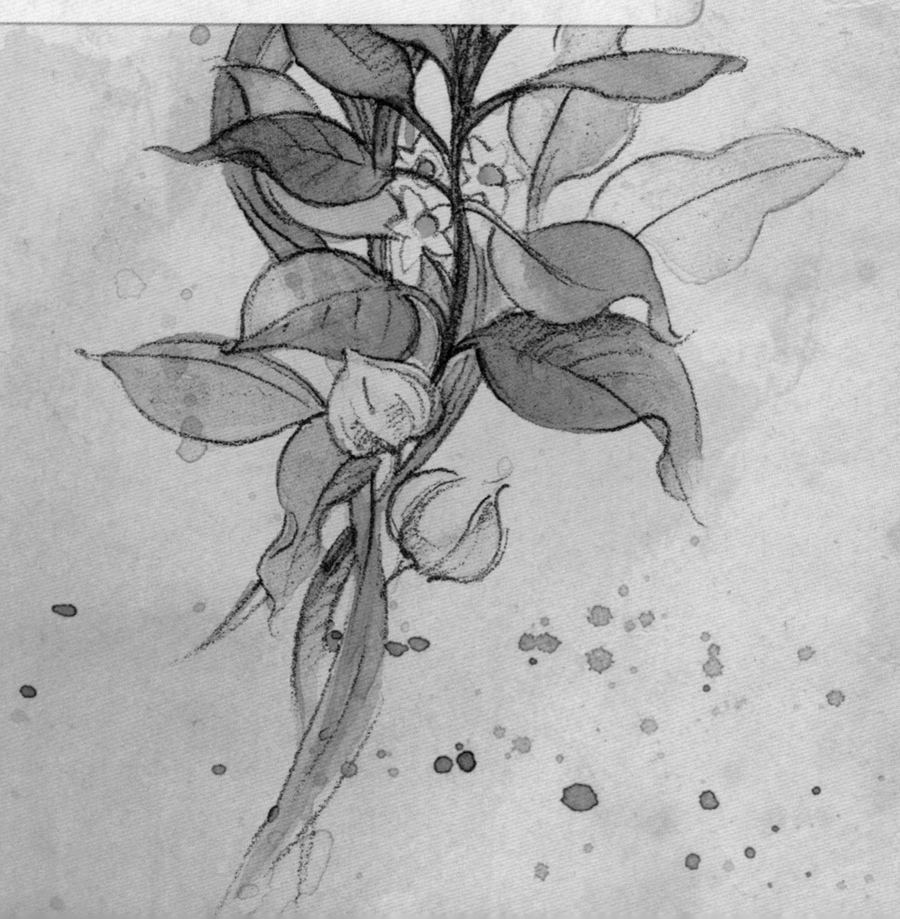

YOU PROBABLY DON'T think much about your thyroid gland. Most of us take it for granted. This butterfly-shaped endocrine gland rests at the base of the front of your neck and regulates the speed at which *everything* happens. It strives to keep the pace of your body in balance with the perceived demands of your day. And you certainly feel *out* of balance when it's not functioning properly, even if you can't exactly place what's wrong.

In typical hormone relay-race style, thyroid signals begin in your brain. Your pituitary gland sends thyroid-stimulating hormone (TSH) down to your thyroid to tell it when to produce more thyroid hormones. Using the amino acid tyrosine in conjunction with the mineral iodine, your thyroid then builds thyroid hormones in the form of thyroxine (T4) and triiodothyronine (T3). These thyroid hormones, especially T3, regulate your metabolism. T3 is sometimes referred to as "active T3" because it has the most impact on metabolism and your body. T4 is the less active "prohormone" form of thyroid hormone, and it is ideally converted into T3 (with the aid of selenium-based enzymes) as needed. Your metabolism not only controls the rate at which you burn calories but also influences the speed at which *every* bodily function takes place. Your thyroid plays a major role in determining your body temperature; the way you digest, metabolize, and assimilate food; your body's ability to make good-quality connective tissue, hair, skin, and nails; and your mood. Thyroid "wobbles" can affect many things, including menopausal symptoms, fertility, and overall vitality.

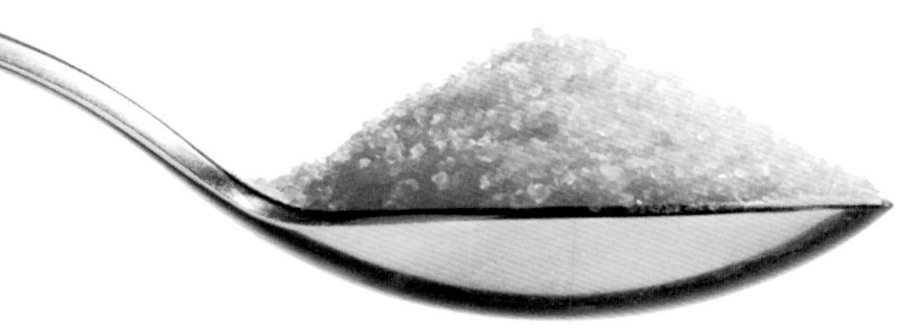

Types *of* Thyroid Imbalance

Thyroid imbalances tilt your body toward either not enough thyroid hormones or too much of them.

Hypothyroidism (underactive/low thyroid) is the most common thyroid imbalance. Things slow to nearly a halt, typically resulting in colder body temperature, weight gain, depression, sluggishness, poor digestion, brain fog, hair loss, dull skin, a crease in the skin around your neck (goiter or thyroid enlargement in advanced cases), and horizontal ridges in the fingernails, among other things. It can look a bit like anemia. Visually, a neck crease would suggest thyroid while pale skin and lips would suggest anemia, but have your doctor run some simple diagnostic tests to be sure. High TSH levels suggest hypothyroid disease because your brain is yelling at your thyroid to keep up the pace, but a full thyroid panel will give you a better picture.

Hyperthyroidism (overactive/high thyroid) is characterized by overdrive: you might feel like a furnace, become rail-thin, toss and turn at night, and feel extremely agitated and anxious. It wears on your whole body. In advanced cases, your eyes might bug out (think: Susan Sarandon in *The Rocky Horror Picture Show*). Both hyperthyroidism and excessive amounts of hypothyroid medications (resulting in hyperthyroidism) can cause heart palpitations, racing heart, atrial fibrillation, and tachycardia, as well as general anxiety.

Autoimmune issues are often at play in either form of thyroid disease, but not always. In Hashimoto's disease (an autoimmune hypothyroid disease), antibodies attack your thyroid gland. In Graves' disease (an autoimmune hyperthyroid disease), autoantibodies activate TSH receptors in the thyroid, causing overproduction of T3 and T4. Antibody tests can diagnose these forms of thyroid disease.

In addition, it's possible for someone to swing from one end of the thyroid spectrum to another, perhaps from hyperthyroid-induced thyroid burnout or overstimulation from inappropriate dosing of hypothyroid medications, thyroid glandular supplements, or iodine supplements.

Even though more and more people — particularly women — have thyroid imbalances, you'd be hard-pressed to find good information about how to take care of your thyroid holistically. Information is scarce and conflicting. Even the experts can't agree on how many people are affected. Estimates of hypothyroid incidence range from 5 to 20 to 40 percent of the population. Part of this discrepancy comes from two different range recommendations used by labs and medical groups. Officially, normal TSH levels run 0.5 to 4.5 or 6.0 microunits per milliliter (µU/mL), but the American Association of Clinical Endocrinologists recommends a normal range of 0.3 to 3.0, which catches millions more cases of hypothyroidism in the earlier (and easier to treat) stages. Labs that rely on older, less conservative recommendations may mark you as "normal," whereas progressive ranges would consider you "borderline hypothyroid." Many Americans, particularly women (although men and children can be affected, too), fall into the subclinical or mild hypothyroid range that might be missed or ignored by doctors.

If you have a thyroid imbalance, you might go see your doctor because you don't feel well, look unhealthy, your weight is off, your mood is shot, and so on. After a series of lab tests, your doctor may come back and say, "Great news! Your lab results came out normal. You're fine!" But is that really comforting when you still don't feel well? You're exhausted and overwhelmed. Are you just getting old? Is it all in your head? What next?

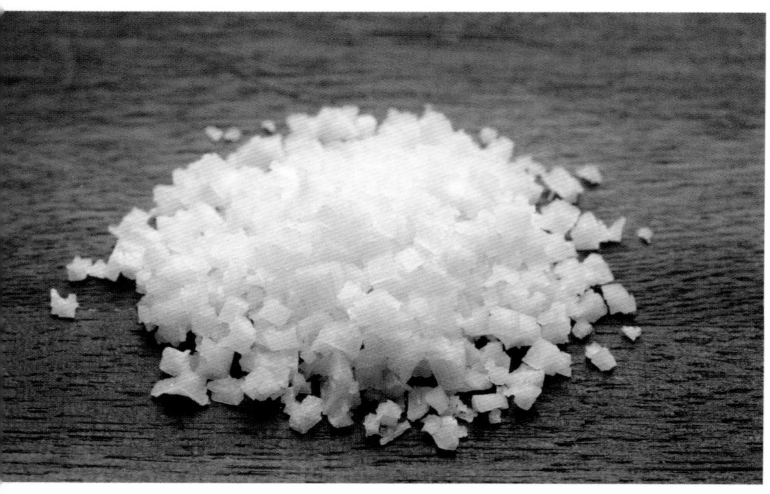

A Holistic Approach *to* Thyroid Imbalance

As with many diseases, the earlier you catch a thyroid imbalance, the easier it is to correct, especially with holistic treatments. First, get a *full* thyroid panel to help get a better picture of what's going on: not just TSH levels but also T3 and T4, with accompanying tests for antibodies to rule out autoimmune complications. Ask for a copy of the results, refer to the ranges mentioned earlier, and take note if your levels are on the edge of normal. Symptom patterns are also important for catching and responding to subclinical thyroid issues. Have your iron levels checked to rule out anemia, and also check for other oddball diseases like Lyme that can throw your whole body into a tailspin. Your tests may come back inconclusive — don't worry, you can still do something about it — but knowing exactly where things stand can help drive appropriate therapies.

Herbal and lifestyle approaches excel at addressing subclinical imbalances, and they're less apt to have negative side effects than some of our thyroid-focused supplements and pharmaceuticals. High-dose isolated iodine supplements, which supply a necessary building block for thyroid hormone production, are often employed to boost thyroid hormone levels. Glandular supplements such as Armour Thyroid, which are made with ground-up animal thyroid glands, also boost thyroid function. Even though high-dose iodine and glandulars are technically natural, think twice before blindly taking them for thyroid management. If used inappropriately, they can make your thyroid problems worse by creating a hyperthyroid storm. Carefully measured thyroid medications prescribed by a doctor may actually be safer. An even gentler route — focusing on lifestyle changes and supportive herbs, especially if you're self-treating — may work just as well in the early stages of thyroid disease. Search around for a practitioner who understands thyroid health and really listens to you. That might be your primary care physician, a naturopath, an herbalist, a progressive endocrinologist, or a team of practitioners who are willing to work together for you.

Underlying Causes *of* Thyroid Problems

The underlying causes of thyroid disease, from a holistic perspective, can be the same for both ranges of thyroid problems, and they vary widely depending on the person. These aggravating factors set into motion chain reactions that favor hypo- or hyperthyroid function depending on the individual's tendency.

- **Stress and grief** often instigate thyroid malfunction, especially if they're severe or long-standing. Your thyroid response is trying to protect you — either trying to slow you down because your body is exhausted or speed you up to meet perceived demands — even though the end result makes you feel worse.

- **Autoimmune disease** might be triggered by gluten in your diet, illness, environmental toxins, or hormonal transitions and imbalances. Try eliminating gluten from your diet for 1 month; then reintroduce it and see how you feel. This can have a tremendous impact for some people.

- **Diet** likely plays a major role in thyroid disease. Besides the aforementioned potential gluten-thyroid reaction, a low-nutrient, high-carb diet rich in chemical additives and leached toxins from packaging probably doesn't help. Certain foods inhibit and simulate thyroid function, too. See the next page for a greater discussion on diet.

- **An indoor sedentary lifestyle** discourages optimal thyroid health. Your thyroid functions better when it's exposed to changing temperatures, regular exercise, and light (especially sunlight in the morning and during the day). If you sit inside all day under artificial lights, at a perfect 68 degrees year-round, staring at a screen, your thyroid gets lazy and cranky. Give it a workout! Multitask with a daily morning or lunchtime walk. Try to spend as much time in a natural environment as you can, including a few hours of sunlight each day.

- **Toxins** may be an underlying factor in triggering thyroid imbalance and autoimmune disease. As best you can, eat organic to avoid pesticides, choose fresh whole foods over processed and plastic-wrapped foods, and store food in glass or stainless steel. Use glass or stainless steel drinking containers rather than plastic. Mercury exposure and other toxins may also be an issue, so do what you can to live a clean and green lifestyle (see page 26), but don't stress about being 100 percent perfect.

- **An emotional connection** can underlie thyroid issues if you feel like you are not speaking or living your truth in life. Is something stuck in your throat that you need to let out? As one of my colleagues, herbalist Maia Toll, who specializes in thyroid conditions, explains, "You have this skinny little neck that connects the head and the heart, and you get a bottleneck there."

GLUTEN AND THE THYROID

OF ALL THE FOOD ALLERGIES and sensitivities, gluten seems to have the greatest connection with thyroid disease, particularly when there's an autoimmune component. The current theory is that the protein compound gliadin in gluten looks a lot like protein in thyroid tissue. If you're sensitive to gluten, your body's gluten antibodies get confused and begin to also attack your thyroid, resulting in Hashimoto's or Graves' disease. It can take several months of complete gluten elimination from your diet to shut those antibodies off and see results.

Diet *and* Your Thyroid

Of course a healthy, whole-foods diet is always important, but certain foods provide the key nutrients that your body needs to make thyroid hormones and can help increase or decrease thyroid function. Before you start taking a bunch of herbs, supplements, or drugs, check in to see if your diet is missing a crucial piece of the thyroid puzzle, or if you're overindulging in foods that could aggravate it.

Foods & Herbs That Boost Thyroid Function

Consider integrating the following foods, herbs, and supplements into your routine if you have hypothyroid issues. Avoid eating excessive amounts if you tend toward hyperthyroid disease.

- **Iodine.** Iodine is an essential mineral for the creation of thyroid hormones, and our key dietary sources include iodized salt, seaweed, seafood, and some multivitamins. Are you getting any iodine? Have you recently switched multivitamins or brands of salt and inadvertently eliminated it from your diet? Lack of iodine can instigate hypothyroid disease and, in extreme cases, goiter. Instead of loading up on isolated iodine supplements (which can swing you into a hyperthyroid state), try integrating a little bit of seaweed into your diet and switch to iodized sea salt.

- **Kelp.** *Laminaria* and *Nereocystis* species — especially digitata kelp — and other types of brown seaweed such as kombu are potent sources of not just iodine but also other minerals, including calcium, iron, and selenium. Studies have shown that seaweed consumption can profoundly increase thyroid function. Add just a little bit of seaweed (i.e., one strip) to soups, broth, and other dishes. Use traditional Asian cuisine as your guide. Combining seaweed with thyroid-inhibiting foods like soy buffers the effects of each. Try taking up to 1 to 2 grams of kelp powder (delivering 200 to 400 mcg of iodine) daily. Seaweed tends to bind to pollutants such as heavy metals and radioactive compounds; purchase from companies, such as those on the Maine coast, that harvest from clean waters and test for contaminants. Keep quantities modest. High doses of seaweed can swing you into hyperthyroid disease. If you have hyperthyroid disease, limit or avoid seaweed, especially kelp and other brown seaweeds. (Learn more about seaweed on page 40.)

- **Selenium.** Another important mineral for thyroid health is selenium, which helps your thyroid more effectively manufacture hormones and facilitates the transformation of inactive T4 into active T3. Preliminary studies suggest that selenium supplementation can treat hypothyroid, autoimmune thyroiditis, and postpartum thyroid disease and also prevent thyroid issues. It may also aid in cases of Graves' disease. Just one or two Brazil nuts a day provides plenty of selenium. Other high-selenium foods include seafood, fish, seeds, meat, and red seaweed (dulse, nori, laver, Irish moss). Work with a practitioner before taking high-dose selenium supplements because consuming more than the recommended daily amount of this trace mineral may cause selenium poisoning and various negative side effects. If you decide to take low-dose supplements, opt for natural yeast-based forms, which appear to be better tolerated than isolated sodium selenite.

- **Ashwagandha.** Ashwagandha gets the nod for hypothyroid clients because it simultaneously calms and energizes, has benefits for autoimmune disease and inflammation, and is one of the few plants (that are common and safe to use) that demonstrate specific thyroid-enhancing effects. Preliminary animal studies show that ashwagandha increases T3 and T4 production, and many herbalists find the herb useful for hypothyroid clients — especially in borderline or

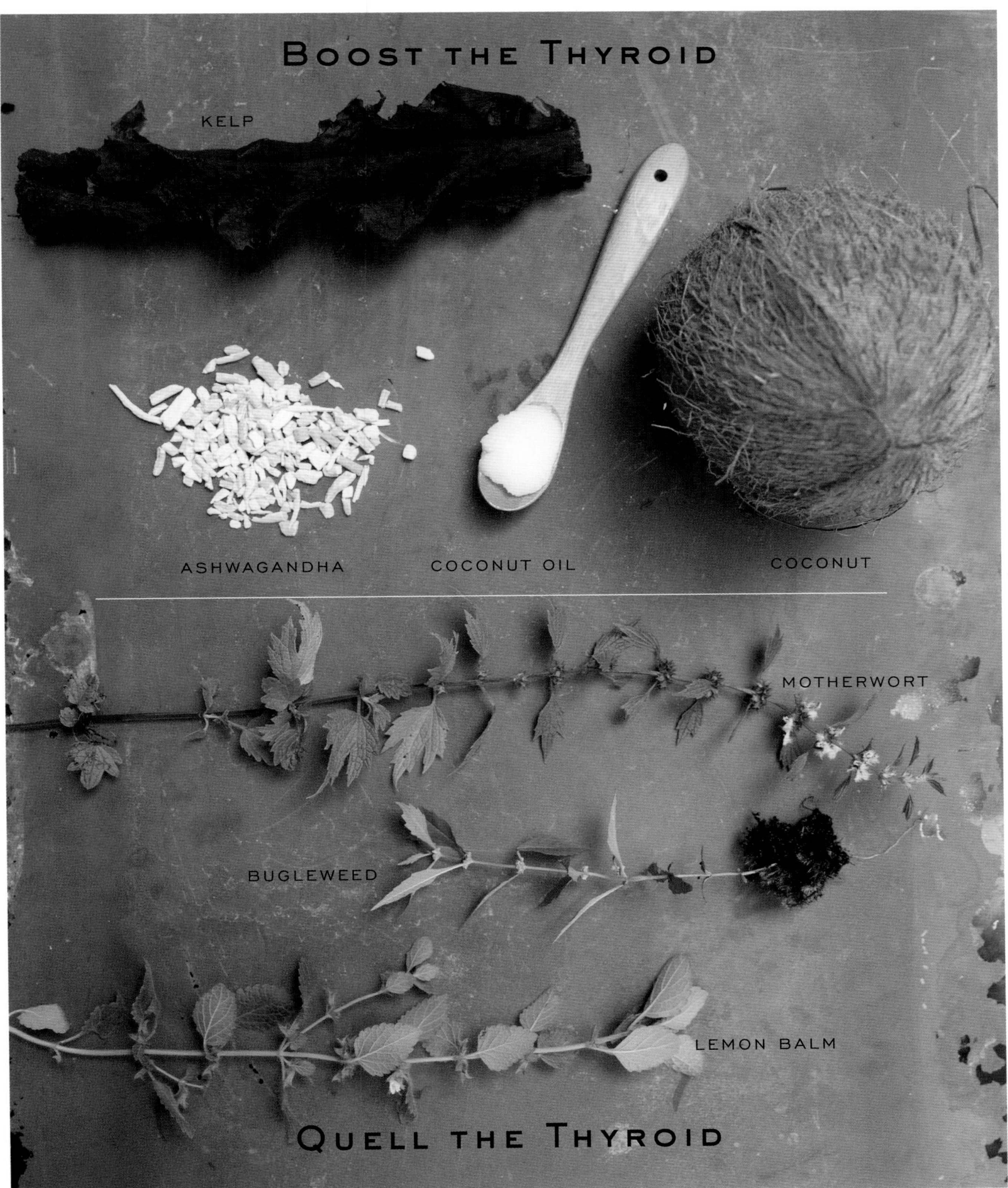
Boost the Thyroid
KELP
ASHWAGANDHA
COCONUT OIL
COCONUT
MOTHERWORT
BUGLEWEED
LEMON BALM
Quell the Thyroid

subclinical cases. The herb's strong safety record and many "side benefits" also make it a good herb to try first. Thyroid imbalance often causes an increased sensitivity to stress, anxiety, fatigue, inflammation, immune malfunction (including autoimmune disease), and low libido, and ashwagandha is traditionally used for all these concerns. It's said to give you the strength of a horse if you take it regularly for a year. To learn more about ashwagandha and how to take it, see page 50.

- **Bacopa and guggul.** These herbs may provide benefit for the hypothyroid or borderline hypothyroid person. The scientific evidence is highly preliminary, but both tend to be very safe and have side benefits that may also be of interest. Bacopa boosts T4 production, but not active T3. This Ayurvedic herb enhances memory and brain function while quelling anxiety. See more on page 177. Guggul, a resin from Ayurveda related to myrrh, seems to improve the conversion of T4 to active T3 and is also traditionally used for weight loss and high cholesterol.

- **Tyrosine.** This amino acid (a component of protein) serves as a building block for thyroid hormones. You should be able to get it from your diet (poultry, fish, cheese, nuts, seeds), and your body can make it from other amino acids. It's rare to be deficient in tyrosine, but if you're having thyroid wobbles, be sure you're eating enough protein and digesting your food well. Digestive bitters (to stimulate digestion, stomach acid, and enzymes) and gut-healing herbs might be helpful if your digestive system is subpar.

- **Medium-chain triglycerides (MCTs).** Coconut oil and other sources of MCTs, like palm kernel oil, gently support thyroid function by decreasing inflammation, boosting metabolism, and improving the function of thyroid hormones. For all the enthusiasm around coconut oil and thyroid health, there is unfortunately almost no research to support it. Yet I know of several firsthand accounts of people who successfully manage hypothyroid disease with a spoonful or two of coconut oil per day. It's worth trying — listen to your body to see if you feel better. Be sure to purchase good-quality unrefined coconut oil. Consider melting it down with equal parts dark chocolate for a tasty "fudge" treat, whip it into smoothies and hot beverages, or use it in cooking or as a butter substitute.

Foods and Herbs That Inhibit Thyroid Function

If you have hypothyroid disease, avoid eating excessive amounts of these thyroid-inhibiting foods and herbs. If you have hyperthyroid disease, they may be a useful part of your regimen. However, you will want to be cautious with soy regardless. People with hyperthyroid disease often feel strung out, so it's handy that herbs that downregulate thyroid hormones also excel at bringing the nervous system down a notch. As always, listen to your body to determine which foods and herbs do or don't help you feel vital.

- **Lemon balm, motherwort, and bugleweed.** Whether as single herbs or a trio blend, lemon balm, motherwort, and bugleweed are frequently used for hyperthyroid disease. Lithospermum may be added to the mix; however, it contains liver-toxic pyrrolizidine alkaloids (PAs) that make its use controversial. Preliminary research suggests that these herbs inhibit hyperthyroid function through a variety of mechanisms, including binding to TSH receptors, inhibiting thyroid hormone production, and preventing thyroid hormone conversion from T4 to T3. Lemon balm also prevents autoantibodies from binding to TSH receptors, making it particularly useful for treating Graves' disease. It's worth noting that lemon balm and motherwort are commonly used for conditions with symptoms similar to those observed in hyperthyroid disease: insomnia, anxiety, agitation, and stress-related cardiac overdrive, including panic attacks, rapid heart beat, palpitations, and tachycardia. Most people take the herbs as fresh plant tinctures, though water extracts (tea) were used in many of the studies. Fresh or dry lemon balm as tea is delightful. Lemon balm and motherwort enjoy widespread use in herbalism — beyond thyroid health — so you may wonder if it's safe to take them in hypothyroid disease. Fortunately, it's not usually a concern. Keep a close eye to see if the herbs agree with you, but herbalists report that adverse reactions are incredibly rare.

- **Soy.** Soy can inhibit and aggravate thyroid function. Of all food-related thyroid issues I see in my practice, soy-thyroid issues are most common. Soy contains goitrogen compounds that inhibit thyroid function. While most often associated with hypothyroid symptoms, it sometimes stimulates the thyroid into a *hyper*thyroid state. Be suspicious if your thyroid issues followed a new supplement or diet switch. Have you recently developed a soy habit? Switched to soy milk or soy-based energy bars? Introduced a food-based multivitamin made in a base of fermented soy? Consider skipping soy for a month, then reintroducing it to see if it's a culprit for you. Particularly avoid processed soy products like isolated soy protein. Interestingly, in Asian cultures where soy is frequently consumed, it's often combined with seaweed, and studies suggest that these two thyroid-active foods balance each other out.

- **Goitrogens.** Other dietary goitrogens are less apt to pose a problem compared to soy. It's rare, but raw cruciferous vegetables — cabbage, kale, broccoli, rutabaga, turnips — occasionally reduce thyroid function. Cassava, peaches, pears, strawberries, spinach, sweet potatoes, and carrots have goitrogenic thyroid-inhibiting effects but are usually not problematic. Cooking negates most of their goitrogenic action, and concern is greatest when the foods represent a large part of your daily diet. I wouldn't worry about these foods unless your raw kale salad and green smoothie binges coincide with increased symptoms. Try backing off and see if you notice a difference.

NATURAL CARE ALONGSIDE CONVENTIONAL THYROID TREATMENT

IF YOU CURRENTLY TAKE MEDICATION for thyroid problems, you can probably incorporate many of the holistic approaches described in this chapter concurrently with the pharmaceuticals, but you should talk with your doctor and your pharmacist first. Ideally, your doctor or practitioner should work with you as you combine therapies. Expect the effects of natural therapies to be slow and building. You'll want to reevaluate every few months to see if they're working for you (and if you're on medications, whether or not the dose can be adjusted or eliminated over time). In conventional thyroid care, doctors may destroy a malfunctioning thyroid with a simple procedure and then prescribe drugs to replicate that function. If you no longer have a functioning thyroid, you will still have to take medications — natural remedies may have a supportive effect but *cannot* replace the thyroid gland. However, herbs, diet, and lifestyle techniques can often be safely used in combination with conventional care. Be aware of signs of an overactive or underactive thyroid (page 205), as these could be a clue that your medication needs to be reduced or increased.

Other Supportive Thyroid Herbs and Nutrients

The following nutrition-based remedies tend to be beneficial for healthy thyroid function, regardless of whether your thyroid needs a boost or to be taken down a notch.

- **Vitamin B complex.** A variety of B vitamins support thyroid and adrenal function and help regulate stress levels. Consider sardines, bee pollen, nutritional yeast, a little wild game or grass-fed meat, and B-complex supplements to increase the Bs in your diet.
- **Magnesium.** This mineral has profound benefits throughout the body, and a deficiency in magnesium may indirectly aggravate an underactive thyroid via calcium balance and hormone production. You can find it in food (blackstrap molasses, nuts, beans, dark leafy greens, cacao) or as a powder or liquid supplement. Magnesium supplements may interact with various medications (including decreasing the effect of Synthroid), but you can often take them at different times of day. Food sources should not be a problem.
- **Bitters and digestive support.** Though not directly thyroid supportive, adequate digestion and assimilation is essential to provide the body with the building blocks it needs to function well. Poor digestion can be an early factor in thyroid problems, and hypothyroid disease compounds the issue by slowing down digestion and metabolism further. You could be eating all the right things but not absorbing them. Herbal bitters are one of our best allies for digestion. Taken regularly just before meals, they turn on digestion by increasing enzyme and stomach acid production, strengthening peristalsis, and boosting bile production and excretion. (For more about bitters, see page 71.) Also try to eat in a way that enhances digestion: choose healthy foods, sit down, relax, and enjoy your meal.

Addressing *the* Autoimmune Connection

In autoimmune-related thyroid conditions, such as Hashimoto's (hypo) and Graves' (hyper) diseases, first look to gluten and stress. Many of our thyroid herbs and nutrients — such as ashwagandha, lemon balm, and selenium — appear to benefit autoimmune disease and are worth trying. Consider adding medicinal mushrooms to the mix as well. Though little research has been done specifically on thyroid autoimmune disease, we know that polysaccharides in mushrooms modulate immune function and are of particular assistance in autoimmune disease. The polysaccharides are best extracted by cooking the mushrooms or simmering them in water (broth, soup, tea); the longer, the better. A double-extraction tincture that includes a decoction may also work. Consider reishi as well as maitake, shiitake, turkey tails, and chaga. Astragalus has similar autoimmune/immune benefits. For more on these remedies, see page 115.

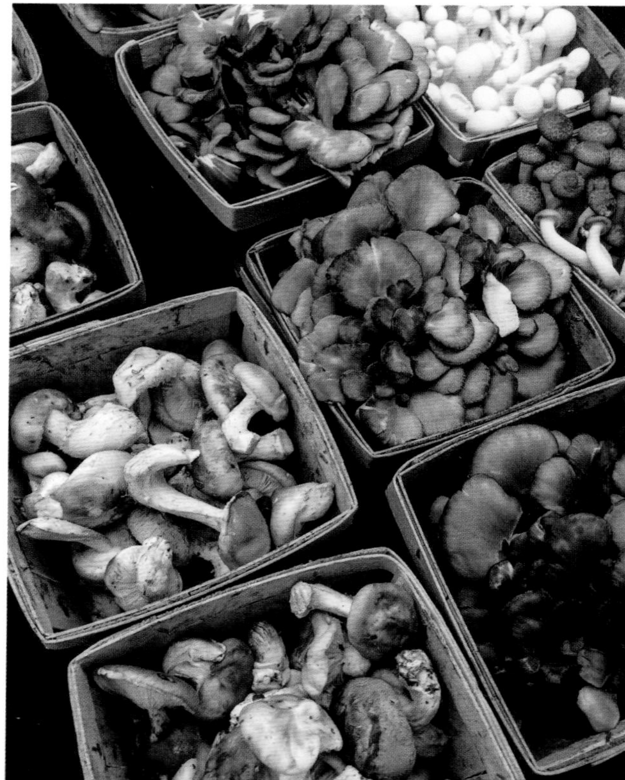

Mushroom Broth for the Thyroid

Consider this broth for regular consumption if you have hypothyroid or Hashimoto's disease. This recipe features immune tonics that aid in cases of autoimmune disease — mushrooms and astragalus — plus nutrient-rich and thyroid-stimulating herbs. Feel free to play around with the ingredients based on your needs, tastes, and herb availability. With a few adaptations, the broth can also be used for Graves' disease: omit the seaweed and ashwagandha, and at the very end, with the heat off, add 1 to 3 tablespoons dried lemon balm leaf (or 1 cup fresh) and let steep, covered, for 15 minutes.

MUSHROOMS

- 1–2 slices reishi
- 1 tablespoon powdered shiitake, or 8 ounces fresh
- 1 teaspoon powdered maitake, 1 ounce dried, or 4 ounces fresh

HERBS

- 2–6 slices dried astragalus root
- 1 tablespoon ashwagandha root
- 1 tablespoon dried nettles
- 2 bay leaves
- 1 strip kelp

BROTH

- 1 gallon water
- 1 grass-fed beef bone (optional)
- Salt and freshly ground black pepper

Combine all the ingredients (except the lemon balm, if using) in a large stockpot. Bring just to a gentle boil, then reduce the heat and let simmer, covered, for at least 3 hours, and up to all day. Remove from the heat. Strain all the solids from the broth. Let cool, then store in the refrigerator. Drink 1 cup of the mushroom broth daily and use it in preparing other dishes. It freezes well.

PROTOCOL POINTS

Hypothyroid and Hashimoto's Disease

Many doctors won't even consider holistic treatment of hypothyroid disease because medications like Synthroid are so effective and generally safe when dosed correctly. However, a holistic approach seeks to address potential root causes of poor thyroid function and provide your thyroid with the nutrients and support it needs to resume normal hormone production on its own. This tends to work best in borderline and early hypothyroid disease and may not be sufficient for severe conditions. You can try most of these holistic approaches alongside medications, too, with attention to a few potential drug interactions, occasional thyroid retests, and adjustment of medication dose as needed.

Diet: Try a gluten-free diet (for at least a few months, and indefinitely if it helps), limit excessive amounts of cruciferous veggies (especially raw), and avoid or limit soy. Check your iodine intake; do you regularly consume it via iodized salt, seaweed, or your multivitamin? Use iodized salt and consider adding small amounts of seaweed to your regular diet, a sprinkle or strip here and there. Iodine intake and thyroid function work in careful balance — too little is problematic, but too much iodine can overstimulate the thyroid. For the same reason, do not take isolated iodine supplements without a practitioner's supervision since it's particularly easy to overdo it. Try adding coconut oil to your diet, and see how that feels for you. Ensure that you're eating adequate amounts of complete protein, especially those that provide tyrosine. Consider eating one Brazil nut or red seaweed daily for selenium.

Lifestyle: Prioritize morning or midday exercise. This gives you a triple whammy of natural thyroid stimulation — exercise, sunlight, and temperature variations — at the most useful time of day to encourage better hormone production as well as sleep-wake cycles. Stress can be a major trigger for all types of thyroid imbalance. Reduce stress, address grief, and incorporate activities for mind-body balance, such as breathwork, yoga, and therapy.

Herbs: Look to thyroid-enhancing herbs, especially ashwagandha and possibly also bacopa and guggul. Combine them with adaptogens for additional stress reduction and energy support, nervines for nerve support, and possibly also medicinal mushrooms and astragalus for autoimmune support. Holy basil makes a particularly nice supportive herb because of its ability to improve energy, reduce the effects of stress, lift mood, and improve immune health.

Hyperthyroid and Graves' Disease

Though less common, hyperthyroid disease can be both more challenging and more dangerous than hypothyroid conditions. Yet natural therapies and herbs are worth considering. From a holistic perspective, hyperthyroid disease has some of the same triggers as hypothyroidism, including stress, food sensitivities, and autoimmune disease. Specific natural approaches aim to reduce thyroid overstimulation and the whole-body overdrive it creates.

Diet: Try a gluten-free diet (for at least a few months, and indefinitely if it helps) and avoid or limit soy to see if this helps. Avoid or limit seaweed and supplemental iodine (unless you're under a practitioner's guidance).

Lifestyle: Prioritize morning or midday exercise outside to stimulate healthy thyroid function and support better sleep-wake cycles. Reduce stress, address grief, and incorporate activities for mind-body balance, such as breathwork, yoga, and therapy. Give yourself extra TLC to improve sleep and relaxation at night (see page 67).

Herbs: Consider drinking lemon balm tea regularly and taking a tincture blend of lemon balm, motherwort, and bugleweed. Add calming adaptogens, sedatives, and nervines as needed, such as holy basil, milky oat seed, passionflower, and skullcap. For autoimmune thyroid disease, consider adding medicinal mushrooms, astragalus, and selenium.

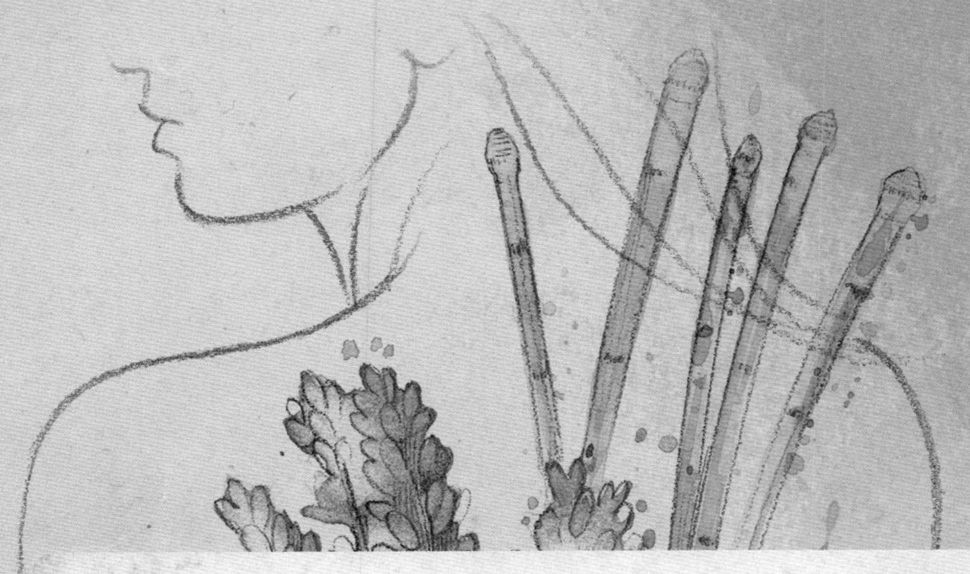

Chapter 14

Your Skin and Connective Tissue: Keepin' It Together

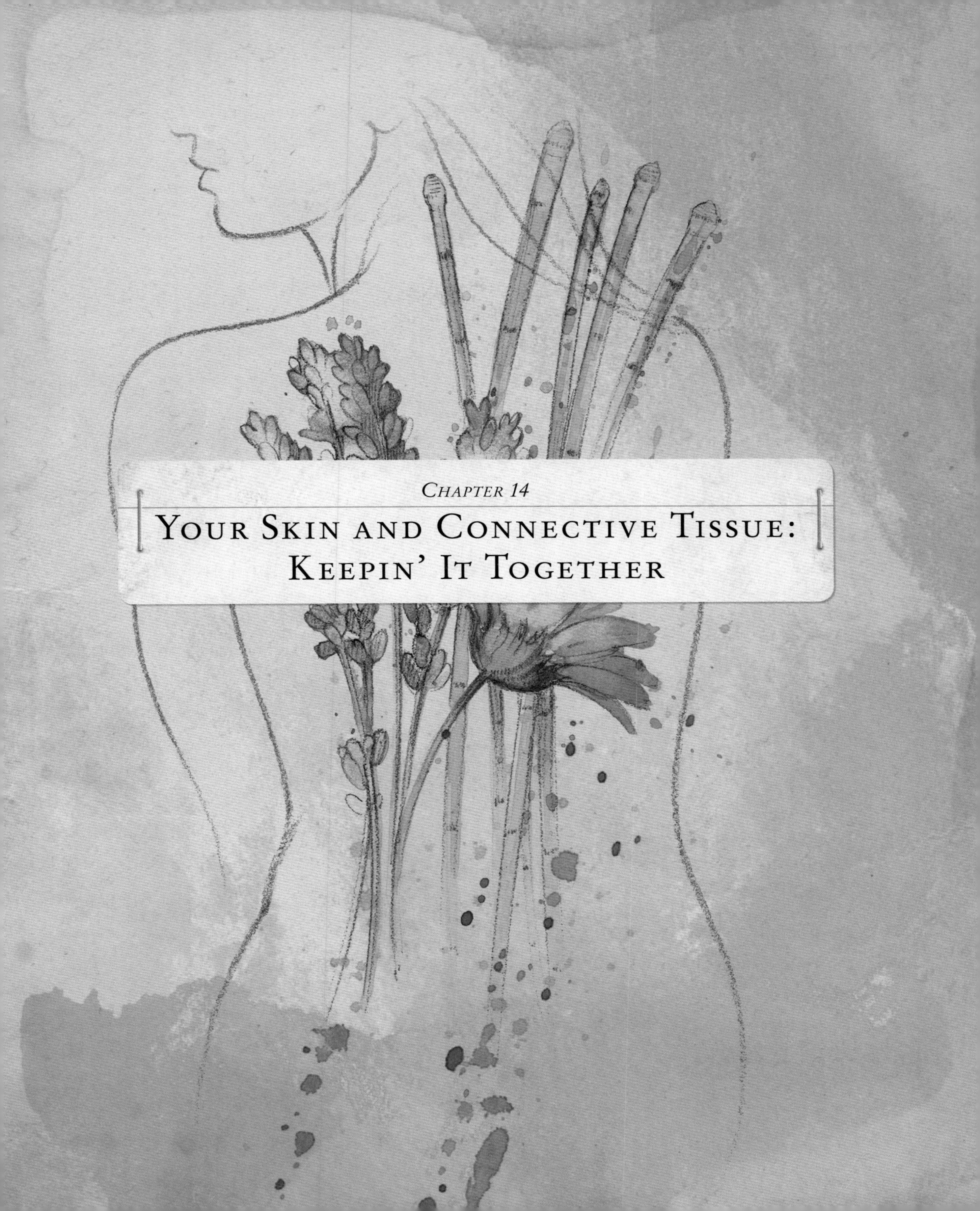

A BEAUTIFUL CANVAS THAT stretches across your body, skin reigns as your largest organ. Like castle walls, it protects you from the elements and invasion while also serving as an important transfer station for moving things in and out of your body — eliminating waste, absorbing compounds, making vitamin D, and so on. The kingdom that is your body works to nourish and maintain its castle walls, completely regenerating the entire skin approximately every month.

Your skin serves as a manifestation of your whole body's health. When everything is in balance, your vibrant skin glows, even as you age. However, it'll crumble if you're not eating (or digesting and assimilating) the nutrients you need, or if your body is bogged down by sleep deprivation, stress, a sluggish or overloaded detoxification system, exposure to harsh elements, or illness.

Healthy Skin *from* the Outside In *and* the Inside Out

Your skin is made up of several layers. New cells rise up from within, come to the surface, and ultimately slough off. Even though your body is mostly water, *all* cells in your body also have lipids (fats) incorporated into their cell lining, which is why the quantity and quality of the fats you eat has a profound effect on your skin *and* total body health. Oil secreted by glands in your skin helps lock in moisture, keeps things smooth, and minimizes wrinkles and dryness, while a deeper lipid layer helps you hold in body heat. The majority of your skin's structure is made up of collagen, a protein-rich connective tissue that helps keep the skin plump, supple, and healthy. Collagen is closely associated with another protein, called elastin, that — you guessed it! — helps your skin remain elastic. As you age, and in certain states of disease, collagen and elastin diminish, creating wrinkles and sags. Another protein-based compound composing your skin is rigid keratin, which helps protect your skin and is concentrated in your hair and nails. Adequate amounts of the mineral silica help your body produce more collagen, elastin, and keratin. (You'll find silica or the silica-rich herb horsetail in most hair-skin-nail formulas.) A thin, slightly acid layer of film on your skin is called the acid mantle, which helps protect you from acid-hating microbes.

You're probably getting the sense that your skin is more than what you slap on it. While topical applications provide targeted care, beautiful skin really comes from within. If you don't have any specific skin woes, you should be able to maintain glowing skin with a simple cleansing and moisturizing routine, good diet, adequate water, and rest. But when things start to go awry, you can get good results with a more intense two-pronged approach: internal remedies and external applications, alongside the usual good diet and lifestyle stuff. Internal remedies address imbalance from within while external herbs deliver healing properties directly to the area affected. You'll usually get fast results from topical remedies, but they often don't totally resolve the issue. In contrast, the internal approach tends to take more time but does a better job resolving the underlying causes. In particular, internal remedies for healthy skin focus on the following:

- Detoxification formulas, to support the skin in its role as an organ of elimination
- High-quality nutrients, like healthy fats and complete proteins, that support the skin and connective tissues
- Avoidance of foods that trigger sensitivities or allergic reactions, which promote inflammation, rashes, and outbreaks
- Stress reduction and nervous system support when it seems connected to outbreaks
- Immune system support when autoimmune disease or pathogen-related skin issues are at play; this can include taking probiotics, limiting sugar intake, and taking herbs that improve your immune function or directly fight pathogens

Topical skin treatments primarily consist of the following:

- Emollient formulas that soften and help protect the skin
- Healing formulas that soothe, protect, and help the body repair rashes, scrapes, and wounds
- Direct application of antimicrobial herbs on bacterial, fungal, and viral infections, from infected cuts to warts

Basic Nutrients *for* Skin Vitality

Ideally, you should provide your body with these basics on a *daily* basis. After all, your skin is in a constant process of total regeneration each month. Key in on therapeutic doses of these nutrients when you know your connective tissue needs a hand: after surgery, during wound healing, and while correcting skin issues.

- **Water** helps keep your skin hydrated, which helps "fluff" collagen and minimize the appearance and development of wrinkles and dry skin. It also improves your body's ability to detoxify more efficiently, which takes a load off your skin and improves its vibrance.

- **Omega-3s, good fats, vitamin D, vitamin A, and carotenoids** all help your skin maintain its moisture, lubrication, and vitality. Eat plenty of orange and dark green produce, calendula petals, liver, and pasture-raised eggs for their antioxidant pigments. Make sure your diet is rich in good fats, including plenty of seafood and fatty cold-water fish, nuts and seeds, and modest amounts of wild or pasture-raised animal products. A fish oil or cod liver oil supplement helps fill gaps but isn't as good as food. (Cod liver oil offers more vitamin A and D.) Vitamin D encourages new skin cell growth and proliferation, especially keratin compounds, and can help correct skin diseases like vitiligo, scleroderma, psoriasis, actinic keratosis, and lupus vulgaris. Besides cod liver oil and sun exposure, other sources of vitamin D include mushrooms (grown with exposure to the sun or UV rays), pastured eggs, fatty fish, liver, fortified foods, and dietary supplements.

- **Silica** strengthens collagen, keratin, elastin, and other forms of connective tissue. Super infusions, decoctions, simmered broths, and capsules of the herb horsetail are particularly rich in silica. Other good dietary sources include whole grains and seeds, including rice, corn, oats, and flax. Nettle and oat straw provide some silica, too. Well-made gelatinous bone broth can also provide a range of supportive nutrients for collagen and skin health.

- **Vitamin C** enhances the quality and healing of connective tissue while improving your absorption of other nutrients. Bioflavonoids, present in all natural sources of vitamin C, improve the action of vitamin C. Herbal sources of both include rose hips, certain types of evergreen needles/branches (white pine, balsam fir, hemlock tree, spruce), hibiscus flowers, amla fruit, citrus, strawberries, tomatoes, bell peppers, and most fresh fruit and vegetables. Fresh, raw, or recently dried forms will be richest in vitamin C; it dissipates quickly during drying, aging, and cooking.

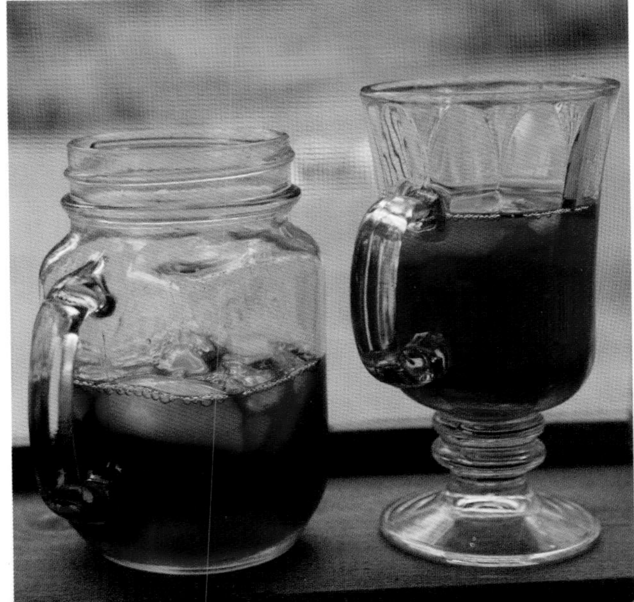

- **Amino acids**, the building blocks of protein, are essential for almost all components of your skin and connective tissue. Be sure to eat complete sources of protein (from animal or combined plant sources), especially those high in the amino acids methionine and cysteine. You'll find these aminos in nuts, seeds, and dark leafy greens — sunflower seeds, pumpkin seeds, Brazil nuts, sesame seeds, wild edible greens (lamb's-quarter, pigweed, purslane), spinach, oats, barley and other whole grains, beans, and lentils.

- **Vulnerary herbs** that support wound and connective tissue repair and vitality include gotu kola, calendula flowers, lavender buds, St. John's wort buds and flowers, and plantain leaf applied topically. Gotu kola also promotes collagen synthesis and capillary strength when taken internally.

Michael Moore recommended eating dishes that combined this range of nutrients when you need extra connective tissue support or repair. For example, you might eat whole corn tacos with dark leafy greens and pepper-tomato salsa and a squirt of lime; steel-cut oats topped with ground flaxseed, slivered nuts, and fresh strawberries; rice and beans cooked with leafy greens and veggies; strong teas and broths with horsetail, oat straw, gotu kola, rose hips, violet leaf, and nettles.

Of course, even if you eat fabulously, it's not going to do much good if your digestive system isn't breaking it down and absorbing it well. Bitter herbs and foods turn your digestive system back on so you get the most out of what you eat. They also stimulate detoxification, which supports skin health. Consider taking bitters before meals or adding them into your remedy blends. Some of my favorites include dandelion root and leaf, burdock root, artichoke leaf, schizandra berries, and turmeric, often combined with some tasty carminative spices like ginger and cardamom. Traditional cultures incorporate bitter, pungent, and aromatic ingredients into their meals, including bitter salad greens, artichoke, tamarind, herbs, and spices. Learn more about your digestive system and the value of bitters in chapter 5.

The Skin-Detox Connection

If you look closely at the ingredients in most teas designed to promote healthy skin, you'll notice that they're loaded with detoxification herbs (perhaps alongside silica- and nutrient-rich herbs). Why? Skin is your *largest* detoxification organ, even if it's not the most efficient compared to, say, your liver. Detox organs can get sluggish or overwhelmed with everyday toxins related to metabolic waste, fighting infections, exposure to irritants, bad diet, food sensitivities (a biggie!), inflammation, and stress. Your skin tries to pick up the slack — and can suffer for it, with poor skin tone, blemishes, and rashes developing as the extra toxins are drawn out.

Traditional alterative herbs that target elimination via the liver, lymph, and kidneys play center stage: burdock, dandelion, yellow dock, red clover, calendula, nettle. These specific alteratives also supply useful nutrients for nourishing the skin while "cleansing the blood" of impurities so that your skin gets some relief. Don't be alarmed if your skin gets worse before it gets better. This happens frequently as a sluggish detox system chugs into life: your body experiences an influx of toxins as they're released from storage in the bloodstream, and the overflow is released through the skin. Your liver, lymph, kidneys, and colon should catch up and remove them from the body; things should clear up within a few days. Slowly building up your dose of detox herbs can minimize the severity of this "healing crisis." See chapter 6 for more on detoxification.

Key Skin Herbs

Although a great many herbs can be used internally and externally for skin woes, I find the following herbs to be the most effective, safe, and commonly available options.

▸ Calendula

Calendula officinalis

Availability: G+ C

Key Properties: These sunny yellow-orange blossoms make a superb oil extraction that you can add to salves and creams for a multitude of skin woes, most specifically dry, itchy, irritated rashes and skin conditions. It's famous for eczema and diaper rash (and other baby skin issues). The effects can be miraculous, often clearing bad rashes within a day or two, and acute allergic skin reactions may disappear within minutes. Think of it as herbal "cortisone cream," even though it works differently. Calendula also speeds healing, decreases inflammation, reduces the risk of scars, acts as a mild antimicrobial, and helps with hemorrhoids.

Additional Benefits: When taken internally, it nourishes the body with carotenoids and moves lymph. See page 41 for more about using calendula internally.

Preparation: You'll get the best results with vibrant, recently dried blossoms and can make an oil infusion via any method. Combining the alcohol intermediary and low-heat techniques makes the most potent oil. Also consider it as a salve, bath, tea, broth, compress, or cream. Apply at least twice daily, or as often as needed. A colorful hue and sticky resin indicate potency.

Cautions and Considerations: Extremely safe, but occasionally people are allergic to this pollen-laden, daisy-family flower.

Similar Herbs: Calendula's herbal ally **St. John's wort** is similarly useful and has added pain-relieving, nerve-healing properties — perfect for shingles, cold sores, and sciatica, as well as the usual skin stuff. The redder the oil, the more potent it will be. Fresh flowers and buds work best, especially if you harvest from a sunny, dry spot after a hot-as-Hades week. Calendula and St. John's wort combine nicely, and every medicine cabinet should have a jar of calendula salve and a bottle of St. John's wort oil. Though St. John's wort interacts with many medications and (in rare cases) causes a phototoxic rash when taken internally, topical use isn't a concern. Learn more about St. John's wort on page 57.

WHAT IS A VULNERARY?

Vulnerary herbs promote wound healing.

General Uses: Use herbs on the skin for wounds and as a component in almost any skin formula to aid regeneration, wound repair, and tissue quality while reducing scars. Internally, vulneraries promote healing in the digestive tract (gut inflammation including IBD, leaky gut, ulcers, heartburn) and respiratory system (cough, irritation, inflammation, bronchitis) in particular but may also target other areas. Consider them after surgery or injury. Many are also cooling, anti-inflammatory, and demulcent in nature.

Examples: Plantain, gotu kola, calendula, St. John's wort, licorice, lavender, yarrow, self-heal, violet leaf and flower, alder, mullein leaf, aloe inner gel (not whole leaf or latex), arnica (low dose/homeopathic, unbroken skin), comfrey (fast-acting, external only), cleavers and chickweed (fresh is best), marshmallow, fenugreek

▸ Lavender

Lavandula angustifolia and other species

Availability: G+ C+

Key Properties: As both an essential oil and a crude herb, lavender can be applied to almost any skin issue: burns, irritations, rashes, bug bites, insect repellent, sunburn, poison ivy, mild infections, and as a disinfectant for wounds. It decreases inflammation, fights germs, and speeds healing. (And thanks to its aromatherapy effects on the brain, it calms your nerves at the same time!) Keep bottles of the essential oil handy for the first-aid kit, car, and bathroom, and use it as an ingredient in salves, sprays, and skin recipes. It's one of the few essential oils that can be applied undiluted to the skin. Lavender-infused disinfectant wipes (available in natural food stores) work great on the go for a "quick wash" and delivery of lavender's healing properties. Most skin types respond favorably to lavender in a toner or cream, especially when acne, irritation, dryness, or redness is involved.

Additional Benefits: Lavender — as aromatherapy, topically, or taken internally — also relaxes the nervous system to quell anxiety and stress while promoting sleep.

Preparation: Essential oil (diluted or not), wipes, infused oil, bath/soak, compress, cream, toner/hydrosol — anything, really, when used topically!

Cautions and Considerations: Topical uses of lavender are generally quite safe; however, I rarely use essential oils for infants and children, preferring gentler remedies made from the crude herb. Lavender has estrogenic and antiandrogen effects (most potent in essential oil form), but it's unclear if this characteristic really poses problems.

▸ Plantain

Plantago spp.

Availability: G W+ C-

Key Properties: This green rosette with its seedy flower stalk pops up from cracks in the pavement and lines woodland trails, just begging to be used for everyday skin issues! Its leaves soothe, heal, provide some slippery mucilage, and — when applied to the skin — help draw out toxins and splinters. They almost immediately stop the itch of bug bites and the pain of bee stings and draw out venom. They even put the itch of poison ivy on hold. They also help wounds to heal and ease skin irritations. Children love and can easily identify this first-aid weed.

Additional Benefits: Use plantain internally in gut, respiratory, and urinary formulas to soothe and heal. Though the leaves are a tad stringy, you can eat them as a foraged green.

Preparation: Fresh leaf poultice — chewed or mashed — works best, but herb-infused oils and salves are handy first-aid remedies year-round. The sooner the herb is applied, the more likely it will work. My mother — who gets awful cellulitis from insect stings — stores a handful of clean, fresh leaves wrapped in a damp paper towel in a container in the fridge for fast medicine making. It keeps for several weeks!

Cautions and Considerations: None known.

Similar Herbs: If you happen to be in a rare spot where plantain can't be found, such as waterways and the Southwest, **alder** leaves can be used as a fresh poultice stand-in. (The bark, twigs, and cones of alder offer complex and useful medicine: vulnerary, astringent, circulation-enhancing, immune-enhancing, antimicrobial . . . But dry the bark and twigs before taking them internally to avoid an emetic effect. Not an issue with chewing a leaf or two.) Clay paste also helps draw out irritants and foreign objects.

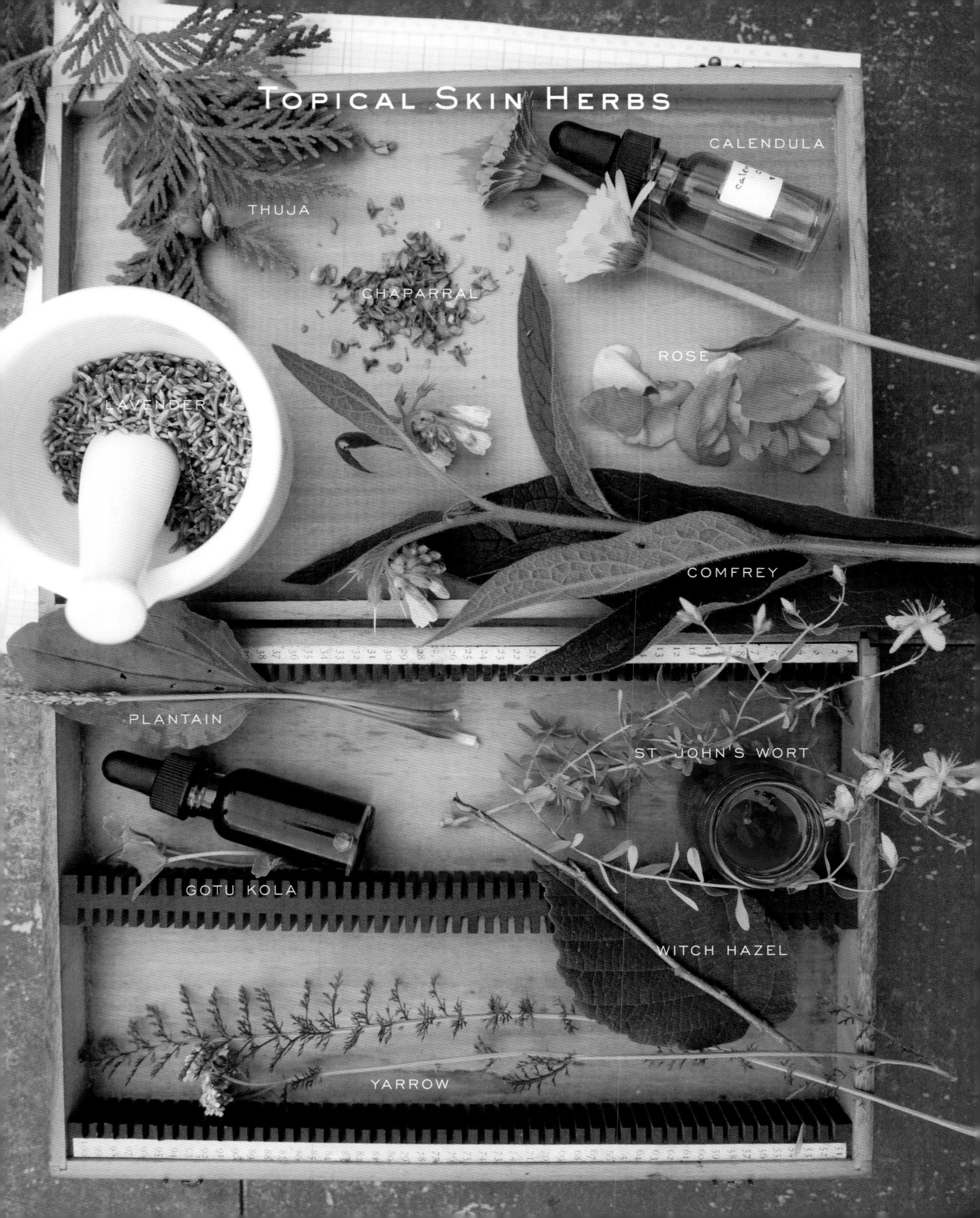

Topical Skin Herbs

CALENDULA

THUJA

CHAPARRAL

ROSE

LAVENDER

COMFREY

PLANTAIN

ST. JOHN'S WORT

GOTU KOLA

WITCH HAZEL

YARROW

▸ Yarrow

Achillea millefolium

Availability: G+ W+ C-

Key Properties: The species name, *millefolium*, translates to "thousand leafed," in reference to its ferny, finely divided leaves, but you can think of yarrow as having a million uses. Best known as a "wound wort" to stanch bleeding, ease injury pain, and speed healing on the battlefield, yarrow's genus name comes from the Greek warrior Achilles. However, this just hints at yarrow's usefulness for the skin and body. As a blood regulator, it helps clot when things need to be clotted, improves circulation and blood flow when needed, and also strengthens the lining of blood vessels and capillaries. This makes it useful internally and externally for hemorrhoids, varicose veins, spider veins, and easy bruising, as well as other cardio-related issues. Yarrow also has some antimicrobial properties (for cuts, colds, stomach bugs, urinary tract infections, and so forth) and astringent-vulnerary abilities (to tighten/tone boggy tissue and improve healing), and it can be applied externally (as a low-alcohol tincture) as an all-natural insect repellent.

Additional Benefits: Consumed or applied hot, it promotes the flow of "juices" in our body — blood circulation, sweat (including to break a fever), and digestive juices. Drinking or applying it cold amplifies the tightening and toning effect on the tissues (e.g., skin, gut, blood vessels). The fresh tea, with ¼ teaspoon salt added per cup, can also be used as an eyewash (as can a tea similarly prepared with rose petals).

Preparation: Simply chew or mash the leaves and apply — you will be amazed! Use the fresh (preferred) or freshly dried leaves and flowers of this common, multipurpose wildflower. The fresh poultice, tincture, and tea are the most common preparations, but you could do just about anything with yarrow. The dried powder, mixed with water into a paste, can be used when fresh leaves aren't available. Standard herb doses (see page 298) apply.

Cautions and Considerations: Generally safe, though large doses aren't necessary nor recommended. Because it is in the daisy family, some people are allergic to it topically, but that's rare. It may interact with some meds.

Similar Herbs: The dried bark, twigs, and cones of **alder** have somewhat similar actions but are less specifically blood regulating.

▸ Witch Hazel

Hamamelis virginiana

Availability: G W+ C+

Key Properties: This medium-size understory tree grows abundantly across the eastern United States. Where I live, almost anyone who takes a walk in the woods will walk by a witch hazel tree, though they usually have no idea unless they see the witchy yellow October blooms. Distilled witch hazel (a hydrosol, often preserved with alcohol) is a classic folk remedy for acne, itches, and disinfecting cuts and scrapes. As a potent astringent, it relieves hemorrhoid and varicose veins.

Additional Benefits: Witch hazel is almost exclusively used topically. Homeopathic witch hazel pills can be taken internally for hemorrhoids, nosebleeds, circulation, and varicose veins.

Preparation: Use the bark or leaves to make hydrosols, topical low-alcohol tinctures, topical teas, oils, salves, and creams. Or simply buy it at the store. Apply topically as often as needed.

Cautions and Considerations: Witch hazel is not generally used internally.

Similar Herbs: The bark of **oak**, and to a lesser extent the leaves, is also high in astringent, antimicrobial tannins and can be used topically, and sometimes internally (short term, in low doses or homeopathic preparations).

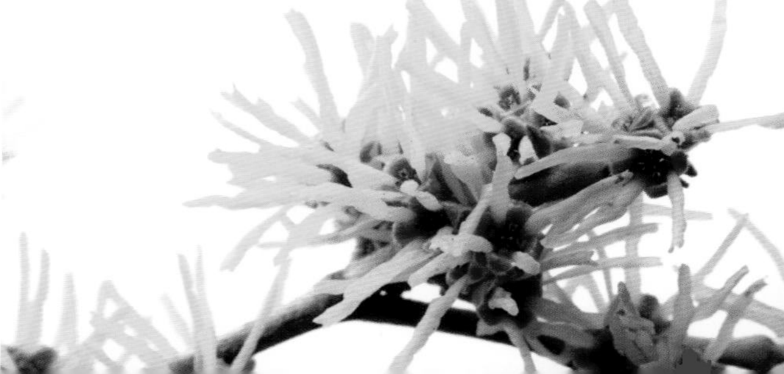

▸ Other Fabulous Skin Herbs

The herbs below tend to have more specific uses than the herbs we've just discussed, but all of them are wonderful allies for healing, nourishing, and strengthening the skin.

- **Gotu Kola**. Though it is often ignored by West-centric herbals, the Ayurvedic herb gotu kola ranks among my favorite skin herbs. It offers potent skin-healing, collagen-repairing, capillary-strengthening, and circulation-enhancing properties, both inside and out. Apply topically for wounds, preventing and healing scars, "anti-aging," spider veins, and varicose veins. Simultaneously taking it internally amplifies the effects. It's better known as a calm-energy adaptogen that enhances mental clarity and memory while quelling anxiety. (Learn more on page 53.) Not bad "side benefits"!

- **Comfrey.** Comfrey leaf and root contain allantoin, a cell proliferative that repairs wounds and broken bones at breakneck speed and may also strengthen skin and connective tissue. Comfrey's slimy mucilage simultaneously soothes as protein in the tissue is bound together. Use comfrey as a stand-in for arnica for bumps and bruises. (**Elder leaf** infused in olive oil works for this, too.) You can also add it to a formula to heal damaged tissue — perhaps with calendula for eczema or alongside antifungals for foot cream. Comfrey can be used in any form, but a low-alcohol decoction tincture (as a liniment or in creams), fresh plant poultice, or decocted bath soak are probably the strongest. The infused oil works well for salves and creams. Comfrey's speed in healing often isn't ideal; it doesn't disinfect and can seal in infections, especially in puncture wounds. It also lacks sophistication of healing response, which can cause excessive scar tissue to develop. **Gotu kola**, **calendula**, **St. John's wort**, and **honey** heal wounds with greater sophistication and less scarring, and I prefer these herbs for healing wounds and preventing scars, with comfrey as a lesser ingredient in the formula. Note: Although comfrey's liver-toxic PAs make it less appropriate for internal use and some PAs may absorb through the skin, periodic topical use should be fine.

- **Rose.** Rose petals and buds heal your skin in two ways: (1) their gentle astringency will tighten and tone, and (2) the aromatic volatile oils nourish and soothe. Rose is a classic herb for aging skin and wrinkles. A drop or two of rose essential oil will take any skin-care recipe to new heights, but unfortunately true rose essential oil can cost $600 per ounce! That's because it takes nearly 1 ton (literally) of rose petals to make 1 ounce of essential oil via natural methods. Rosewater hydrosol makes a more affordable stand-in. Add a few drops of the essential oil to recipes or use rosewater hydrosol (homemade or store-bought) for toners, creams, and so on. Beware of adulteration in both the essential oil and hydrosols, and be sure you're buying medicinal-quality roses (not potpourri), preferably organic. You can add petals (or tea made from them) to your bath. You'll get more aromatics from a long-steeped cold infusion and more astringency with hot water. Learn more about rose on page 158.

- **Thuja.** An evergreen with scalelike growth and small brown cones, thuja grows abundantly in pockets across the Northeast (*Thuja occidentalis*, also called eastern white cedar and arborvitae) and Northwest (*T. plicata*, also called western red cedar and incense cedar). Eastern thuja is the official medicinal species, though the western can be used similarly. Thuja has the greatest reputation for fighting warts when applied externally or taken homeopathically or in drop-doses internally. However, it can be used with great effect for almost any icky skin "critter," including fungal, bacterial, and viral infections. I have seen it work quickly for ringworm, athlete's foot, toenail fungus, and other fungal issues, though continued use to fully resolve the issue is recommended. In low or homeopathic doses taken internally, thuja can be used to stimulate immune function, which has made it useful for both internal and external infections, the common cold, and possibly cancer. Harvest the newest green growth, and use the needles fresh or dry to make infused oil, salve, tincture, vinegar, or a soak. Apply frequently, ideally two to four times daily until the issue has been resolved for several weeks. Thuja blends well with other common antimicrobial herbs like **chaparral** and **tea tree.**

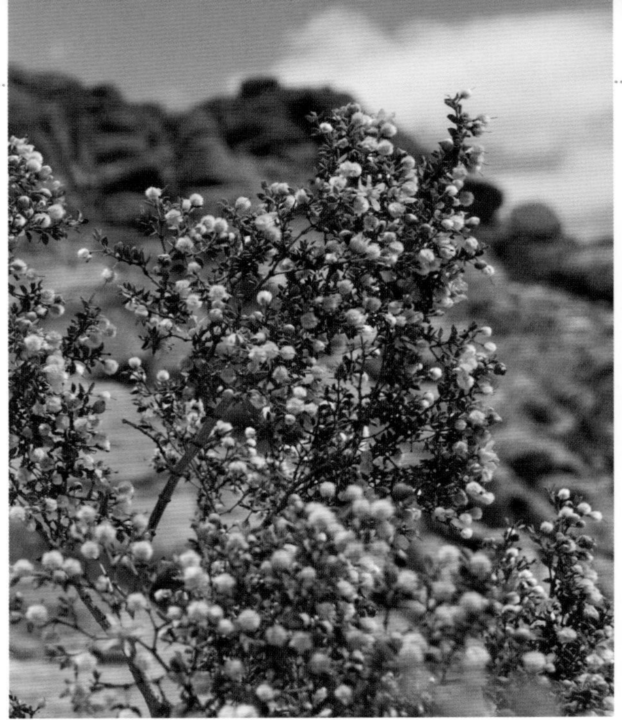

- **Chaparral.** A shrubby tree that grows in vast swaths throughout much of the American desert, chaparral has a potent fragrance that fills the air when it rains, garnering the love of southwestern herbalists. These same aromatics play a role in the herb's potent antioxidant, anti-inflammatory, antimicrobial, antivirals, and wound-healing properties. It is most noted for its ability to quickly heal wounds with minimal scar formation while discouraging and fighting skin infections of all types. You'll find it in almost every Southwest-made antifungal formula. It relieves itching and knocks the infection back within just a day or two, but fungal infections (which have a way of creeping back as soon as you get complacent) require long-term repeated applications to fully resolve. Herbalists who specialize in first aid, including 7Song and Sam Coffman, find chaparral invaluable and broadly useful in their medic kits. Thanks, in part, to chaparral's antioxidant profile, the infused oil offers light protection against sunburn and sun damage and can also be applied in a variety of forms (oil, bath, compress) postsunburn to soothe the burn and reduce damage. Apply topical chaparral remedies as often as needed. Although you will find people who use chaparral internally for a variety of uses, including cancer, I would not advise it due to potential liver toxicity. If you're processing and drying large quantities, work in a well-ventilated area; otherwise you may find the fragrance overpowering.

TAKE A BATH

DID YOU KNOW THAT a good soak in the tub delivers herbs directly to your skin *and* inside your body? You can absorb herbs' healing properties so well through the skin during a bath that French herbalist Maurice Messegue often recommended herbs in bath form — including hand and foot baths — for a wide range of ills with great success. This is a particularly effective way to deliver herbs to babies and children (so small and thin-skinned), but it also works for adults. Make a strong pot of tea and add it to the bathwater, or fill a stocking with dried herbs and hang it under the faucet as the tub fills.

Sparkling Skin Super Infusion

This tea blend includes therapeutic doses of nutritious, detoxifying, anti-inflammatory, and nervine herbs, all of which support healthy skin. Feel free to play around with the ingredients based on your needs, tastes, and what you have on hand.

- 2 tablespoons burdock root
- 1 tablespoon horsetail
- 1 tablespoon lemon balm
- 1 tablespoon nettles
- 1 tablespoon oat straw
- 1 tablespoon red clover
- 2 teaspoons peppermint or spearmint
- 1 teaspoon calendula
- 1 teaspoon yellow dock root
- Sprinkle of rose petals or buds

Combine the herbs in a 1-quart glass jar or French press. Add enough boiling water to fill the container. Stir, cover, and let steep for at least 4 hours and up to overnight. Strain, pressing on the herbs to remove as much liquid as you can. Drink hot or cold throughout the day.

Calendula-St. John's Wort Salve

This simple recipe handles so many skin woes! Rashes, itches, eczema, bug bites, wounds, cracks, diaper rash, hemorrhoids, and more. I keep it in large jars as well as lip balm tubes for on-the-go care (roll it up and wipe what you need off the top with your finger or a tissue). A potent salve comes out deep orange-red. For instructions on making the infused oils, see page 313.

- 1 ounce beeswax, smashed into bits
- 3 ounces calendula-infused olive oil
- 1 ounce St. John's wort–infused olive oil
- 20 drops lavender essential oil (optional)

Melt the beeswax in a double boiler over low heat. Add the infused oils. Stir until everything is melted and combined. Remove from the heat and stir in the lavender essential oil (if using). Then pour into containers. Let cool, then cap the containers. This should keep at least 1 year, often several years.

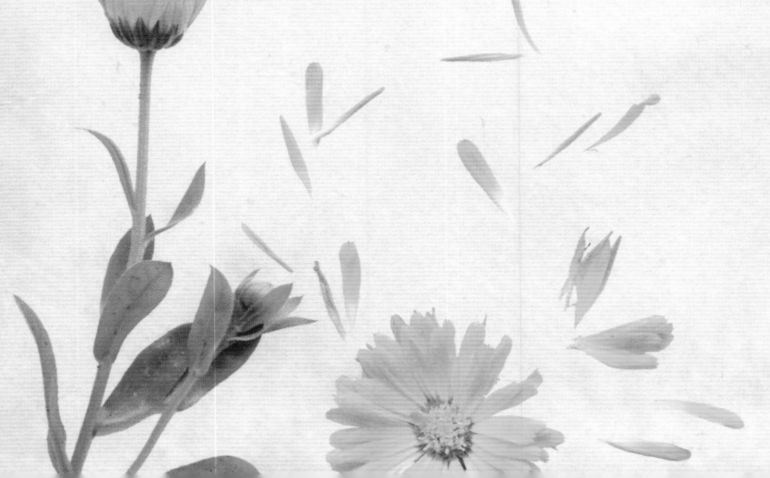

Specific Skin Woes: Considerations *and* Protocols

Although skin-care protocols can be tricky and highly individual, here's a quick guide to the most useful internal and external approaches.

Itches and Rashes: Eczema, Psoriasis, Poison Ivy, and Co.

Anytime you see chronic itchy rashes, take a close look at (1) food sensitivities, (2) topical irritants, and (3) stress. Chances are, one or more is taking its toll. Try to go as natural and gentle as possible in all aspects of your life, and also look at underlying factors including inflammation, irritation, and poor detoxification and digestion. See the protocol for eczema (below) for more.

In cases of poison ivy and itchy bug bites, plantain tends to work better, as do salves and compresses made with fresh chickweed or cleavers. Jewelweed, grindelia, and sweet fern are classic remedies for poison ivy — apply the mashed plant, tincture, ice cubes made of the concentrated tea, or a cool wash. Also consider witch hazel or lavender. A clay paste or plantain poultice helps draw out irritants of various sorts. A few drops of lavender or peppermint essential oil (pure peppermint burns the skin, so dilute it well) can counter the itch.

Practice identifying poison ivy and its relatives to avoid it in the future; those irritating oils can hang out for years! Awful mystery rash? If fresh juices of parsley-family greens (carrots, parsnips, wild carrot, celery) get on your skin and bake in the sun, they burn, blister, and create a nasty rash.

If your rash gets worse or spreads under whatever remedy you place on your skin, get to the doctor. You may have a staph infection, which can get dangerous quickly.

PROTOCOL POINTS

Eczema

Eczema is a form of dermatitis that often coincides with allergies, asthma, migraines/headaches, sinus problems, and gut issues. Inflammation and irritation are common themes.

Diet: Sleuth out and avoid sources of food allergies and sensitivities; gluten/wheat and eggs are common culprits. This alone will "fix" most cases of eczema. Also eat a whole-foods diet that is low in sugar and bad fats. Focus in particular on skin-supportive nutrients (see page 217), being sure to get omega-3s and probiotics, whether from food or supplements.

Lifestyle: Sleuth out and avoid any topical irritants including soap, lotion, laundry detergent, softener, and other personal-care and cleaning products. Seek out all-natural products or make your own. Try to avoid scratching the itch — it only makes the rash more itchy and damages the skin.

Herbs: Develop a skin-care routine that soothes and moisturizes with ingredients like calendula, olive oil, oatmeal, aloe, lavender, rose, plantain, and goat's milk soap. Calendula oil, salve, or cream can be miraculous. Address underlying internal factors including stress, inflammation, and detoxification with herbs like holy basil, nettle, lemon balm, turmeric, burdock, and red clover. Try the Sparkling Skin Super Infusion (page 225).

Wounds and Poor or Damaged Skin

Whether you have a chronic skin issue or a recent wound, you can really boost the healing response with herbs. Most chronic skin issues, ranging from rashes to acne, weaken the vitality of connective tissue and skin. Alongside the usual — good diet, sleep, et cetera — focus on the skin nutrients and apply wound-healing herbs such as gotu kola, calendula, St. John's wort, yarrow, plantain, and perhaps some comfrey.

In an acute injury, you can pack the wound with mashed fresh yarrow or chaparral leaves to help stanch bleeding, disinfect, and relieve pain. If the wound is deep, keep it clean and avoid infection with antimicrobial herbs and a careful eye. Honey makes an excellent wound healer, and a few drops of lavender essential oil may also help. Oil-based remedies are generally not recommended until the initial stages of healing have taken place. Compresses, diluted tinctures, and poultices tend to be more appropriate. Little infections become dangerous if not attended to; seek medical attention if you're unsure or see increasing redness.

For chronic poor wound healing — let's say you often get sores on your skin or are not recuperating as you should after surgery — first get checked out by a doc to rule out conditions like diabetes or other underlying issues that need addressing. Then amp up on skin nutrients and address inflammation and stress. Consider gotu kola (vulnerary) and holy basil (anti-inflammatory, stress-buster, and whole-body tonic) to support healing from within.

Acne

Acne develops when your skin doesn't rejuvenate properly and a pore gets clogged with oil, dead skin, and possibly bacteria. Poor detoxification tends to be an underlying factor. Most conventional acne therapies take a harsh antimicrobial approach, but acne has many underlying patterns, and the antimicrobial approach can be harsh on the skin. If you can figure out which factors are contributing to your acne, you can choose herbs appropriate for addressing your triggers. In general, look to alterative herbs such as yellow dock, dandelion, burdock, red clover, turmeric, schizandra, and alder. Tea blends are

ALL-NATURAL BUG SPRAY

YES, YOU CAN MAKE YOUR OWN BUG SPRAY to repel mosquitoes, ticks, and other biting insects, and it's super easy.

- 5 drops lavender essential oil
- 5 drops rose geranium essential oil
- 5 drops citronella or lemon eucalyptus essential oil
- 5 drops catnip essential oil (optional; it's hard to find)
- 2 ounces yarrow tincture or plain vodka

Combine all the ingredients in a spritzer bottle and shake well. Apply as needed to keep the bugs away. You can also use sweet fern as a smudge to chase off pesky insects, or just add it to your campfire.

If the bugs win out over your best efforts, see page 220 for postbite care. My favorites: lavender essential oil and plantain leaf as a poultice or salve.

nice; however, capsules and tinctures can work, too. Remember, your skin might get a bit worse for a few days before it gets better. Alterative herbs often aid hormone-related acne, too, but you may also need herbs specific to your hormone issues, like vitex.

People with acne often suffer from an inability to properly digest and process fats and general digestive-liver sluggishness. As much as possible, enjoy a whole-foods, nutrient-dense diet and avoid excess sugar, bad fats (pizza, fried food), alcohol, and drugs. Eat lots of veggies and bitter and fiber-rich foods regularly. Drink plenty of water.

In acne-prone skin, pores become clogged and skin irritated easily. Avoid this with a hands-off approach: don't touch, rub, poke, or pick at problem points. Additionally, try to keep hair, and more specifically the products used in styling it, away from acne-prone skin. Change bedsheets often, especially pillowcases, and wash clothing that is worn frequently (pajamas, baseball caps, and coats/jackets) to help minimize breakouts. Treat your cell phone to a wipe now and again. Get plenty of sleep, and address stress as it arises.

Develop a comprehensive yet gentle skin-care routine that includes a thorough (but not too harsh) cleanser and a light moisturizer like filtered jojoba oil or Rosemary Gladstar's well-loved "perfect cream" (you can find the recipe in her books and online). Applying a light coat of noncomedogenic moisturizer helps discourage your skin from producing more oil. Antimicrobial additions include tea tree, lavender, oregano, bee balm, or calendula. Once or twice a week, exfoliate with cornmeal (harsh) or coarsely ground oatmeal (gentle). Also consider a weekly honey pat (smear a teaspoon of honey over your face and pat for about 10 to 15 minutes, letting it get really sticky — this helps clean pores, invigorate skin, and balance microbes).

Infections, Warts, and Fungi

When it icks, turn to the antis! Antimicrobial herbs kick back skin fungus, bacteria, and other microorganism-related skin woes surprisingly well. Although herbs may not be as hard-hitting as conventional medications, they have a more multifaceted approach. One herb can target multiple types of germs — bacteria, fungi, et cetera — while also healing the skin. The variety of antimicrobial constituents and actions in plants discourages drug resistance, too. Hit it hard and stick with it until you've been clear for a few weeks to a month. Fungal issues have a way of creeping back if you let them.

In an acute situation like an infected cut, you can probably stick with topical antimicrobial herbs. However, for chronic issues the problem lies deeper, and you'll want to look internally. Bacteria and fungi love sweet stuff. Cut out most — preferably *all* — sugars, sweeteners, and refined carbs (the white stuff) and take it easy on high-glycemic fruits, potatoes, and grains. Add in herbs that discourage microbes: garlic, pau d'arco (fabulous with chai spices!), ginger, cinnamon, cloves, cardamom, oregano, bee balm, thyme, and alder. Taking probiotics and fermented foods like kimchi can help rebalance the good guy/bad guy playing field.

Fungal and Bacterial Infections

Fungal and bacterial infections generally require antimicrobial herbs applied topically — liberally, regularly, and without pause. Thuja and chaparral are the real stars, able to handle almost any skin germ that comes your way. Berberine-rich herbs including goldenseal, Oregon grape root, barberry, or *Coptis* also work well for a range of microbes, even staph (but be careful since staph infections get dangerous quickly). Berberines stain yellow, and be mindful of ethical overharvesting concerns (buy organically cultivated herbs, rather than wildcrafted). Don't underestimate the value of backyard antimicrobials, including alder bark and twigs, *Monarda* species leaves, and oregano, garlic, and thyme, which tend to work best as soaks, compresses, vinegars, and liniments. Generally, alcohol-, vinegar-, and water-based remedies work better for microbial infections, though chaparral and thuja often work well as oils and salves, too. Antimicrobial essential oils make potent additions to your blends: tea tree, spruce, lavender, eucalyptus. As a formula "extra" consider adding an herb that promotes the growth of healthy tissue, such as comfrey, horsetail, or gotu kola, and make sure you're covering all the bases of skin nutrition.

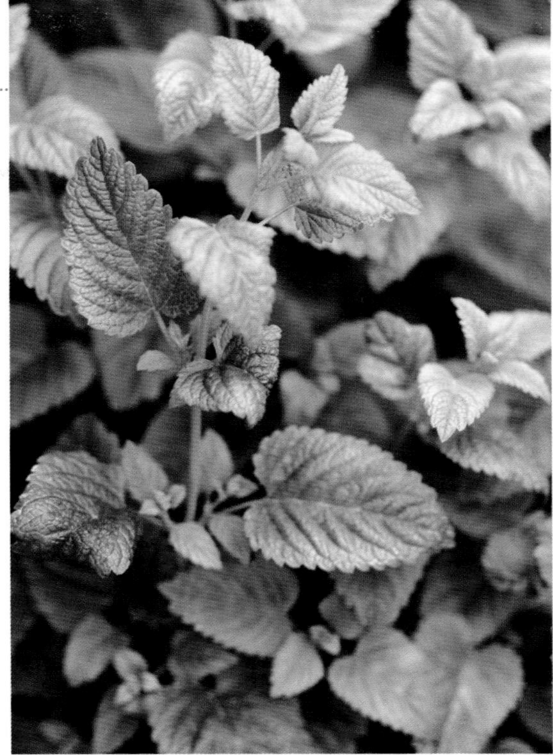

Warts

Warts have a couple of fierce foes: thuja and celandine. Thuja works well in almost any form. For celandine, the fresh bright orange latex, applied topically, works best. Try mashing it up and applying a bandage on it overnight — this often completely eliminates warts in a matter of days! Also consider low-dose or homeopathic thuja internally. This virus-based condition is benign yet contagious, and outbreaks tend to be tied to the health of your overall body, immune system, and general good health habits. The virus can be spread by contact with a wart and particularly thrives in moist environments like sweaty shoes and public showers.

Herpes

Herpes, a family of viruses that causes cold sores, genital herpes, shingles, and chicken pox, requires a slightly different approach. Halt its spread with speedy application of lemon balm leaf, which contains compounds that help block herpes from breaking into your cells and replicating, while simultaneously encouraging healing. Also take it internally to soothe nerves and support overall health. The fleeting essential oil of lemon balm is our key player, so use fresh plant material or freshly dried herb, or purchase the essential oil (expensive!) or cream. Try a few squirts of fresh plant tincture (not more than a few years old), then dab some more on location. Self-heal oil or salve quells itching. St. John's wort oil (the redder, the better) simultaneously fights the virus, soothes nerve pain, and promotes healing, which is great at any stage of outbreak, even postshingles nerve pain and crankiness. In chronic herpes issues like cold sores and genital herpes, consider taking the amino acid supplement lysine and reducing your intake of arginine-rich foods like nuts, seeds, soy, and shellfish if they seem to be triggers (they're otherwise healthy foods).

BEAUTY SLEEP

LIVING IN A HIGH-STRESS STATE shuts down attention to the skin, and skin-friendly nutrients get sent elsewhere. Your body gives extra TLC to your skin while you sleep, eliminating toxins via an interconnected detoxification system, repairing damage, and generating new skin cells. Signs of sleep deprivation, including dark rings under your eyes and a gaunt, grayish, wrinkled appearance, will show on the skin in just *one* night, worsening as the deprivation continues. So make sure to get your beauty sleep!

AT A GLANCE: TOPICAL SKIN-CARE HERBS AND FORMULAS

Use this chart as a quick reference for the topical herbs discussed in this chapter and other common herbs with similar uses. You can use herbs singly or in formula.

	Vulnerary (Wound Healing, Scars)	Anti-Itch, Rashes, Eczema	Poison Ivy	Bug Bites/Stings	Burns/Sunburns	Mild Sunscreen/Sun Protection	Dry Skin	Oily Skin/Acne	Aging Skin/Wrinkles	Varicose/Spider Veins and Hemorrhoids	Bleeding	Pain	Antifungal/ Antibacterial/Disinfect	Antiwart	Antiherpes	Baby Skin	Natural Preservative
Topical Herbs																	
Aloe leaf/gel	X	X	X		X				X				X			X	
Calendula flower	X	X					X			X			X			X	
Cayenne pepper*											X	X			X		
Celandine aerial parts														X			
Chaparral leaf	X				X	X							X		X		X
Chickweed aerial parts	X	X	X	X	X											X	
Cleavers aerial parts	X	X	X	X	X											X	
Comfrey leaf/root*	X					X	X		X								
Dandelion flower								X				X					
Goldenseal/berberines root/leaf				X							X		X				X
Gotu kola aerial parts	X								X	X							
Green tea leaf	X				X	X			X	X							X
Grindelia flower/bud		X	X	X													
Horsetail aerial parts	X								X								
Jewelweed aerial parts			X														
Lavender bud	X	X	X	X	X		X	X	X				X	X		X	X
Lemon balm aerial parts	X	X			X			X							X	X	
Licorice root		X													X		
Oatmeal		X	X				X	X	X							X	
Oregano/bee balm aerial parts	X												X				X
Plantain leaf	X	X	X	X												X	
Rose petals	X				X			X	X	X	X					X	
Self-heal aerial parts	X	X			X		X		X						X	X	
St. John's wort bud/ flower (fresh)	X	X			X	X						X			X	X	
Sweet fern leaf		X	X	X													
Thuja leaf													X	X			
Witch hazel bark/leaf	X	X	X	X				X	X	X	X		X				
Yarrow aerial parts	X	X		X						X	X		X				

	Vulnerary (Wound Healing, Scars)	Anti-Itch, Rashes, Eczema	Poison Ivy	Bug Bites/Stings	Burns/Sunburns	Mild Sunscreen/Sun Protection	Dry Skin	Oily Skin/Acne	Aging Skin/Wrinkles	Varicose/Spider Veins and Hemorrhoids	Bleeding	Pain	Antifungal/Antibacterial/Disinfect	Antiwart	Antiherpes	Baby Skin	Natural Preservative
Bases																	
Alcohol	X		X	X						X		X	X	X	X		X
Clay		X	X	X				X			X						
Oil/cream	X	X		X			X		X	X		X			X	X	
Rose hip seed oil	X								X								X
Shea butter		X					X		X								
Vinegar	X		X	X	X								X	X			X
Vitamin E oil	X						X		X								X
Water	X		X		X	X										X	
Essential Oils*/Hydrosols																	
Citrus*								X									X
Lavender	X	X	X	X	X		X	X	X			X	X		X		X
Lemon balm	X	X						X	X						X		
Oregano/thyme													X	X			X
Peppermint		X	X	X								X					
Rose	X						X		X								
Rose geranium							X	X	X								
Rosemary/spruce/eucalyptus													X				X
Tea tree								X					X	X			X
Wintergreen/birch*												X					

*These herbs have potential side effects and should be researched more thoroughly before being used.

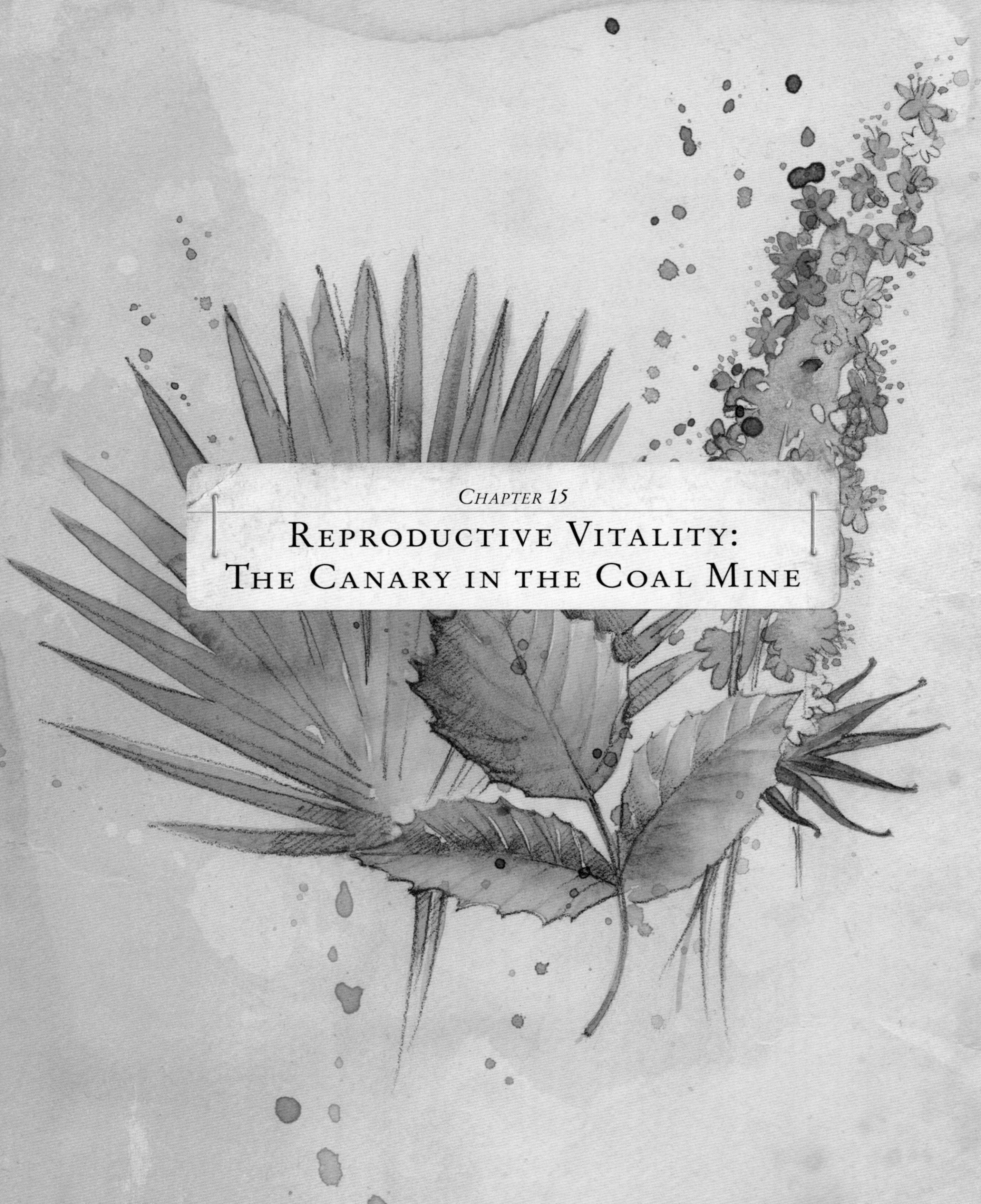

Chapter 15

Reproductive Vitality: The Canary in the Coal Mine

REPRODUCTIVE HEALTH serves as a barometer for your overall health in at least two ways. First, your reproductive system comes last in the pecking order of your body's priorities. You need to be able to breathe, circulate blood, digest, detoxify, et cetera, in order to survive. The ability to make babies (the ultimate purpose of the reproductive system) is superfluous, something to do when everything else is going great. After all, making and raising babies taxes your body and mind and certainly isn't necessary (from a pragmatic perspective) for your survival. For this reason, reproductive issues can be the canary in the coal mine for bigger-picture problems. Stress, sleep deprivation, nutrient deficiencies, thyroid wobbles, obesity, cardiovascular disease, and blood sugar issues are just a few things that can send your hormones swinging and muck up the reproductive wiring.

In a slightly different yet connected way, your reproductive system functions as a loudspeaker for your body's overall health. This is particularly true for women, whose complicated and difficult-to-ignore cycles expand and contract each month and are easily thrown awry. Imbalances elsewhere amplify during weak points in the monthly cycle, most commonly the days just before you get your period. Men are equally affected, but because their hormones and cycles are a little less obvious — at least until middle age, when they manifest as prostate and sexual problems — it's easy to ignore the warning signs.

Hormonal Overview: Conversations between Your Brain *and* Gonads

At its simplest, your reproductive system's goal is to make babies to propagate the species, but of course it's so much more than that. Your reproductive hormones affect your mood, energy levels, libido, detoxification, elimination, bone strength, skin, and more. They naturally kick into overdrive during adolescence, normalize during your early adulthood, then wobble and taper off later in life. Most reproductive hormones are produced in the ovaries and testes, prompted by hormones from your brain that tell your gonads what to make and when. (It's kind of like the childhood game Operator: gonadotropin-releasing hormone in your hypothalamus prompts the release of various "stimulator" hormones in your pituitary, which then signal hormone production in your reproductive glands. Those hormones are then released into the bloodstream to instruct the reproductive organs and exert effects throughout your body.) Your liver clears old hormones from the bloodstream.

If your reproductive hormones start to falter, your brain starts to "yell" at the reproductive system to pick up the pace, and eventually those brain hormones may begin to waver as well. As people age, both men and women begin to accumulate more "old, cranky" versions of their primary reproductive hormones. They tend to wreak more havoc on the body than "young, happy" hormones, most notably increasing the risk for certain cancers, including breast, ovarian, and prostate, but also contributing to benign prostatic hyperplasia (BPH) and fibroids. We'll delve more deeply into those cranky hormones in the separate male and female sections of this chapter.

Basic Needs *and* Tonics *for* Both Sexes

As with any body system, a good diet, adequate sleep, and regular exercise set the stage for vibrant health. But one area that *really* demands your attention when balancing reproductive health is stress. Even though stress and reproductive hormones are produced by different endocrine glands, the signals that trigger their production start in the brain. Your brain has an amazing capacity for multitasking, but it can only do so much. If you're living in fight-or-flight mode, reproductive hormones get put on mute while stress does all the talking. Also, stress and reproductive hormones have similar building blocks, and when push comes to shove, guess which get those nutrients?

This is why most holistic reproductive protocols include a foundation in nourishment — in the form of nutrient-dense herbs, diet, or specialized dietary supplements — and stress management. Adaptogenic herbs that help your body adapt to stress and manage the stress response, as well as nervine herbs that bring things down a notch and nourish the nervous-endocrine system, make great supportive herbs in a reproductive formula.

Maca, ashwagandha, schizandra, ginseng and ginseng-like herbs (codonopsis, eleuthero, and others), holy basil, oat straw and milky oat seed, and nettles are just a few favorites that cross these categories, serving as nutritives or stress modulators. Lifestyle approaches are also ideal: meditation, yoga, spending time in nature, and regular exercise are just a few ways to bring your body out of fight-or-flight mode and back into rest-repair-and-reproduce mode.

Alongside these approaches, we use specific reproductive herbs to nudge and fine-tune hormone output. They're incredibly effective solo, but they work even better in a broader, more holistic program. In most cases, reproductive herbs don't actually contain any hormones, but they seem to alter and improve the way your body produces and eliminates hormones. In many cases, they're amplifiers. For example, vitex enhances the function of progesterone greatly, but if you aren't making any progesterone at all, it's not likely to do much. This is in contrast to both conventional and naturopathic medicines' use of hormone drugs, including birth control pills and bioidentical creams, that literally *contain* hormones and put them into your bloodstream to *do* the job. The drugs put your body in the backseat and drive it around. The herbs sit next to you while *you* drive, reminding you how to do it yourself.

So now that you have some basic understanding of reproductive health, let's delve into male and female reproductive health.

Men's Reproductive Health

Truth be told, only two reproductive issues tend to bring a guy to my office door: loss of libido or sexual function and benign prostatic hyperplasia (BPH). But it'd be unfair to men (and the ladies who take care of their men) to say that's all the male reproductive system is about.

Male genitalia has an inside-outside layout, with the penis and scrotum (home to testicles, also called testes) outside the body and a few other glands hanging out nearby, just below the bladder, with some important tubing to connect it all. They primarily focus on sex and fertility, with the majority of the glands relating to semen production.

Semen

Semen production requires a perfect interplay of nutrients, hormonal stimulation, and clear runways so that you can make strong swimmers and get them where they want to go. As with your entire body, you are what you eat, and your diet plays a major role in semen quality: amino acids from protein, fructose from carbs, fatty acids from good fats, antioxidants, vitamins, and minerals. Folic acid, omega-3s, vitamins E and C, selenium, and zinc are key players. It's not surprising to hear that recent studies show a nutrient-dense diet improves sperm quality, reverses fertility issues, and improves the likelihood of not just conception but also a healthy pregnancy and healthy baby.

Male Hormones

On the hormone front, testes do the bulk of the work, producing various male hormones — collectively called androgens — that include testosterone as well as dehydroepiandrosterone (DHEA), androsterone ("andro"), and others. The all-important testosterone is an anabolic steroid and major sex hormone. Besides encouraging sperm production, sexual desire, and fertility, testosterone encourages the body to increase bone mass, muscle mass, and body hair and leads to an overall sense of vitality and virility. (Men and women *both* have testosterone *and* estrogen, but each gender favors one.) In men, the pituitary's release of luteinizing hormone (LH) in the brain stimulates the production of testosterone in the testes. Follicle-stimulating hormone (FSH) from the pituitary *plus* testosterone *together* stimulate sperm production. A little bit of "young, happy" testosterone gets converted into "old, cranky" dihydrotestosterone (DHT) via normal body processes, but as you age, the tendency for this to occur increases. DHT offers three to ten times the potency of testosterone, but not always in a good way, especially if the DHT/andro ratio goes off kilter. High DHT levels correlate with balding and prostate problems. High estrogen (estradiol) levels also pose problems and may put men at an even greater risk of prostate issues, including BPH and cancer.

The Penis and Erectile Function

From a practical perspective, the main job of this phallic focal point of male anatomy is to get sperm where it wants to go. From an anatomy and physiology perspective, it's all about circulation. Although the penis contains some muscles, cartilage, and tubing, sexual and reproductive tasks are highly dependent on the penis's blood vessels that create rigidity. Although overall sexual vitality relates primarily to testosterone, the parasympathetic nervous system (the "relaxation response") controls sexual arousal, while the fight-or-flight sympathetic nervous system shuts down the erection, ideally after it's done its job. So you can see that both your nervous and cardiovascular systems play a major role in a happy, healthy sex life. Sexual problems tend to be related to one or both. Erectile issues tend to be the canary in the coal mine for a man's overall health. Underlying issues that may need to be sleuthed out and addressed include heart disease (especially atherosclerosis), diabetes and blood sugar issues, depression, psychological stress, post-traumatic stress disorder (especially from sexual abuse, which is incredibly common among women *and* men), and medication side effects. Depending on the situation, you may want to incorporate adaptogen, nervine, anti-inflammatory, or circulation-enhancing herbs into your treatment protocol.

PROTOCOL POINTS

Low Libido in Men

Loss or diminishment of libido is worth a checkup to rule out underlying causes that may necessitate medical attention. If you have difficulty attaining or maintaining an erection, look at cardiovascular health, diabetes, blood sugar imbalance, and drug side effects. Stress, abuse history, emotional and relationship issues, or hormone imbalance may also be at play, especially in climax and arousal issues.

Diet: Eat a healthy whole-foods diet. Indulge regularly in aphrodisiac foods, including shellfish, cayenne, chocolate, rosemary, and garlic.

Lifestyle: Stress management, mind-body balance, adequate sleep, regular exercise, and communication and connection with your partner are all important. Enlisting the aid of a specialized therapist may also help.

Herbs: Libido herbs can be zippy or chill, depending on what you need. Zippy libido herbs include ginseng, rhodiola, codonopsis, cordyceps, tribulus, and eleuthero. More balancing libido adaptogens include schizandra, ashwagandha, damiana, and maca. If you're a stress case, consider calming and nervine herbs like passionflower, skullcap, lemon balm, damiana, roses, hawthorn, linden, and milky oat seed. For cardiovascular involvement, consider garlic, hawthorn, and cayenne. For specific erection support, consider red ginseng, muira puama, cordyceps, or low-dose yohimbe (with caution).

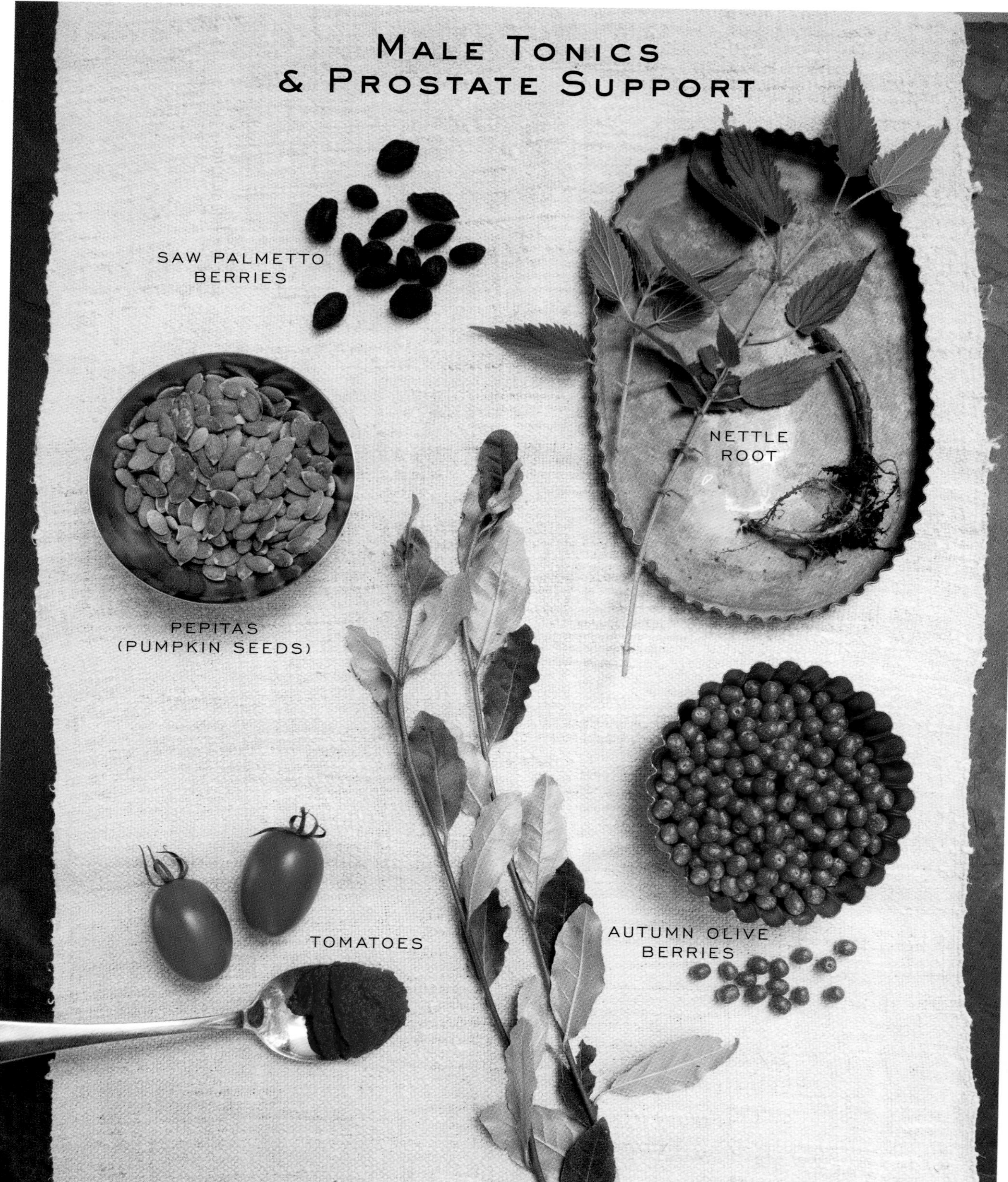
Male Tonics
& Prostate Support
SAW PALMETTO
BERRIES
NETTLE
ROOT
PEPITAS
(PUMPKIN SEEDS)
TOMATOES
AUTUMN OLIVE
BERRIES

Prostate Woes

The walnut-size prostate gland that wraps around the male urethra near the bladder tends to cause the most issues as you age. Its main goal is to produce the nutrient-rich fluid that transports and nourishes sperm. Unfortunately, it can get inflamed, sometimes due to infection (prostatitis), or it can develop cancer — and both conditions require treatment by a doctor. Prostate cancer is by far the most prominent cancer in men and second only to lung cancer in causing death, but it's almost 100 percent treatable if caught early. So be sure to get regular prostate-specific antigen (PSA) tests and rectal exams (however unpleasant) as directed by your doctor.

Benign prostatic hyperplasia (BPH), or prostate enlargement — the most common prostate woe — affects most men over the age of 50, and your risk increases as the decades continue. It's usually easy to manage or treat with natural therapies. Abnormal, noncancerous growth causes BPH. The enlargement pinches on the urethra and puts pressure on the bladder, causing frequent, painful urination; discomfort; and feeling like you can't completely void your bladder. Fortunately, several herbs show promise for their ability to manage the condition.

▸ Saw Palmetto

Serenoa repens

Availability: G- W- C+

Key Properties: The awful-tasting berries of this shrubby palm may be your best defense against BPH. Remember the "old, cranky" testosterone known as dehydrotestosterone (DHT)? High DHT levels encourage the prostate to become enlarged. Saw palmetto appears to help reduce DHT's damaging effects in a couple of ways. First, it reduces the amount of "young, happy" testosterone that gets converted into DHT. Then, it makes it harder for DHT to bind to prostate cells and cause problems. Research suggests that it also normalizes the endocrine gland's reproductive hormone function and discourages estrogen, another culprit in prostate issues. Although it may be appropriate in prostatitis and prostate cancer protocols, it's not sufficient alone to treat these more severe conditions, and working with your doctor is essential. Though research is mixed, saw palmetto may be the most effective, safest remedy for alleviating simple BPH. It also reduces inflammatory compounds related to BPH, promotes overall prostate and bladder health, and fights cystitis.

Additional Benefits: Less commonly, we use saw palmetto to balance hormones in women, particularly to reduce excess testosterone and as part of a protocol in polycystic ovarian syndrome.

Preparation: The fatty components of saw palmetto responsible for its activity aren't well extracted as tea (and it tastes terrible!) or tincture, though a fresh berry tincture in high-proof alcohol may work. Most often saw palmetto is taken as soft gel capsules, 160 mg twice per day, standardized to 85 to 95 percent fatty acids and sterols.

Cautions and Considerations: Although generally safe, it may cause stomach upset (take it with food) and may make PSA scores appear better than they are. PSA scores determine the likelihood of prostate cancer, so scrutinize even slight increases if you're taking saw palmetto.

Similar Herbs: Saw palmetto works even better if it's combined with other prostate-friendly herbs and nutrients. It's commonly combined with **pygeum**, which seems to be exceptionally beneficial for BPH but is unfortunately unethically overharvested in Africa. **Nettle** root is a more sustainable, local substitute. Also consider men's health tonics (see page 238), including pumpkin seeds, pumpkin seed oil, lycopene, pomegranate, and anti-inflammatory herbs.

Men's Health Tonics *and* Key Nutrients

Your reproductive vitality interlinks with other body systems and patterns, particularly circulation, inflammation, stress, and nutrition. For this reason, herbs that address these issues often manage male reproductive issues and prevent disease, solo or in combination with more traditional "men's herbs."

▸ Zinc and Pumpkin Seed Oil

Zinc, pumpkin seeds, and pumpkin seed oil provide important nutrients for your reproductive organs' function, disease prevention, and treatment. Even though you don't need a lot of zinc — just 11 to 15 mg per day — it's essential for semen production, fertility, and your prostate. In fact, semen contains a good deal of zinc, and you lose a little bit with each ejaculation. Adequate amounts of this mineral help prevent cancer and reduce BPH symptoms. High-dose supplements aren't necessary and may even be problematic; modest doses from food and supplements are preferred. Oysters are *loaded* with 27 to 50 mg of zinc (hence the aphrodisiac reputation), and you'll get 1 to 5 mg from shellfish, most meat/poultry/fish, yogurt, cashews, pumpkin seeds or pepitas, and other nuts, seeds, and dairy. A handful of raw pumpkin or pepita seeds provides the added benefit of pumpkin seed *oil*, which helps tighten and tone the bladder and prostate tissue while reducing BPH symptoms. Studies suggest that it works at least in part by inhibiting damaging effects of testosterone and DHT on the prostate.

▸ Lycopene

This deep red carotenoid pigment gains high marks as an antioxidant that specifically targets the prostate to prevent cancer. It's most famously high in tomatoes but can also be found in autumn olives, a common invasive berry with up to 18 times more lycopene than tomatoes, as well as watermelon, pink grapefruit, pink guava, lycii/goji berries, rose hips, and carrots (especially red ones). As a fat-soluble nutrient, lycopene gets a bioavailability boost when cooked, concentrated, or served with a little bit of oil or fat. That's why, ironically, ketchup has at least triple the lycopene content of a raw tomato (even though it's obviously *not* the healthiest food overall). Tomato paste and sauce provide a happy medium, ideally stored in glass instead of cans or plastic to reduce your exposure to bisphenol A (BPA) and related plastic compounds that cause cancer and disrupt hormones. Tomato-heavy and high-lycopene diets are associated with a reduced risk of prostate cancer, possibly because this fat-soluble antioxidant targets fat-rich organs — such as the prostate and testes — and fights the oxidative damage that can lead to cancer.

PROTOCOL POINTS

BPH

This condition is incredibly common and relatively benign, yet also uncomfortable for those whom it afflicts. A healthy lifestyle and certain herbs can reduce your risk of developing BPH and may alleviate symptoms.

Diet: Stick to a healthy whole-foods diet. Add a daily handful of pumpkin or pepita seeds. Enjoy these regularly: tomato products or autumn olives (lycopene), pumpkin seed oil for drizzling and dressings, and antioxidant-rich anti-inflammatory foods like pomegranate, rosemary, turmeric, ginger, and green tea.

Lifestyle: Hit the streets! Physically active men tend to have fewer and less severe BHP issues, possibly because exercise decreases inflammation and helps normalize stress and reproductive hormone production. Just walking a few hours a week can cut your risk by 25 percent.

Herbs: Saw palmetto forms the backbone of your herbal BPH formula, but you can also include other prostate-supportive herbs, including anti-inflammatories (turmeric, ginger, rosemary, holy basil, green tea) and prostate-specific herbs and nutrients (nettle root, pumpkin seed oil, zinc).

▸ Adaptogens

Adaptogens address and prevent a range of male complaints. In fact, most adaptogens historically entered common use as virility, fertility, and longevity herbs for wealthy, powerful men. They generally strengthen male hormone production, at least in part by regulating the nervous-endocrine system via stress and reproductive hormones. This improves the overall sense of energy and vitality while also improving fertility, libido, and disease resistance. Although any adaptogenic herb may be of service (learn more about adaptogens in chapter 3), the following specific adaptogens offer particular benefit for men:

- **Ginseng.** Ginseng improves the weight and health of male sex glands, boosts fertility, and specifically addresses erectile dysfunction (red Asian ginseng is particularly potent). Ginseng's zippy energy enhances mental and physical energy, which can help with depression, fatigue, and "feeling old." More sustainable and less expensive substitutes such as codonopsis, jiaogulan, and eleuthero may provide similar benefits.

- **Ashwagandha.** In Ayurvedic medicine, ashwagandha has a similar reputation. Ashwagandha tends to be more gentle and restorative to the nervous system, providing calm energy while quelling anxiety and stress. Studies support its ability to decrease inflammation and pain and improve fertility and sperm vitality, and it's well tolerated by many. True to the modulating aspect of adaptogens, studies suggest that ashwagandha restores normal hormone levels in men with testosterone deficiencies. Infusing it in milk or a similar creamy substitute helps drive it to the nervous system and fat-rich organs. Taking it regularly for a year reportedly gives you the strength and, ahem, stamina of a stallion for the decade to come.

- **Maca.** The adaptogen of choice in the Andes, maca serves as a staple food crop (a nutrient-dense root related to turnips), libido tonic, and energy booster. Studies note that it enhances fertility and sexual interest without affecting hormones directly. Even though maca tastes great, it gets so slimy in tea that it's impossible to strain. Consider just adding the powder to food and smoothies, taking it in capsules, or using a tincture (the last being the form used in most studies). Some people find that the raw powder causes digestive upset and thyroid inhibition (as would eating other raw cruciferous roots), but problems are rare and not an issue with tincture.

▸ Circulatory Herbs

Circulatory herbs increase blood flow to your reproductive organs and specifically target the penis and erectile function. This was cemented in my brain when a colleague pointed to a bottle of hawthorn-garlic-cayenne heart pills on the shelf in a local shop and enthused, quite loudly, on how pleasantly surprised he was when his heart tonic perked up other things! When it comes to men's health, we're specifically interested in herbs that improve blood flow and blood vessel lining. You'll find more details on cardio herbs in chapter 10; some of the best for reproductive health include the following:

- **Hawthorn.** One of the best-researched heart tonics, hawthorn benefits almost every aspect of cardiovascular health, including blood flow from the heart, blood pressure, endothelial health, and more. Energetically, it's useful for emotional issues that are felt in the heart, including grief and heartbreak.

- **Garlic.** Acting as a tonic to the entire cardiovascular system, garlic has modest effects on cholesterol and blood pressure numbers. It also has a reputation as a sperm booster, cancer fighter, and aphrodisiac.

- **Cayenne.** This pepper is a blood mover, blood vessel dilator, and heart tonic, reportedly able to dissolve blood clots and even stop a heart attack in its tracks (though high-dose cayenne capsules taken for weight loss have actually *caused* heart attacks in two otherwise healthy men). Cayenne breaks down fibrin and plaque and inhibits platelet aggregation, which makes blood less sticky and better able to move through the vessels. Add some extra sprinkles to your food or a pinch to your formula as a "mover and shaker" synergist. The kick of heat also pumps up mood-boosting endorphins. Ever lick a sliced hot pepper? It's exciting!

- **Cacao.** Despite its aphrodisiac reputation, cacao hasn't achieved as much attention as a functional restorative for men, but it's an excellent candidate. Research on dark chocolate and pure cacao show that it has multiple benefits for endothelial and heart health as well as the ability to boost endorphins and mood.

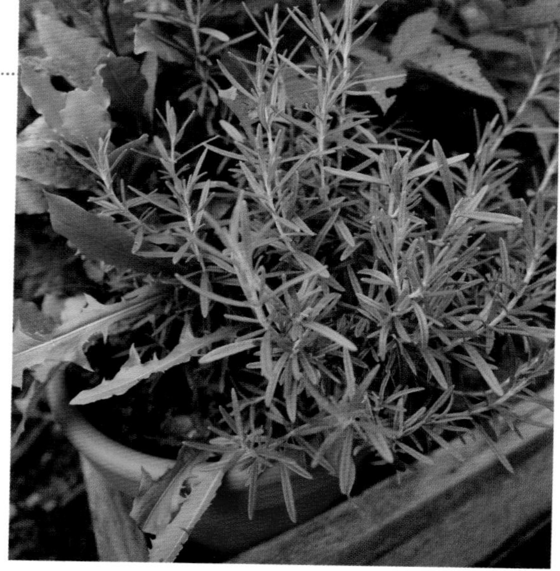

Anti-inflammatory Herbs

Anti-inflammatory herbs benefit both circulation and cancer prevention while offering many other benefits throughout the body. Studies suggest that squelching inflammation decreases BPH symptoms and prostatitis (though prostatitis still demands medical attention). Turmeric, ginger, holy basil, green tea, and rosemary are notable anti-inflammatory herbs, most of which also benefit blood flow and mood. They're excellent supportive herbs in formulas for the prostate, libido, and more.

WHAT IS A PHYTOESTROGEN?

"Phytoestrogen" refers to specific plant chemicals that act like estrogen or the herbs that contain these chemicals. Phytoestrogen herbs and foods bind preferentially to estrogen receptor sites (bumping out some stronger natural estrogen and xenoestrogen), yet they exert a much weaker estrogenic activity, perhaps 2 percent of what your body's natural estrogen would do.

General Uses: Phytoestrogens help modulate estrogen levels in the body, reducing estrogen overload and providing some estrogen activity when estrogen levels would otherwise be low (e.g., menopause). Estrogens tend to support bone health and perimenopause symptoms, including hot flashes and night sweats. They also appear to reduce the risk of estrogen-dependent cancer, though most doctors recommend avoiding them, erring on the side of caution. Consuming phytoestrogen foods starting early in life seems to offer more protective benefits. Drug interactions are possible.

Examples: Legume family: soy (the richest source, though it does not agree with everyone and is best used in traditional whole-food forms), beans, legumes, red clover blossoms, alfalfa, licorice, fenugreek. Also lignan-rich foods: flaxseeds (richest), sesame seeds. Mint family: sage, motherwort, lavender, mint. Other sources include hops, shatavari, kudzu, and marijuana.

PROTOCOL POINTS

Cancer Prevention for Men and Women

Even though genetics play a role in your risk of developing cancer, diet and lifestyle are much bigger players. Be proactive and get regular screenings. The earlier cancer is detected, the easier it is to treat.

The following recommendations specifically reduce your risk of reproductive cancers (prostate, breast, and ovarian); however, they may decrease your risk of other cancers as well. It's a fine line between cancer prevention and cancer treatment. Cancer cells are often present in the healthy person, and it's the uncontrolled, rapid proliferation of those cells (and resulting damage to the body) that indicates disease. Therefore, herbs, mushrooms, and lifestyle approaches that prevent cancer can also be used as adjuncts to more specific cancer treatment, with the guidance of a qualified practitioner.

Diet: Focus on a nutrient-dense, low-glycemic, whole-foods diet low in animal products and rich in plants. Try to avoid sugar, processed food, processed meat, and excessive alcohol. Limit or avoid animal products, especially red meat and dairy. Phytoestrogenic foods such as beans, soy, flax, and sesame appear to have a protective effect against cancer, but they (particularly soy) are also discouraged by some experts.

Specific nutrients that target and protect male and female reproductive organs include antioxidants in general, particularly vitamin E, selenium, cruciferous vegetables, garlic and onion family plants, medicinal mushrooms (reishi, maitake, shiitake, turkey tails, chaga), vitamin D, turmeric and spices, bioflavonoids, and red-purple pigments (anthocyanins in berries and pomegranate, betacyanin in beets). Lycopene (tomato paste, autumn olives) protects against prostate cancer.

Studies suggest that modest quantities of these protective nutrients, taken in combination, are better than high-dose silver bullets. This is yet another example of how your body prefers nature's whole package over drugs or even supplements. In prostate health studies, isolated selenium supplements increased cancer risk while those in a more foodlike matrix decreased risk. Another study illustrates this fact even better: In an animal study, isolated lycopene diminished tumors by 18 percent, powdered tomato by 34 percent, powdered broccoli by 42 percent, and the combination of tomato and broccoli by 52 percent.

A diet rich in these nutrients may fight active cancer (ideally under an oncology specialist's care), but prevention is always easier than treatment. Mediterranean and vegan diets seem particularly good at preventing various types of cancer, including prostate and breast, as well as improving heart health and other body systems.

Lifestyle: Exercise and mindfulness meditation reduce your risk of cancer and relapse. Also, go natural! Limit or avoid endocrine-disrupting chemicals in your personal-care products, including parabens, fragrances, and other synthetic compounds. According to some studies, endocrine-disrupting chemicals are responsible for 20 percent of male infertility and testicular cancer cases. Exposure to plastics (especially in food and drink: beverage containers, food packaging, can lining) is another source of endocrine-disrupting chemicals that can increase the risk of testicular, prostate, breast, and ovarian cancers.

In addition to a variety of plant-based antioxidant-rich and phytoestrogenic food-herbs and medicinal mushrooms, astragalus, adaptogens (holy basil, codonopsis, ashwagandha), and turmeric are some of our most promising and safest preventive remedies.

If cancer is detected, work with an oncology specialist to determine how alternative and conventional care can work together for your benefit. Self-treatment is *not* recommended; however, there are many things you can do to support your body. Mushrooms (especially turkey tails and reishi), adaptogens, and immunomodulator herbs (astragalus) tend to improve outcomes while decreasing side effects, and ginger or medical marijuana can reduce therapy-related nausea. You should work with your holistic oncology expert before combining these remedies with conventional therapy.

Women's Health Tonics *and* Key Nutrients

Compared to the male reproductive system, the female cycle is a tad more complicated, and a bit more obvious. During your reproductive years, the female body expands and contracts, ebbs and flows, on an approximately 28-day cycle. Though at times exhausting, that cycle also offers a measurable biofeedback loop to gauge the vitality of your whole body. Adolescence and menopause amplify the effect. Slight imbalances scream through the megaphone of haywire hormones. It's interesting to note that women in many other cultures rarely suffer the hormonal extremes that Americans endure. We all have the same hormones, but many factors — including stress, cuisine, sleep, activity level, obesity rates, pharmaceutical interventions, and exposure to endocrine-disrupting hormones — influence our hormone levels and how they make us feel.

When the female cycle operates in balance, it's a beautiful thing, a monthly symphony of hormones that help maintain other aspects of health, including bone strength, mood, and immune function. Paying attention to and nurturing that cycle is an opportunity to connect daily with your body and the rhythms of life.

Before we jump into the intricacies of the female hormone cycle and its effects throughout the body, let's cover some of the basic herbs and foods that nourish the female reproductive system. These herbs rarely have overt hormonal effects but instead provide important nutrients and tone up the tissue and structure of your reproductive system.

▸ Iron and Iron-Rich Food and Herbs

Iron helps the body recover from monthly blood loss (and, hence, iron loss) during monthly menstruation. How much iron you actually need to replenish will depend on diet, iron absorption, overall body health, and the amount bled during menses. Don't take iron supplements without first getting a simple blood test. Though low iron levels are common, unnecessarily pumping yourself with iron increases the risk of heart disease. You're at a greater risk of iron deficiency (anemia) if you are overly thin, vegetarian or vegan, have a digestive or malabsorption disease, or bleed heavily during menses. Signs of anemia include fatigue, anxiety, brain fog, heart issues like tachycardia, cold hands and feet, headaches, and pale lips and gums. The interplay of various compounds — folic acid, vitamin B_{12}, vitamin C, stomach acid, and intrinsic factor — improve iron assimilation. Food first: animal-based foods are more easily absorbed than plant-based iron and include liver, beef, shellfish, poultry, and fish. Vegetarians can get more out of plant-based iron by taking it alongside vitamin C–rich produce and making sure to have adequate B_{12} (only available in animal-based foods) supplements. Plant sources of iron include dark leafy greens, legumes, soy, and seeds, and most of our nutritious herbs, including nettle, yellow dock, dandelion, and raspberry leaf. Yellow dock and dong quai roots don't contain a lot of iron, but they "build blood" by encouraging your liver to release iron from storage into the bloodstream and support hormone health. Cooking, simmering, and superinfusing foods and herbs will improve iron's bioavailability.

▸ Bone-Supportive Food and Herbs

Calcium helps build bone strength, which is especially important for women. Estrogen protects bones from calcium loss until menopause. Without it, bone loss accelerates, putting women at greater risk of osteoporosis and bone fractures. While it's never too late to support your bones, starting as young as possible helps ensure strong bones postmenopause. Calcium, vitamin D, and weight-bearing exercise *together* encourage your body to lay down bone. Calcium-rich foods and herbs include nettle, dairy (especially Parmesan), canned fish with bones, bone broths, seaweed, horsetail, oat straw, alfalfa, raspberry leaves, legumes, and fortified tofu. Phytoestrogens in the diet — soy in whole-food

ESTROGENS: THE GOOD, THE BAD, THE UGLY

HORMONES CAN BE COMPLICATED, and estrogen is no exception. This "one" hormone comes in many forms and is present in women and to a lesser extent (balanced with higher levels of testosterone) in men. Three main forms of estrogen are produced by the body:

- Estrone (E1), secreted by the ovaries and fat tissue
- Estradiol (E2), produced in various ways but primarily in the ovaries of women, and in small amounts in the male testes
- Estriol (E3), produced by the placenta during pregnancy

Modest amounts of estradiol help improve bone strength, mood, skin elasticity, and overall hormone and reproductive health. High doses and more "cranky" forms like estrone interfere with healthy hormone function in both men and women and increase the risk of cancer and erectile dysfunction. Obesity increases your exposure to cranky estrone, and it's also the dominant estrogen postmenopause.

Phytoestrogens, or plant estrogens, occur naturally in the form of various compounds in legume (e.g., beans, soy, licorice, red clover), lignan-rich (flax, sesame), and mint-family aromatic (lavender, motherwort, sage, spearmint) plants. Phytoestrogens bind preferentially to estrogen receptor sites in the body but have a much weaker action (approximately 2 percent of what natural estrogen can do). Therefore, phytoestrogens in their natural form of crude herbal medicine and food tend to have a balancing effect on estrogen-related issues. They mellow out estrogen excess but provide at least some estrogen when levels are low (for example, after menopause). For more on phytoestrogens, see page 240.

Xenoestrogens are hormone chemicals that mimic estrogen and often also have antiandrogen effects. Often called "endocrine disruptors" or "hormone disruptors," these chemicals are often present in plastics (including but not limited to BPA, PCBs, phthalates, PVC), agricultural chemicals (atrazine, DDT, insecticides, livestock growth promoters), and dioxin (related to bleach). Dairy and fish exposed to these chemicals can concentrate and deliver the compounds to you when you eat them. We are all exposed to xenoestrogens, and high levels of exposure are linked to early puberty, reproductive organ cancers, feminization in males, fertility issues in both sexes, and more. You can drastically limit exposure by reducing your reliance on plastic (especially for food, drink, and the household), going organic, and choosing more naturally made products whenever possible for your home, garden, and food. Phytoestrogens, cruciferous vegetables, and liver-moving herbs may also limit the damage and increase the elimination of the chemicals from your body, but there's still a lot we don't know.

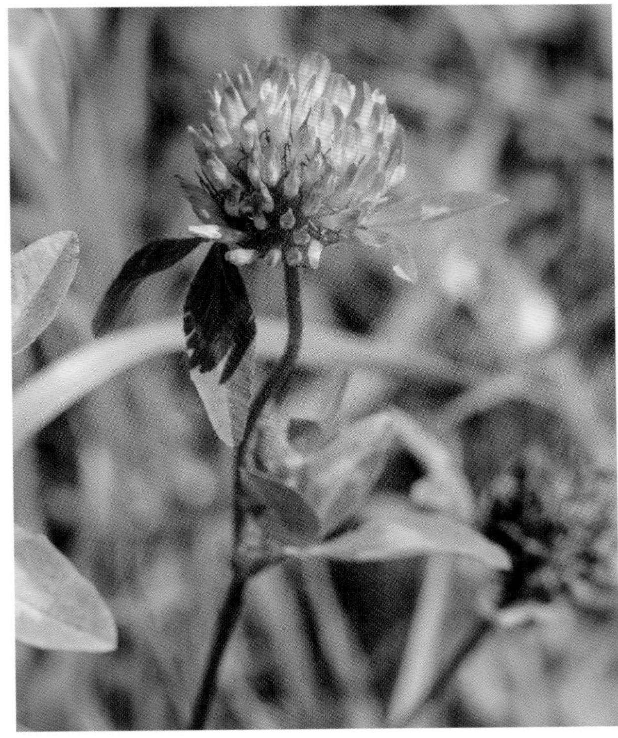

forms (edamame, tofu, miso, tempeh), flaxseeds, sesame seeds, red clover blossoms, legumes — encourage hormone balance that can decrease the rate of bone loss while increasing the body's ability to build bone. For a more extensive discussion of bone health, see page 270.

▸ Cabbage-Family Plants

The cabbage family plays a special role in preventing breast cancer and detoxifying "cranky estrogen" that circulates through the body and wreaks havoc after menopause. Plants in this family (particularly broccoli) are rich in indole-3-carbinol (I3C), which, when digested, turns into diindolylmethane (DIM). Both I3C and DIM are available as supplements. They help transport this cranky estrogen out of your body more efficiently via the liver. Another compound in these foods, sulforophane, protects you from cancer by improving immune response and sophistication. Aim for two servings per day of cabbage-family vegetables and greens, such as broccoli/sprouts, cabbage, Brussels sprouts, arugula, kale, turnips, cauliflower, bok choy, and watercress. Note: Although it's rarely an issue, the cabbage family contains goitrogens, which may inhibit thyroid hormones. Cooking helps to destroy most of these compounds, but you may not want to overdo the cabbage family (especially raw) if your thyroid function is low.

PROTOCOL POINTS

Yeast Infections

This may or may not be a hormone-related issue. Some women are more likely to get cycle-related yeast infections if both progesterone and estrogen levels are low. (Levels can drop at midcycle if you don't ovulate or just before your period if stress disrupts progesterone balance.) Birth control pills make yeast infections more likely by depleting important nutrients like B vitamins and weakening immune function. You may want to get tested to determine if you're dealing with yeast or something else, like bacterial vaginosis — holistic/herbal approaches are pretty much the same in either case, but medications differ.

Diet: First and foremost: ditch sugar, white flour/food, and alcohol, all of which feed yeast. Indulge in antimicrobial foods and spices, including ginger, garlic, cinnamon, and oregano. Boost your intake of fermented foods (especially veggies like kimchi) or take a probiotics supplement to help the good guys shove out the bad.

Lifestyle: You may want to limit sex for a bit. Not only can it irritate already sensitive lady parts, but it may also encourage infection due to semen alkalinity (the vagina is generally more acidic, which is less hospitable to yeast and bacteria) and partner-to-partner transmission (especially if your partner is a lady or uncut guy). Be aware of anything else that goes into your nether regions, including funky lubes, oil-based formulas, and less-than-clean toys, that could throw good flora off or introduce a pathogen. Wear breathable panties and go commando at night.

Herbs: Antifungal/antimicrobial and probiotic-supportive herbs include garlic, ginger, rose petals, chaga (technically not an herb, but quite nice as tea!), oregano, bee balm, alder, pau d'arco, and low-dose thuja. Consider taking them as tea, tincture, capsule, or food. If the issues seem cycle-related, then you should also include herbs that help balance those aspects of the cycle.

Topical Treatments: Inserting a garlic clove (wrapped in clean cloth) may help, but garlic may irritate sensitive vaginal lining. Consider specialized suppositories with ingredients like tea tree, borax, and homeopathic remedies. Topical remedies may be sufficient in a one-time infection, but internal remedies and diet/lifestyle changes are usually needed for chronic infections.

Woman's Nutri-Tea

This recipe bridges the basic infusion and super infusion methods of steeping tea. It's rich in nutrients and other compounds that benefit a woman's body and tastes great. Feel free to tinker with the ingredients based on what's in your herb closet.

2 tablespoons nettles
2 tablespoons oat straw
2 tablespoons red clover
1 tablespoon lemon balm
1 tablespoon peppermint
1 tablespoon raspberry leaf
1 tablespoon spearmint
Sprinkle of calendula petals
Honey (optional)

Combine all the herbs. Pour 4 cups boiling water over the herbs and let steep, covered, for 1 hour or longer. Strain, squeezing as much tea as you can from the herbs. Enjoy one to two cups daily, or as desired.

Lady T

Pleasantly tasty and nice for toning and nourishing the tissues in your lady parts. Welcome additions include oat straw and red clover blossoms.

1 teaspoon lady's mantle leaf/flower
1 teaspoon raspberry leaf
A few rose buds or petals
1 teaspoon honey (optional)

Combine the herbs. Pour 1 cup boiling water over the herbs and let steep, covered, for 15 or more minutes. Strain and enjoy. Also nice iced.

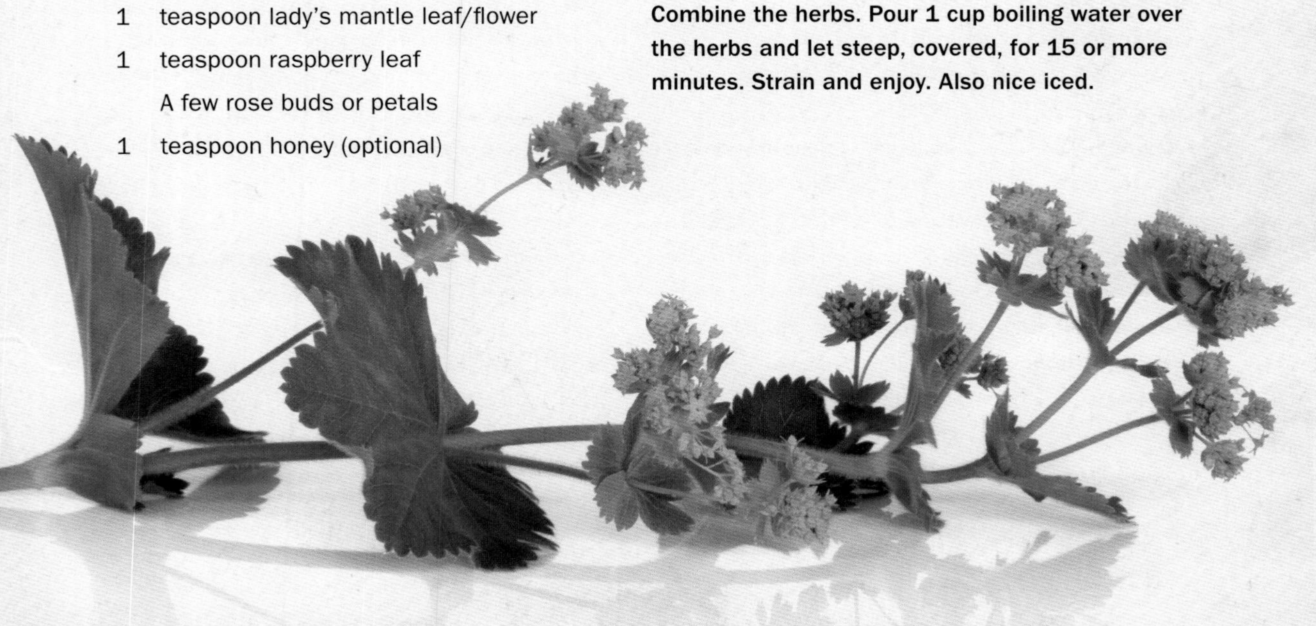

▸ Rose-Family Tissue Toners

Members of the rose family are noted for their gentle astringent action, and they strengthen the tone of various tissues in the body while being safe enough for daily use. Raspberry leaf remains the most popular of the "female" rose-family herbs for good reason. Studies show that it strengthens the uterine lining and muscles, which not only facilitates a swift, easy birth but also supports the general well-being of your lady parts. Raspberry leaf is one of the few herbs with widespread acceptance as safe for use (as a standard infusion) during the last two trimesters of pregnancy. Women of all ages can benefit from the herb. Raspberry leaf is also rich in many of the nutrients women need, including calcium, iron, vitamin C, and magnesium. Learn more about raspberry on page 36. Other rose-family astringent tissue toners include lady's mantle, rose petals, cinquefoil, strawberry leaf, avens, and agrimony. These are common weeds and garden herbs. At least one of them is probably already growing in your backyard.

The Female Cycle

Unlike the male reproductive system, women keep almost all their organs hidden. Your two ovaries provide a nourishing home for eggs-in-waiting, also called follicles. You're born with a set number of follicles that have the potential of becoming the star egg of a cycle. About 4 months prior to the cycle, a follicle is chosen and "groomed" for her role. The two major female hormones, estrogen (estradiol) and progesterone, are produced in the ovaries under the direction of pituitary hormones: follicle-stimulating hormone (FSH) and luteinizing hormone (LH), respectively. The production of FSH and LH come at the urging of the hypothalamus's gonadotropin-releasing hormone (GnRH). During each cycle, an egg is released from one of the ovaries, travels down a fallopian tube, and enters the uterus, where it hopes to meet up with some sexy sperm to create a baby. If that occurs, the uterus becomes an incubator. On the other side of the uterus, through the cervix, lies the vagina, the entrance to the more intimate lady parts.

While you probably have some understanding of the basic woman's cycle, getting to know it on a deeper level tends to produce a few "aha" moments, both in identifying negative patterns and in understanding which herbs will best support you. No two women are exactly identical, so don't fret if your cycle doesn't quite follow this time frame. Many women's cycles run a tad shorter or longer or fluctuate a little bit from month to month.

Day 1 to 14: Estrogen Dominance

The first day of your cycle begins on the first day of menses. In the absence of pregnancy, progesterone will have just dropped, oxytocin surges, and your uterine lining begins to slough off. In your ovaries, a follicle awaits her crowning moment in the beauty pageant of eggs. In the 4 months since she was selected from the pool of follicles, she's (hopefully) been pampered with vitamins, nutrients, and hormones so that she's now at peak vitality and just about ready to meet the guy of her dreams. This lucky follicle (and soon-to-be egg) produces estrogen in your ovaries via stimulation from FSH in the brain. The estrogen she secretes triggers the body to begin rebuilding uterine lining once the old

HOW DO HERBS AFFECT MY HORMONES?

MOST OF OUR "REPRODUCTIVE HERBS" don't *contain* hormones. Think of them as a megaphone: they encourage your hormones to work better. They may stimulate hormone production, improve hormones binding to receptor sites on cells, or otherwise synergize with hormones.

HORMONES AT WORK: AN OVERVIEW

Here is a quick overview of the hormones involved in the female cycle and the herbs that lend a hand in normalizing their production and function:

Day 1–14 GnRH ► FSH ► estrogen ► tissue building and egg development
Helpful herbs: black cohosh, phytoestrogens (soy, beans, flax, clover), dong quai, shatavari

Day 14 Oxytocin (from the brain) ► release of egg/ovulation or release of uterine lining/menstruation
Helpful herb: cotton root bark (also helpful is sex/orgasm, which stimulates oxytocin production and release)

Day 14–28 GnRH ► LH ► progesterone ► specializes uterine lining tissues, boosts mood, promotes healthy menstruation timing, duration, and flow
Helpful herbs: vitex, damiana, partridgeberry

stuff has been removed. In addition, the estrogen secreted by your follicle strengthens and lubricates vaginal tissue, protects against bone loss, keeps your mood humming, and bolsters your immune health. Women often find it easier to lose weight and manage appetite during this part of the cycle (after menstruation), too.

Day 14: Ovulation

The special day has come! A surge of oxytocin — the "releasing hormone" — releases your follicle from the ovary, and she becomes an egg (*the* egg!) that travels down your fallopian tube into your uterus to either meet up with some swimming sperm or be released from the body. Oxytocin has profound effects throughout the body and most notably gets you in the mood. Did you notice that *everyone* looked good to you this week? That's your body encouraging you to get down and make a baby at this perfect time. Oxytocin increases libido and aids climax, and sex and foreplay, in turn, increase oxytocin action. At this time, estrogen dips down and progesterone kicks into gear. You'll notice that your basal body temperature dips just a bit before ovulation and then rises a few tenths of a degree afterward. Also in the days preceding ovulation, your body boosts its production of cervical mucus to make the entry friendlier for sperm and the organ that delivers it.

Day 14 to 28: Progesterone Dominance

Now that this month's egg has left the building, progesterone (stimulated by LH) is produced by the corpus luteum, the empty throne that the egg departed in the ovaries. Like estrogen, progesterone also keeps mood and the immune system humming, but its primary goal is to finish the job that estrogen began and prepare the uterine lining to either grow a baby or slough off nicely in the next cycle. Your body temperature remains a tad higher through this portion of the cycle, and you might notice that you're hungrier and don't lose weight quite as easily. Don't worry: that's the body's way of holding on to nutrients in case you need them for a fetus. If conception occurs, you'll notice your basal body temperature rise another few notches (due to a pregnancy-related progesterone surge), as well as a lot of other changes including breast swelling and mood changes. If pregnancy is not achieved, basal temp will drop when the corpus luteum ceases to excrete progesterone. Oxytocin surges, and the cycle begins anew.

If only it always went so smoothly! You'll experience some normal teeters in hormones during adolescence and perimenopause as your reproductive system kicks on and off baby-making mode. But a great many other factors influence your cycle during the reproductive years and affect how manageable adolescence and menopause are for you.

Estrogen Woes

High, low, dwindling, or the wrong kind of estrogen can all make your reproductive system a bit cranky.

Perimenopause

Perimenopause naturally occurs when follicles (and, thus, estrogen) begin to taper off during the final reproductive years. The beauty pageant of follicles continues, but the candidates become fewer and farther between, and not quite as young and vital. As a result, your follicle doesn't produce as much estrogen, and your brain may "yell" down to your ovaries (increased FSH levels), begging your follicle to step it up. These hormone wobbles cause night sweats, hot flashes, moodiness, and more. Once the wobbles have passed and menopausal estrogen levels remain low, you lose estrogen's protective effect on bones and its nourishing effect on reproductive tissues, which may lead to vaginal dryness. You can use estrogen-supportive herbs and a phytoestrogen-rich diet to smooth things out during this natural body transition. Officially, menopause is the moment at which your reproductive cycles cease completely (usually diagnosed after 1 full year without a period), and perimenopause is the transition time before menopause.

Weak Estrogen and Low Vitality

Weak estrogen activity and low vitality during the reproductive years can be due to many factors, but most often it coincides with a "deficient" or "yin" constitution: thin, possibly anemic, anxious, fatigued, malnourished, stressed, and sleep deprived. Symptoms may also include patchy, light periods that are more brown than red and a lack of fertility. Cravings can help us sleuth out what nutrients are missing: chocolate (magnesium), sweets (balanced carbs and blood sugar support), fried food (omega-3s), meat (iron, protein, B vitamins), milk (calcium), shellfish (trace minerals). A nutrient-dense diet is key, as are herbs that nourish the nervous-endocrine system, improve sleep, decrease the stress response, and improve blood flow to the reproductive organs. For fertility, dietary supplements including basic nutrients, adequate folic acid and vitamin B complex, calcium, vitamin D, and iron, and omega-3s can gradually build the vitality of follicles-in-waiting. It may take up to 4 months for the effects to become fully evident. Digestion-enhancing herbs, nutritives, and herb-infused bone broths may be appropriate, too. Also consider herbs that support estrogen, especially dong quai and shatavari, which are often used in combination with warming adaptogens like ginseng, codonopsis, and ashwagandha.

PROTOCOL POINTS

Perimenopause

The years leading up to menopause are called perimenopause, and this transition time can be difficult for some women. Understand that this transition is normal; however, it shouldn't feel like hell. Here are some considerations:

Diet: Eat a good-quality diet, high in cabbage-family plants and phytoestrogen foods, including flaxseeds, sesame seeds, beans. Consider adding modest amounts of traditional whole-food forms of soy like miso, tempeh, edamame, and tofu; however, they can be hard to digest, a source of food allergies or sensitivities, and thyroid inhibiting for sensitive people.

Lifestyle: Stress management and regular exercise are key. Weight-bearing exercise specifically supports bone strength (in combination with calcium and vitamin D intake). Work hard to maintain a good sleep schedule, giving yourself more bedtime if needed.

Herbs: Black cohosh and phytoestrogens (including red clover and sage) for help with hot flashes. Vitex for help with mood swings and cycle irregularity, especially during the earlier years of perimenopause. Supportive herbs for stress, mood, mental clarity, libido, et cetera, as needed, combined with the reproductive herbs. Shatavari for improved cervical mucus and relief of vaginal dryness.

Estrogen Overload

Too much of the wrong kinds of estrogen is a common issue in the industrialized world. There are several forms of estrogen available from your body, from food, and from other outside influences. The most problematic forms of estrogen are estrogen stored in fat cells (cranky estrone) and xenoestrogens from various chemicals (see page 243). Animal-based foods like meat and dairy naturally have small amounts of hormones that may upset your own hormone balance, especially if they're produced in a factory-farm environment where additional hormones are pumped into the animals to increase weight and milk production. Remember, it's all about balance. Just enough estrogen is great, but too much estrogen increases your risk of breast and ovarian cancer, impairs fertility, aggravates fibroids, and also encourages thick but less specialized menstrual lining (especially if you're not ovulating and producing progesterone). Balancing your weight, eating whole organic foods and a more plant-based/vegan diet, and avoiding chemicals as much as possible are important. Especially limit your use of plastic for food and drink by using glass and stainless steel materials and limiting plastic-packaged items. Phytoestrogens may decrease the damage of more problematic estrogen sources by bumping them out. Fiber and foods or herbs (like those cabbage-family wonders!) that support detoxification can help your body eliminate problematic estrogen from the body more effectively.

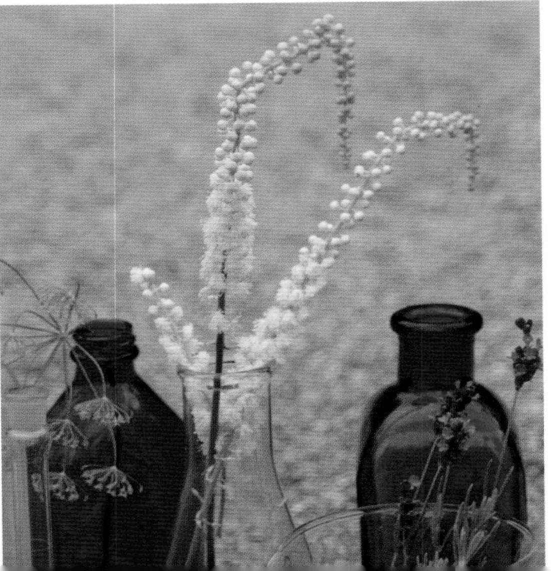

Herbs *to* Support Estrogen Balance

These herbs help increase or modulate healthy estrogen production. Although they're most commonly used to offset the natural dwindling of estrogen during perimenopause and after menopause, they can also be used for irregular cycles in younger women.

▸ Black Cohosh

Actaea racemosa, syn. *Cimicifuga racemosa*

Availability: G W- C+

Key Properties: This perimenopause ally supports the body as it begins to produce less estrogen. Unlike many herbs, black cohosh root has been widely researched in more than 200 studies and is commonly prescribed for menopause symptoms in Europe. Though we're still figuring out how black cohosh works, it appears to increase estrogen levels without directly supplying estrogen to the body. It may also lower levels of luteinizing hormone, which tends to be high in postmenopausal women. Although no one herb works for every woman, black cohosh is the most reliable bet for hot flashes and night sweats.

Additional Benefits: Black cohosh also relieves rheumatic pain, lifts black cloud depression, and helps decrease bone loss. It relaxes uterine muscles and is sometimes used for menstrual cramps and labor support.

Preparation: For hot flashes and perimenopause, consider Remifemin standardized capsules, the form most researched and prescribed; follow the dosage instructions on the product label. Otherwise, consider crude herb capsules or tincture. It's not so tasty as tea. Use standard herb doses (see page 298), or slightly less.

Cautions and Considerations: Modest doses of black cohosh are generally safe, but high doses aren't necessary and may cause side effects. Although research suggests black cohosh decreases the risk of breast cancer, most doctors don't recommend taking it if you have an increased risk for estrogen-dependent cancer. A few cases of liver toxicity with black cohosh have popped up worldwide — a very small number considering how widespread its use is, and no cases have involved Remifemin. The liver toxicity appears to stem from rampant adulteration of black cohosh with Chinese *Actaea* and *Cimicifuga* species. Be sure to buy black cohosh products that you can trust, such as Remifemin or from a company that properly sources and identifies their cohosh roots, which is easiest in the whole plant/root form. Black cohosh is often unethically harvested. Purchasing certified organic black cohosh both ensures sustainability and is an extra safeguard for identity, thanks to the paper trail necessary for certification. Don't use black cohosh during pregnancy without supervision. It may interact with medications, especially those with hormonal influence.

▸ Dong Quai

Angelica sinensis

Availability: G- C

Key Properties: Dong quai has a celery-like flavor that indicates its place in the parsley family, with a bit of smokiness thanks to the traditional processing method of the root. Though less useful in menopause, dong quai is the premier Chinese tonic herb for estrogen deficiency. Consider it if you're a younger woman who needs support in the first half of your cycle. Indicating patterns include being thin and anemic with light periods (perhaps spotty and brown), fertility issues, and a tendency toward anxiety. Dong quai builds blood and strengthens the effects of your natural estrogen, acting like a megaphone while increasing circulation and blood flow to the uterus, and indirectly fortifying iron levels.

Additional Benefits: Dong quai is considered a nourishing tonic for women to improve energy and vitality, often in combination with ginseng and other adaptogen or qi tonics.

Preparation: Consider it as a tincture, decocted tea/broth (not tasty but traditional in Chinese medicine), or with other herbs in capsule form. Standard herb doses (see page 298) apply. In traditional Chinese medicine, dong quai is rarely prescribed alone. Blend it with herbs such as codonopsis, ginseng, and licorice that tone and nourish your body and help balance stress hormones.

Cautions and Considerations: The herb can increase bleeding and is not recommended during the first days of your period, if you have a tendency toward heavy periods or a bleeding disorder, or if you are on blood-thinning medications. Do not take it during pregnancy without supervision. May aggravate reflux and photosensitivity.

▸ Herbs for Extra Estrogen Support

Motherwort, **sage**, **shatavari**, and **maca** can be helpful for mood swings and menopause-related hot flashes. For the best results, blend reproductive herbs with adaptogens like **ginseng** and **eleuthero** because these herbs simultaneously balance stress and reproductive hormones while also enhancing libido. Uplifting mood herbs can be useful for women who are depressed or experiencing mood swings. Consider **damiana** or **St. John's wort** in a formula. St. John's wort interacts with many pharmaceuticals, so check with your pharmacist before taking it.

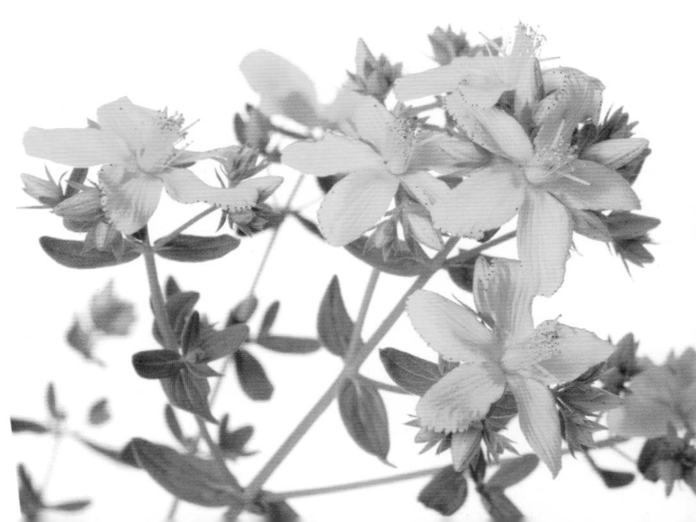

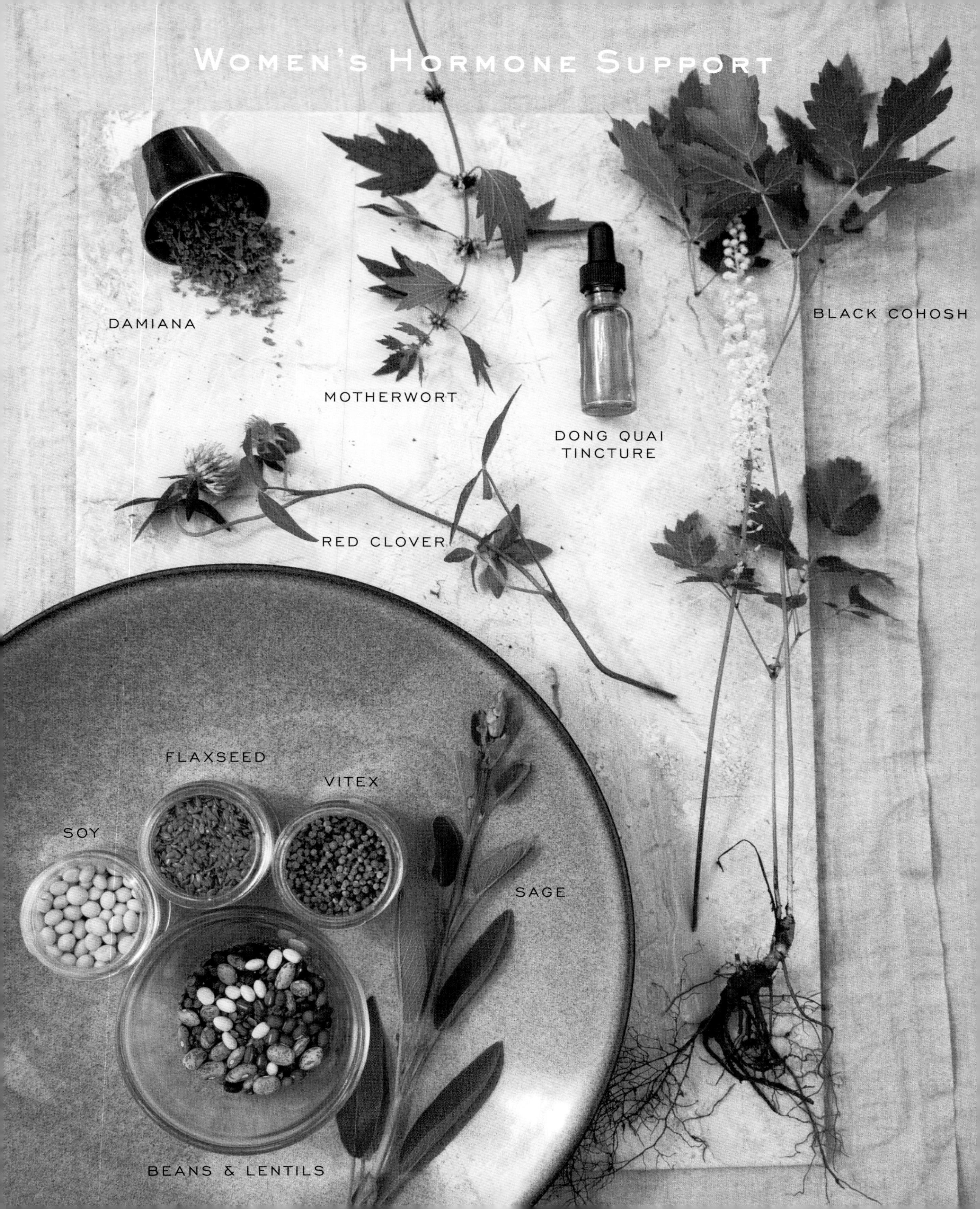
Women's Hormone Support
DAMIANA
MOTHERWORT
DONG QUAI TINCTURE
BLACK COHOSH
RED CLOVER
FLAXSEED
VITEX
SOY
SAGE
BEANS & LENTILS

Ovulation *and* Progesterone Woes

Two major things upset progesterone balance: stress and lack of ovulation. In turn, progesterone imbalance causes or worsens fertility issues, PMS, mood swings, depression, sensitivity to stress, cycle-related migraines, systemic inflammation, cramps, immune weakness and infections (cold, flu, yeast), and fibroids.

Stress puts your brain hormones into overdrive, which encourages a faster release of progesterone to get its mood-boosting benefits. The corpus luteum has a finite amount of progesterone, and blowing it all before you reach the end of your cycle means that you spend a few days before your period with low levels of both estrogen (already naturally low during this time) *and* progesterone. This really messes with the areas of the body that progesterone and estrogen normally benefit: mood, immune function, pain. Everything seems to fall apart around the same time each month, just before your period.

Lack of ovulation can occur naturally during perimenopause and (of course) after menopause, or it may also occur if your body isn't healthy and reproductive hormones get out of whack. If you don't ovulate, there is no corpus luteum, and you don't get the benefits of progesterone during the second half of your cycle. You may or may not get your period. Your reproductive system becomes estrogen dominant, so the uterine lining builds and builds, but it doesn't specialize. This makes conception quite difficult (and impossible during cycles where you don't ovulate). Cycle length may vary widely. When you *do* get your period, especially if it happens to be during a cycle where you finally ovulate, menstruation tends to be very heavy because the tissue has been building over several cycles and doesn't slough off nicely. The blood loss can lead to anemia. You may also experience the symptoms of progesterone deficiency, except that without ovulation, the symptoms tend to start midcycle and last longer. As one of my clients described it, "Around day 15, my world goes black." Once you've fully entered menopause, your body will need to adjust to the constant lack of progesterone. (Over-the-counter progesterone creams and prescribed bioidenticals deliver progesterone and might make you feel great, but they delay the inevitable.)

Supporting Oxytocin Release and Ovulation

Most reproductive protocols — herbal or conventional — completely ignore oxytocin and ovulation. Oxytocin is a "releasing hormone" that surges to stimulate menstruation, ovulation, birth and labor contractions, the let-down reflex in breastfeeding, orgasm during sex, and those feel-good cuddly sensations you experience when snuggled up with someone you love. Stress and a general lack of nutrition and body vitality can inhibit oxytocin's production and effects. In addition to addressing that, you may want to give oxytocin a nudge during certain points with herbs that improve your body's own oxytocin effects. This might be just what you need to retain a cycle, ovulate, bring on a late period, and so on. My favorite oxytocin synergist herb is cotton root bark, though some herbalists also use blue cohosh.

Unpublished research that my teacher, herbalist Michael Moore, helped conduct on cotton root bark found that it didn't contain oxytocin but seemed to increase the strength of the body's natural oxytocin. Although it is classically used as an abortifacient, his research found that it was more apt to simply bring on a late period. I don't use it to bring on late periods (nor to encourage labor), but it could be used this way with a practitioner's guidance. I prefer it for amplifying oxytocin to encourage ovulation. It's relatively safe and can be given, a milliliter of tincture or so a day, for a few days during the desired ovulation time.

Blue cohosh may have similar activity to cotton root bark; however, as an at-risk plant, it's not ethical to wildcraft it. Blue cohosh is most famously combined with black cohosh to induce labor by stimulating the contract-relax cycle in the uterus. I do not recommend this practice for various reasons, including potential damage to the fetus. In extreme situations, it *may* be appropriate, but only under the skilled care of an herbalist midwife.

Cumulatively, cordyceps may also act as an oxytocin synergist and is classically used to boost libido/climax, boost mood, and stimulate milk flow during nursing.

Enhancing other aspects of your cycle, as well as your overall health, can profoundly affect the quality of your eggs and your ability to ovulate and have a normal cycle. Even simple nutritive supplements like a multivitamin, vitamin D, omega-3s, vitamin C, and B vitamins including folic acid can enhance the physical vitality of your reproductive system over the course of 4 months or more. Also try to reduce stress in your life; stress hormones directly inhibit oxytocin and other reproductive hormones. This can support fertility and the likelihood of a smooth pregnancy and healthy baby as well as your own overall reproductive well-being. Well-timed sexual stimulation can also improve oxytocin production and release, including its extra benefits for ovulation.

Herbs *to* Support Progesterone Balance

Remember that progesterone issues aren't *just* about progesterone. If stress is an issue — and it usually is — you should address it. If the health and vitality of your follicles have faltered, do what you can to support them, including a nutrient-dense diet and dietary supplements. That said, there are some phenomenal herbs that enhance the progesterone part of the cycle and bring cycle fluctuations to normalcy.

▸ Vitex

Vitex agnus-castus

Availability: G W C+

Key Properties: Also called chaste tree berry, this is the most useful herb I know to directly increase progesterone. It tends to be quite effective in perimenopause, serious PMS, irregular periods, fibroids, and fertility issues related to progesterone deficiency. It tends to lengthen or normalize cycle length, often within just one or two cycles of tak-

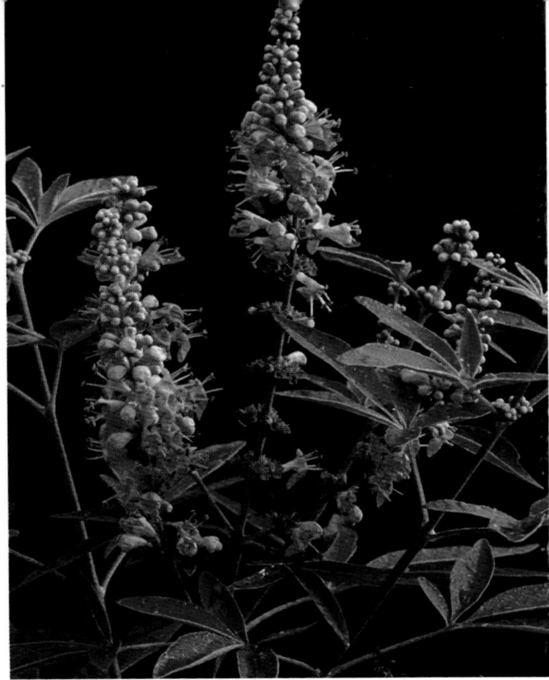

ing the herb (though sometimes it takes months). In a protocol, vitex helps retrain an awry cycle. Although vitex doesn't contain progesterone, research suggests that it indirectly increases progesterone levels in the body. It may also normalize or increase the pituitary's production of LH.

Additional Benefits: Vitex appears to inhibit prolactin yet (paradoxically) also can be used as a galactagogue to increase milk flow while nursing. It was traditionally used to reduce libido in men (hence the name "chaste berry"), but its efficacy is unclear, and it does not have this effect in women.

Preparation: This shrub can be cultivated in all but the coldest climates. Use the dry berry tincture, preferably in combination with supportive and stress herbs. Capsules may also work. Tea tastes nasty. Standard herb doses (see page 298) apply.

Cautions and Considerations: Although I've had great experiences with vitex in my practice, it doesn't work for everyone and may aggravate depression in some women. Be particularly cautious if birth control pills made you feel cranky or crazy. Vitex can be taken ongoing for several years during perimenopause. In other cycle issues like PMS, I prefer to use vitex temporarily to bring the body into balance. In either case, slowly wean off it so that the body can maintain balance without any herbal support.

▸ Damiana

Turnera diffusa

Availability: W- C

Key Properties: This yellow wildflower dots the Southwest and Mexico and has a reputation for enhancing libido and mood, simultaneously calming, uplifting, and energizing the spirit. Consider it both aphrodisiac and nervine. You'll find it in fun herbal libidinous products, often combined with chocolate, vanilla, sweets, or spices (which improves its flavor dramatically). Not much research has been done on damiana, but what we do have suggests it supports testosterone and LH in men. For women, LH support means better progesterone balance. Although it doesn't affect progesterone as overtly as vitex, damiana is worth adding to formulas where libido and mood support are also desired. It's a delightful plant for men and women alike.

Additional Benefits: Beyond its reproductive benefits, damiana may also be used for lifting yet calming mood.

Preparation: Tincture, capsule, or tea, but most often blended with chocolate, spices, and sweeteners for a better-tasting cordial or elixir. Standard herb doses (see page 298) apply.

Cautions and Considerations: Don't use it during pregnancy.

▸ Additional Progesterone Support

Adaptogens are important ingredients in a formula to normalize progesterone indirectly, particularly if stress is a factor. I almost always blend vitex with **schizandra**, an herb that supports the liver (potentially helping to clear waste and "old" hormones out of the body), the nervous and adrenal systems, libido, and mood. Other stress-relieving adaptogens like **holy basil**, **gotu kola**, and **ashwagandha** may be helpful. A daily **multivitamin** or **vitamin B complex** supplement can also help support the nervous-endocrine system during times of stress. I add **pulsatilla**, just one drop per dose (it's toxic in standard doses), to ease symptoms for women who feel hysterical during PMS.

Also watch your carb intake and boost activity level. You may notice that your cycle improves just by changing your diet. See chapter 9 for a greater discussion on blood sugar balance. Polycystic ovary syndrome (PCOS), which is linked to insulin resistance, can wreak havoc on the progesterone phase of your cycle. For PCOS, a protocol that combines progesterone, stress, and blood sugar management tends to work best. Don't hesitate to seek professional guidance.

PROTOCOL POINTS

Low Libido in Women

With women, stress is often the underlying factor in a libido of zilch, and menopause or lack of ovulation can also make it difficult to get in the mood.

Diet: Eat a healthy whole-foods diet.

Lifestyle: Stress management, mind-body balance, adequate sleep, regular exercise, and communication and connection with your partner are all important! Think of your libido as a muscle. If it's been awhile, you might need to do a few practice runs to get things back into gear. Enlisting the aid of a specialized therapist may also help. If there has been a history of abuse, consider therapy and flower essences.

Herbs: Specific libido herbs include the zippy and the chill, depending on your needs. Zippy libido herbs include ginseng, rhodiola, codonopsis, tribulus, and eleuthero. More balancing libido adaptogens include schizandra, ashwagandha, and maca. Shatavari specifically improves libido and cervical mucus. If you're a real stress case, consider adding calming or nervine herbs to the mix like passionflower, skullcap, lemon balm, damiana, roses, hawthorn, linden, or milky oat seed. Don't be afraid to indulge in aphrodisiac foods including shellfish, cayenne, chocolate, and garlic.

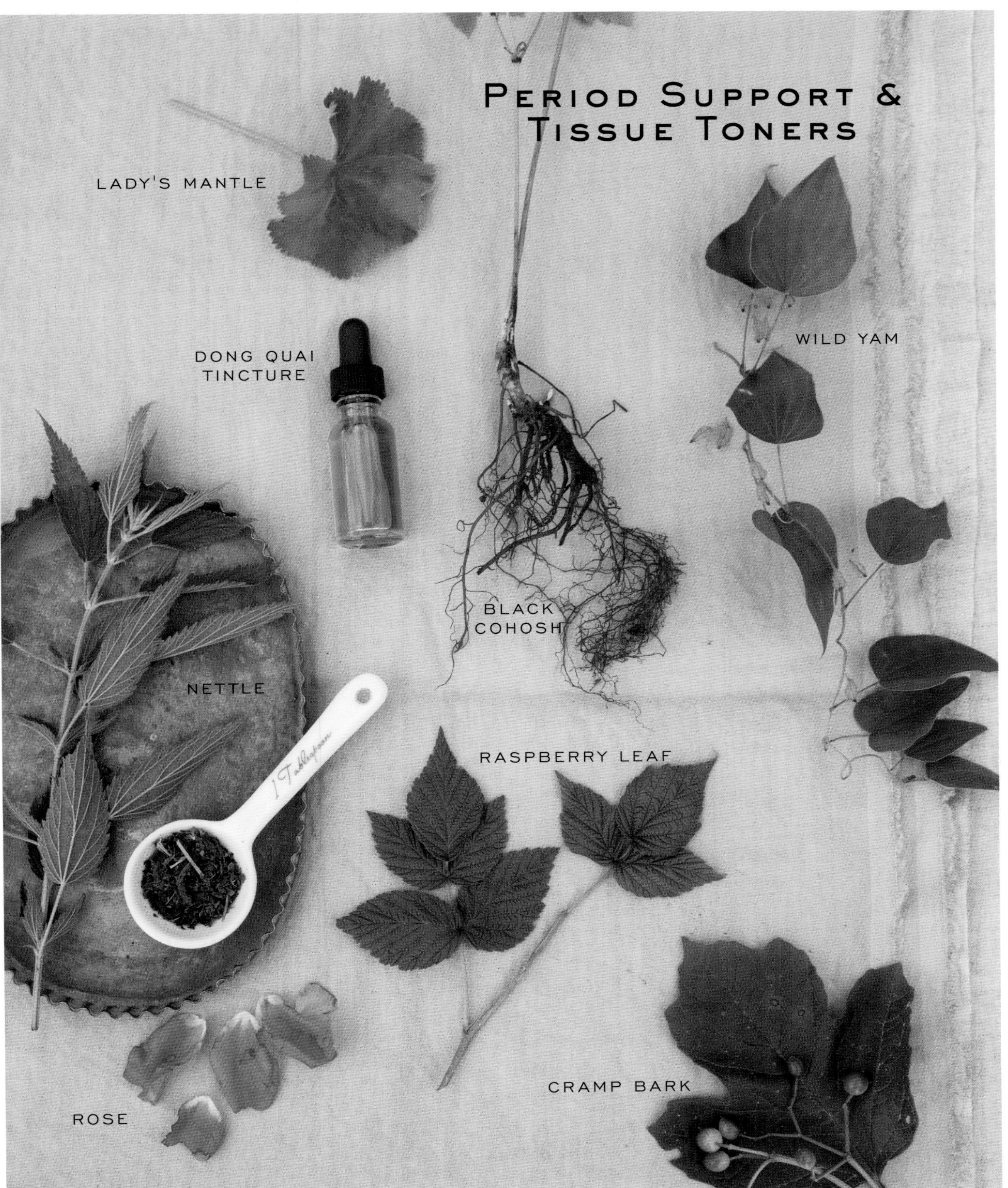
Period Support &
Tissue Toners
LADY'S MANTLE
DONG QUAI
TINCTURE
WILD YAM
BLACK
COHOSH
NETTLE
RASPBERRY LEAF
CRAMP BARK
ROSE

Period *and* Pain Support

Alongside a protocol of herbs that support a better cycle, these remedies can directly address menstrual cramps as well as other causes of uterine pain, like fibroids or ovarian cysts. If you are having difficulties with your period or uterine pain, be sure to also get a full gynecological checkup.

▸ Cramp Bark

Viburnum opulus

Availability: G W C

Key Properties: Cramp bark will symptomatically relieve cramps for most women. The tincture, taken every 15 minutes, will usually abate symptoms within half an hour with fewer side effects than conventional pain relievers. Teas and pills may not work as quickly. Cramp bark can be a godsend for some women, but it doesn't get to the underlying issue. You may find that normalizing your overall cycle with herbs relieves cramps. If not, you should see a qualified holistic practitioner such as a naturopathic doctor or uterine massage therapist for long-term relief.

Additional Benefits: Cramp bark may also work for gut spasms, back pain, leg cramps, et cetera, applied topically or taken internally. Midwives use it to delay labor contractions. This relaxing herb also offers some sedative and hypotensive properties.

Preparation: Harvest the bark in spring or fall. Use a fresh or dry plant tincture (replaced every few years, because it loses potency after a while); take two to four squirts every 15 minutes as needed. Also consider capsules or tea. Standard herb doses (see page 298) apply.

Cautions and Considerations: May upset gastroenteritis and hypotension. Don't use with blood thinners or bleeding disorders. Use during pregnancy only with supervision.

▸ Additional Period Support

Viburnum species (*Viburnum* spp.) grow wild across the country, and most have been used by Native Americans for similar uses to cramp bark. **Black haw** is also popular in commerce. Other in-the-moment cramp relief herbs that relax uterine tissue include **angelica, dong quai, wild yam, black cohosh,** and **ginger.**

Nettle is loaded with calcium, magnesium, iron, and other nutrients that are helpful for almost any woman. During menstruation, it can build the blood and help slow and stop heavy bleeding. It may slowly correct cramps related to nutrient deficiency. It's best taken as a strong infusion of 1 ounce of herb infused in a quart of hot water for 30 minutes to 4 hours.

Also consider taking **magnesium** and a **vitamin B complex supplement**; deficiency tends to increase the likelihood of muscle and menstrual cramps. Other supportive remedies include **iron-rich food** and herbs during heavy bleeding and daily use of tissue-toning herbs like **raspberry leaf tea.** See page 242 for more herbs rich in iron and page 86 for astringent herbs.

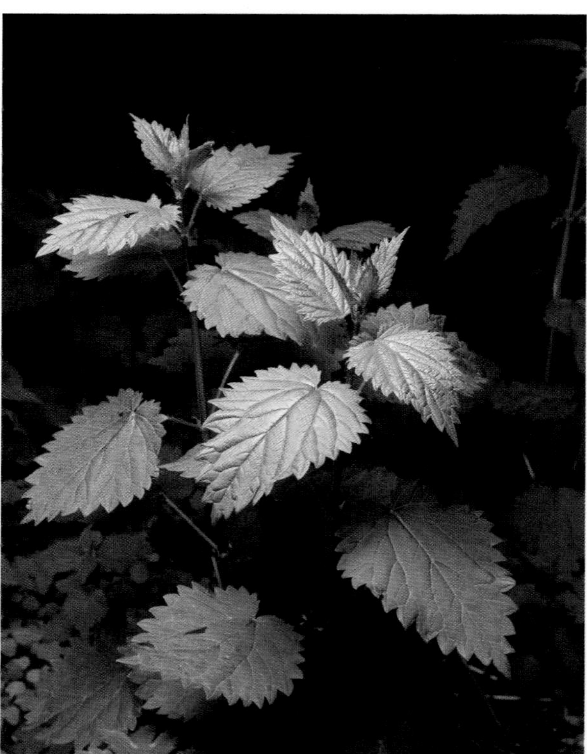

PROTOCOL POINTS

Menstrual Cramps

One of the most common reproductive issues, period. Modern medicine treats it with massive NSAID use, and you'll need to increase doses as your body adapts, which can put you at high risk for ulcers while actually worsening cramps. The underlying issues can include hormone imbalance, structural issues, endometriosis (hard to treat), and nutrient deficiency (easier to treat). If menstrual cramps persist or become unbearable, get checked to ensure nothing more serious is going on.

Diet: Eliminating coffee, both decaf and regular, as well as black tea and excessive amounts of chocolate helps women who are sensitive to the xanthine compounds (including but not limited to caffeine) that aggravate cramps and pain. Green and white tea don't tend to be as problematic. Also boost dietary magnesium and B vitamins: leafy greens, nuts, seeds, small servings of red meat. Some women find that their cramps may go away when they eliminate meat and dairy or eat a vegan diet, perhaps due to the inflammatory nature of these foods or the hormones that may be present in them.

Lifestyle: Uterine massage, in the schools of Maya Abdominal Therapy or visceral manipulation, can address a range of issues related to the uterus, including cramps, fibroids, and fertility issues. A lack of circulation or poor organ alignment can increase the likelihood of problems, and uterine massage aims to bring the uterus into proper alignment and increase blood flow to the reproductive system. Find a practitioner at www.arvigotherapy.com.

Herbs and Supplements: Magnesium with B vitamins, taken regularly, will gradually reduce or eliminate cramps for many. Cramp bark tincture often offers quick, symptomatic relief. Also consider the wild yam, dong quai (note that it can increase bleeding), or angelica root. Ginger makes a nice anti-inflammatory, pain-relieving synergist (high doses may increase bleeding). Recent studies have found that both ginger and cinnamon (encapsulated) reduce the severity of menstrual cramps and other symptoms, especially if you start taking them a few days before your period. Ginger tends to increase blood flow, while cinnamon may lessen it.

PMS

Progesterone issues are likely at play.

Diet: The usual whole-foods diet. Some women do better on a vegan diet or one low in animal products, while others do best with animal products, including meat. Tinker with your diet and see what feels best to you. Be sure to get enough B vitamins from diet or supplements. Omega-3 fatty acids improve mood and decrease inflammation.

Lifestyle: Stress management and adequate sleep are incredibly important. Daily activity boosts mood and improves hormone regulation.

Herbs: Key in on progesterone support (vitex, damiana) alongside stress support herbs (adaptogens, nervines). Herbs that support estrogen and ovulation may be used simply to bring the whole cycle into better balance, especially if cycle lengths vary widely.

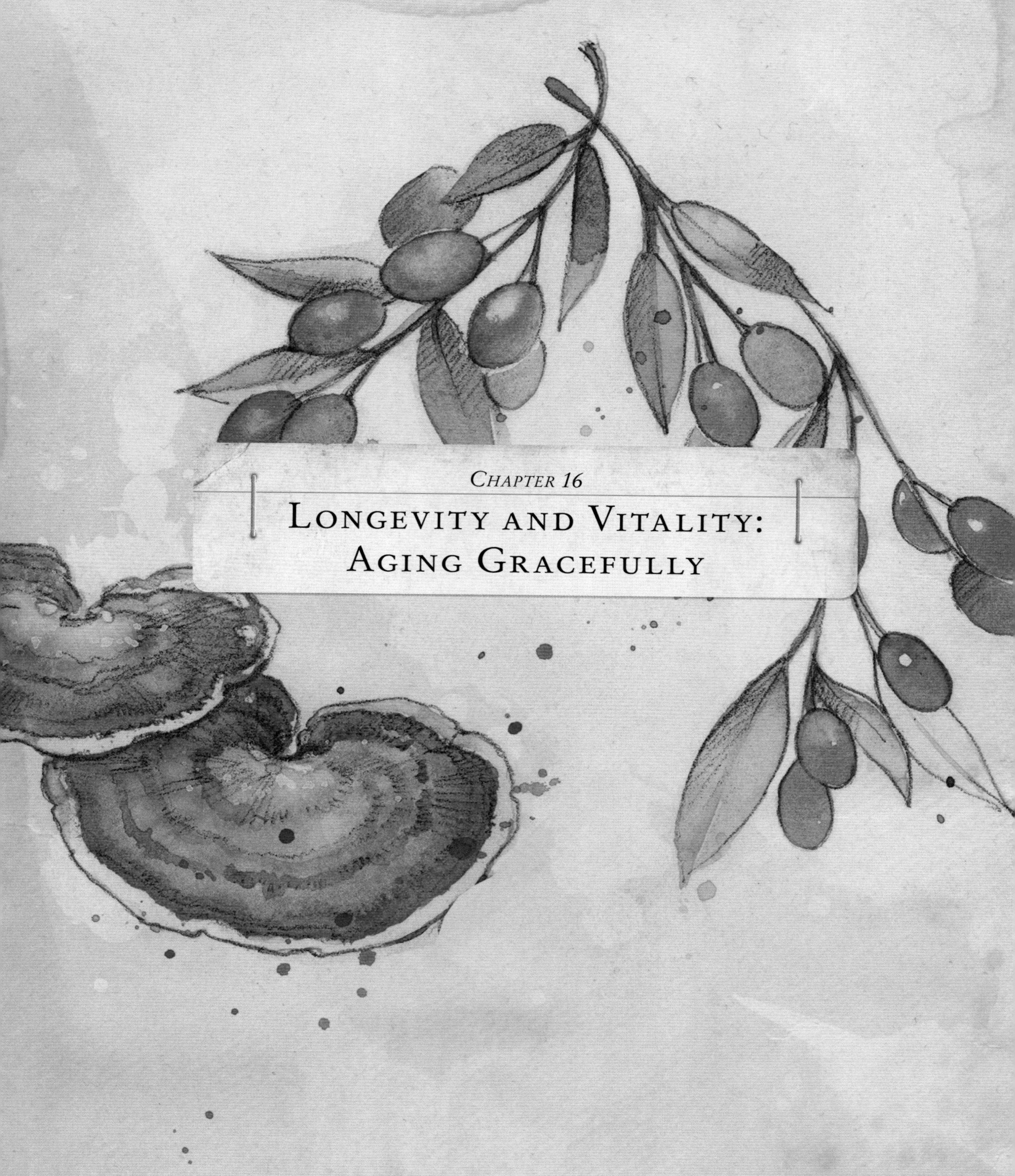

Chapter 16

Longevity and Vitality: Aging Gracefully

THOUGH THE PRECEDING chapters cover many aging-related topics, "aging well" is such an important topic that it warrants special attention. If you want to live a long, productive life in good health and with good energy, and to enjoy your golden years with minimal fuss and maximum vitality, a holistic approach to health and wellness is essential. No matter your age, it's never too early or late to make beneficial changes in your life. The younger you begin, the better off you'll be. Signs of aging will likely begin to manifest in your forties and fifties, as the effects of imbalance accumulate and symptoms become more noticeable. Maybe your energy levels aren't what they were, your body doesn't recuperate as quickly from injury or illness, or you find yourself more susceptible to various diseases. Making positive changes *now* can both improve your current health and increase your odds for a longer, better-quality life. It's not just about reaching your hundredth birthday but about being able to enjoy every day of your life as much as possible.

A broad category of tonic herbs, mushrooms, and foods serve as your primary allies in longevity and vitality. They have various actions — nutritious, antioxidant, anti-inflammatory, circulation enhancing, adaptogenic, immune modulating, anticancer, detoxifying — but as a group these tonics share some general qualities: They're extremely safe. They often benefit multiple body systems. They tend to be gentle yet profound when taken on an ongoing basis. Choose the ones that key into your personal aging concerns and consider adding them into your daily routine for the best results.

Fighting *the* Free Radicals

You've likely heard of free radicals (the agents of oxidation) and antioxidants (the heroes that fight them). Free radicals are molecules (or atoms) with an odd number of electrons — they have an unpaired electron in an outer ring. Electrons normally exist in pairs, and when that free radical encounters another molecule, it may steal an electron from it to pair with its own odd electron. The second molecule, having lost an electron, itself becomes a free radical. A chain reaction of free radical production — that is, oxidation — begins.

When this happens in your body, it's like pulling blocks from a Jenga game. You'll stay standing for a while, but as damage accumulates, things fall apart. Your body will do its best to fight the damage (making and putting new puzzle pieces back in), but eventually oxidation overwhelms the body's healing response. As you can imagine, oxidation accelerates the aging process.

Antioxidants squelch grabby free radicals by giving them electrons, stabilizing the molecules and preventing oxidative chain reactions. Different types of antioxidants, from different sources, act on a variety of free radicals and replenish spent antioxidants. The more antioxidants, the merrier! What does this have to do with aging? Research suggests that your body's rate of oxidation and degeneration begins to outpace repair in your late twenties (yikes!), but you can stretch that tipping point out *much* later in life by consuming antioxidant-rich food and herbs, exercising, and living a good lifestyle. Stress, inactivity, junk food, and excessive exposure to toxins (the usual "bad guys") all increase your level of oxidative stress and the number of free radicals your body must address.

Inflammation is technically a different chemical process, but there's a lot of crossover with oxidation in its causes, as well as the herbs, diet, and lifestyle changes that help the body control it. For example, new research suggests that antioxidants (as well as healthy lifestyle habits), renowned for their oxidation-fighting power, also encourage the body to kick up its anti-inflammatory activities. Both inflammation and oxidative damage tend to accumulate as you age and are inexorably linked to the diseases and unpleasant aspects of aging: wrinkles, cancer, heart disease, diabetes, chronic pain, and memory/cognition issues, including Alzheimer's and dementia.

ADDRESSING SPECIFIC AGE-RELATED DISEASES

THE FOLLOWING HERBS are not so much cures for disease, as they are support for body systems associated with disease, and they help to prevent and sometimes manage disease. Nothing is a guarantee — we are individuals and complex — but you can at least reduce your risk factors. Some of these herbs are controversial — always do your research and consider seeing a health professional to decide if they are right for you.

Heart disease: Consider hawthorn, gotu kola, rosemary, CoQ10, ginger, turmeric, berries, hibiscus, rooibos, garlic, onions, green tea, lots of antioxidants, low-glycemic/low-carb/high-fiber/vegan or Mediterranean diet, exercise (especially cardio, but start slowly if you have heart problems), mind-body balance. See chapter 10 for more details.

Diabetes: Consider holy basil, cinnamon, blueberry or bilberry leaf and fruit, fenugreek (large doses), chromium or brewer's yeast. Adopt a low-glycemic/low-carb/high-fiber/high-protein diet with lots of antioxidants, and get adequate exercise (especially weight bearing). See chapter 9 for more details.

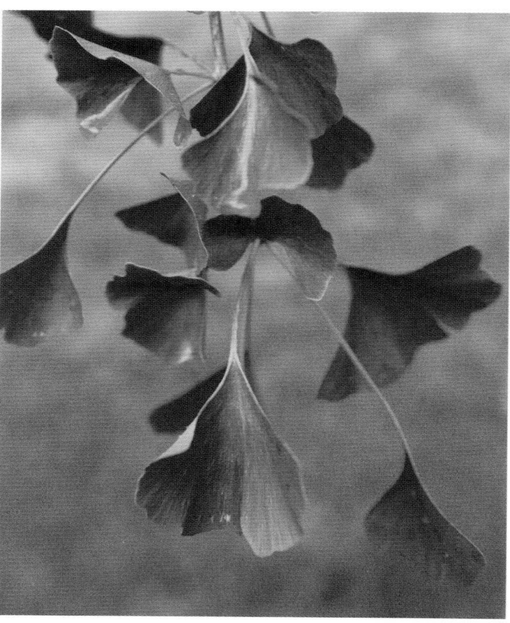

Autoimmune disease: Possibilities include nettle, gentle detox herbs (like burdock), medicinal mushrooms, astragalus, ashwagandha and other adaptogens, schizandra, turmeric, ginger. Adopt a vegan/low-glycemic/high-fiber/plant-rich diet with lots of antioxidants. Focus on mind-body balance and gentle exercise. Avoid problem foods and toxins. See chapter 7 for more.

Cancer: A plant-based/vegan or Mediterranean diet, regular exercise, stress reduction, mind-body balance, and a hopeful and proactive attitude are crucial. Consider medicinal mushrooms, green tea, turmeric, red clover, garlic and onions, saw palmetto, cruciferous vegetables, lots of antioxidants. For detoxification support, you might turn to Essiac, a tea mixture made with sheep sorrel, burdock, slippery elm, and turkey rhubarb. Please do not self-treat for cancer! Some of these herbs are highly controversial, and conventional treatment may still be needed. See page 241 for specific prostate and breast cancer prevention tips.

Chronic pain: Consider nettle, turmeric, ginger, holy basil, rosemary, green tea, magnesium, cherry, gentle detox herbs, anti-inflammatories, and alkalizing herbs. Eat a healthy diet full of antioxidants, avoid problem foods and sugar, and focus on gentle exercise and mind-body balance. See chapter 12 for more.

Alzheimer's and dementia: Supportive herbs include gotu kola, bacopa, ginkgo, rosemary, turmeric, ginger, holy basil, lemon balm, sage, spearmint, lion's mane mushroom, and rhodiola. Your approach should also include adequate sleep, challenging activities, stress reduction, meditation, toxin avoidance, regular aerobic exercise, lots of antioxidants, and all that other good stuff. See chapter 11 for more.

If you are in an advanced disease state, work with a practitioner, let your doctor know all the natural remedies you're taking, and also check with your pharmacist about interactions with medications.

FITNESS AND LONGEVITY

THE SINGLE MOST IMPORTANT thing you can do to improve your life span and stave off the effects of aging is to exercise regularly. All forms of exercise are beneficial. Cardio (aerobic) improves heart and brain health, weight-bearing exercise increases bone density, and activities like yoga and tai chi improve balance and mind-body well-being. As you age, you lose valuable muscle mass, and strength training helps counter that while providing other benefits, including blood sugar balance. Stretching decreases your risk of injury. Aim to be active 5 to 7 days a week for 20 to 30 minutes each day, but *any* exercise is always better than no exercise at all. If you're not sure where to start, consider walking.

The Longevity Diet: Eat Your Antioxidants

Key in on nutrient-dense, antioxidant, and anti-inflammatory foods to fortify your body against the effects of aging. Start with the general healthy diet detailed in chapter 1, and center it around these foods:

- **Berries** and similarly pigmented fruits and herbs — blueberries, bilberries, cherries, autumn olives, cranberries, dark purple grapes, pomegranate, jujube dates, hawthorn, rose hips, goji/lycii, hibiscus, rooibos — contain loads of antioxidants. They also help protect heart health, improve blood sugar balance, boost brain function, and strengthen capillary and blood vessel lining.
- **Leafy greens and cruciferous veggies** are the nutrient-dense antioxidant powerhouses of the vegetable world. They include spring nettle tops and other wild greens like dandelion and lamb's-quarter. Of course, *all* vegetables are good!
- **Garlic, onions, and other alliums** contain antioxidant sulfur compounds that protect your body from a wide range of damage, target and protect your immune and cardiovascular systems, aid detoxification, and help modulate blood sugar.
- **Omega-3 fatty acids** do double-duty because they encourage your body to *make* anti-inflammatory compounds while also offering essential fatty acids (EFAs) that create healthy cell linings, which improves your hair, skin, and nails, nerves, brain, mood, heart health, reproductive hormone balance, immune health (especially in autoimmune disease), allergies, and more. Sources include wild-caught fatty fish (salmon, sardines, herring/kippers, mackerel, trout, anchovies), fish/cod liver oil supplements, flax, hemp, chia, walnuts, purslane, grass-fed/wild meat and eggs. Other good fats can be found in olive oil, olives, coconut, avocado, nuts, and seeds.
- **Culinary herbs,** including basil, rosemary, parsley, oregano, mint, thyme, sage, lemon balm, and *Agastache* species, are loaded with antiaging, antioxidant, and anti-inflammatory compounds. Don't be shy — pile them on!
- **Tea, chocolate, and spices** contain more antioxidants per ounce than perhaps *any* other consumable. Turmeric and ginger may be your most valuable spices and can be used in ample amounts, but don't forget an extra sprinkle of coriander, cumin, cayenne, caraway, cardamom, cloves, or nutmeg.
- **Eat the rainbow.** A variety of pigments offers a variety of antioxidant nutrients and compounds. Challenge yourself to make the brightest, boldest, most colorful dishes!

Of course, you'll also want to limit or avoid the usual bad guys that also accelerate age-related symptoms and diseases: sugar, high-glycemic foods, processed food, excessive meat and animal products, factory-farmed foods, grilled or browned food (especially meat and carbs), pesticide and herbicide exposure, excessive alcohol, cigarettes. Unfortunately if you're on certain pharmaceuticals, like blood thinners, you have to be careful about consuming large amounts of otherwise healthy foods that tinker with blood coagulation. These include garlic, omega-3s, leafy greens, green tea, and certain spices. Your doctor may be able to work with you to adjust your medication dose accordingly. Check with your doctor before making any big dietary changes, especially if you have serious health conditions or take pharmaceuticals.

Herbs to Combat Free Radicals

By decreasing the aging effects of grabby free radicals and bringing down your body's overall anti-inflammatory response, you can expect the following herbs and foods to directly benefit your heart health, brain function, and blood sugar balance, to reduce your cancer risk, and to relieve pain. As an added benefit, they're all tasty enough to incorporate into your daily routine of food and tea, though certainly specialized supplements are an option, too.

NUTRIENT DENSITY AND DIGESTION AS YOU AGE

AS YOU AGE, poor diet and digestive function inadequacies begin to add up. Weak digestive function is widespread in our modern culture: indigestion, gastritis, reflux, leaky gut, low stomach acid and enzyme production, poor peristalsis, pharmaceuticals that reduce nutrient absorption or slow gut motility, et cetera. For a more detailed discussion about digestion and digestive herbs, see chapter 5.

If you have inflammation and damage to the gut lining (reflux, leaky gut, gastritis, inflammatory bowel disease, ulcers), first focus on healing your gut. This includes eating good food and avoiding less healthy foods as well as foods that you're sensitive or allergic to. Specific herbs that soothe and heal the gut include licorice root (and its safer deglycyrrhizinated form called DGL), slippery elm bark, marshmallow root, aloe inner gel, cabbage juice, and plantain leaf. Slowly work in fiber from whole foods like seeds, grains, vegetables, and fruit while also increasing your beneficial bacteria with a probiotics supplement and fermented foods like kimchi. Once your gut lining is in a better place, it's time to improve digestive function.

If your digestive function is weak (indigestion, difficult time with fats, gas, bloating, constipation), turn to bitter, aromatic, and carminative herbs such as dandelion, artichoke leaf, catnip, lemon balm, chamomile, ginger, and cardamom. These herbs kick up digestive juices so that you can better absorb the nutrients in your food while also improving how food moves through your digestive tract. If you're on antacid medications like Prilosec, it will be difficult, if not impossible, to attain good digestive health, and you're likely to end up with diseases related to nutrient deficiency with long-term use. Signs of nutrient deficiency or malabsorption include osteoporosis, poor hair/skin/nail health, weak connective tissue, low vitamin B_{12}, dry skin, anemia, and fatigue. Talk to your doctor to see if you can be weaned off the medications; DGL may suffice for wobbles and flare-ups during the transition.

▸ Garlic

Allium sativum

Availability: G+ C+

Key Properties: Garlic is as fond of your heart and immune system as it is of olive oil, rosemary, and dinnertime. While garlic won't necessarily chop numbers off your cholesterol or blood pressure, it can make modest improvements over time and strengthen your entire cardiovascular system, thin blood, improve blood vessel lining, and mellow blood sugar spikes. Garlic fights all the bad guys; it's antioxidant, anti-inflammatory, and antimicrobial and improves your body's ability to remove toxins and metabolic waste.

Additional Benefits: Eating or applying raw garlic wards off modern-day vampires like bacterial, viral, and fungal pathogens, parasites, and even biting insects, while strengthening your immune function and response to these invaders. Meanwhile, your good bacteria thrive on steady doses of garlic, onions, and leeks.

Preparation: The more it stinks and makes you cry, the more powerful it is. Mince or chop up fresh garlic to release its juices, wait 10 to 15 minutes, and you have food medicine at its peak. Though best raw, it will retain some of its benefits if cooked after this point. A clove or two a day should do it. If you want something less odiferous, try aged garlic capsules, which have performed well in studies, too.

Cautions and Considerations: Generally safe, but garlic can interact with several medications, including blood thinners, when taken in regular therapeutic doses. May cause indigestion, gas, garlic/onion breath/body odor, and allergies for some. Garlic oil may irritate skin and mucous membranes.

Similar Herbs: Other **alliums** — onions, chives, leeks, ramps, et cetera — offer similar benefits.

▸ Lycii Berries

Lycium barbarum, L. chinense

Availability: G W C

Key Properties: Also known as goji berries, lycii are rich in antioxidant pigments called carotenoids, particularly red lycopene and yellow zeaxanthin, and useful polysaccharides. Long revered in traditional Chinese medicine as a pleasant-tasting, nourishing longevity fruit, lycii has recently gained renown as a superfood in the West. Studies support its ability to enhance sexual function and immune health, fight cancer, improve physical endurance, promote heart and blood sugar health, and improve eye health.

Additional Benefits: According to Himalayan herbal traditions, regular intake of lycii gladdens the spirit and increases cheerfulness.

Preparation: Use approximately ½ ounce (15 grams) daily in tea, food, and smoothies. Add the dried berries to porridge, granola, and trail mix much as you would raisins. Mix the powder into smoothies. Because carotenoids are fat-soluble, a little heat and fat in the dish should improve bioavailability.

Cautions and Considerations: Lycii is a very safe food herb. Allergy is rare but possible. It is in the nightshade family (as are tomatoes, peppers, potatoes, eggplant), so it may not agree with you if you're sensitive to these foods. It may lower blood sugar levels. Though probably fine during pregnancy and lactation, seek professional guidance.

Similar Herbs: Various ***Lycium* species**, often called desert thorn or wolfberry, grow wild throughout the United States; some but not all can be used similarly.

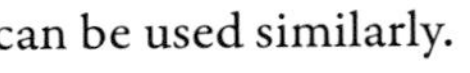

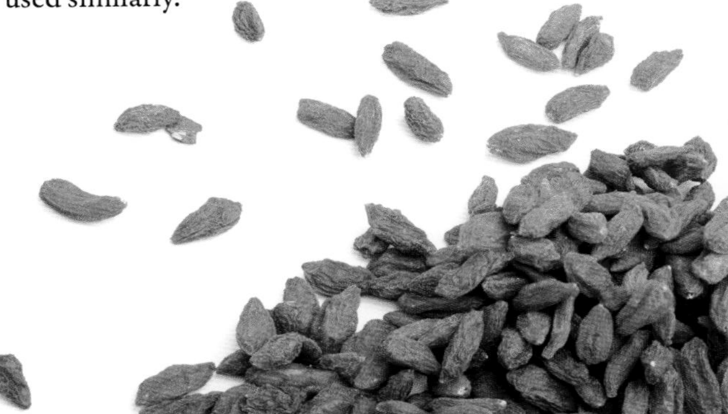

Antioxidants & Anti-inflammatories

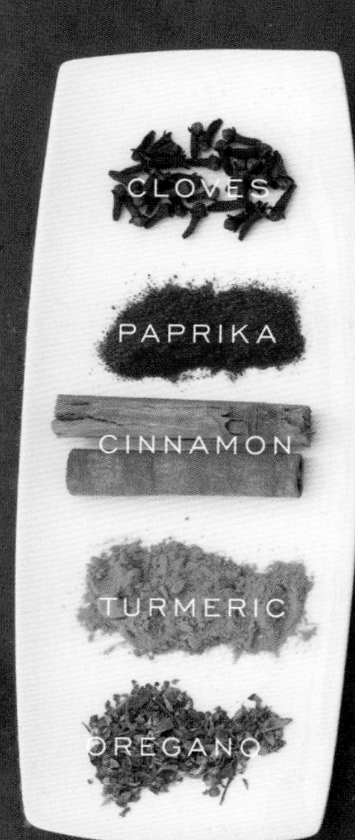

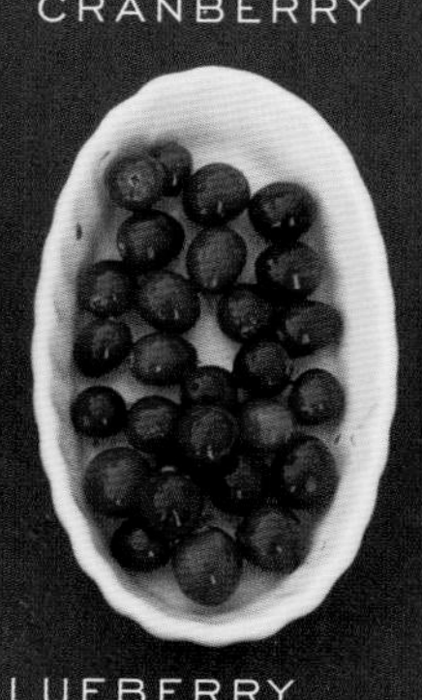

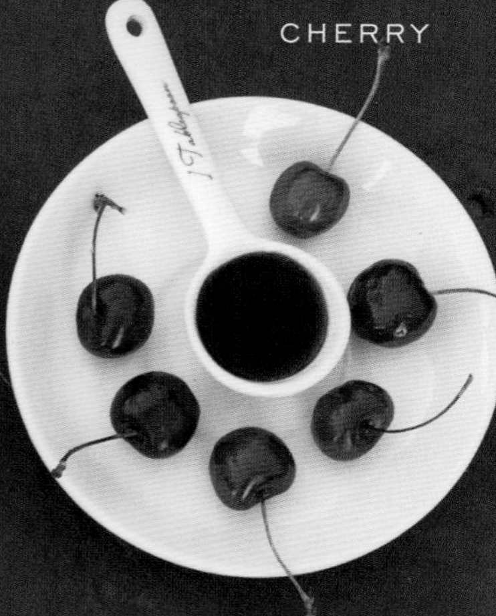

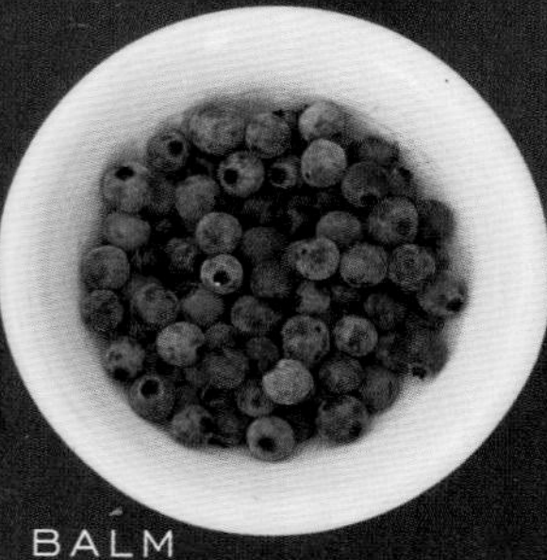

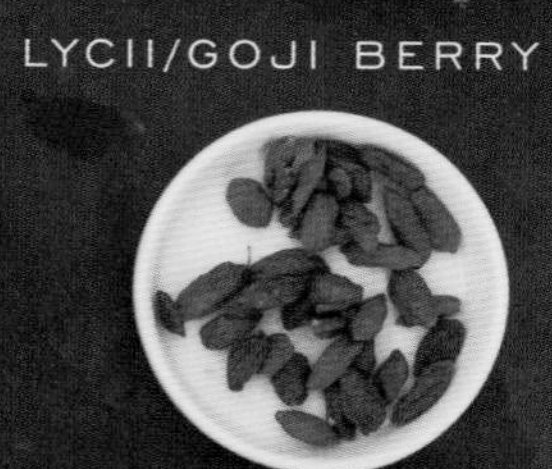

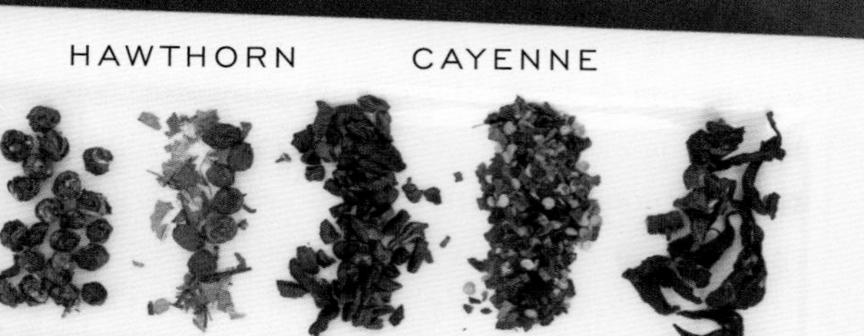

▸ Other Powerful Antioxidants

The antiaging clout of **blueberries** stems from more than a decade of research by scientists at the U.S. Department of Agriculture (USDA) Human Nutrition Research Center on Aging and other leading scientific organizations. These berries improve brain signaling, memory, coordination, blood sugar levels, and night vision, combat venous insufficiency and other circulation-related issues, help prevent cataracts, and stave off similar age-related issues. The closely related **bilberry** is nearly identical in appearance and use, and there's also a bit of crossover with its cousin the **cranberry**. The darker and brighter the deep blue-purple anthocyanin pigments, the better. Other classic superfruits include **tart cherries** (noted for their beneficial effects on pain, sleep, and heart health) and **pomegranates** (noted for protecting the heart, lowering cholesterol levels, fighting cancer, and even increasing bone strength). Enjoy them daily fresh, frozen, as pure juice, or in quality powdered/capsule formats. Aim for ½ to 2 cups daily — or a quart or more a week — of the fresh fruit or equivalent amounts. Learn more about these red-blue-purple tonics on page 157.

Rooibos and **hibiscus** offer berrylike antioxidants and often appear in fruity herbal blends. Recent research has found that they promote heart health by lowering cholesterol, blood pressure, and possibly blood sugar, and that they also support the body's own antioxidant production and liver health. Aim for 3 to 6 cups of tea daily. Learn more on page 155.

Hawthorn has an amazing capacity to heal the heart. When taken regularly, this gentle tonic strengthens the pumping ability of the heart, relaxes blood vessels, lowers blood pressure, repairs damage, and fights oxidative stress. It's particularly useful for hypertension, congestive heart failure, angina, and heart attack prevention and recuperation. It can be taken in any form, and the solid extract is particularly tasty and concentrated. Be patient: it's a slow-acting tonic, not a heart drug. Learn more on page 153.

Leading the pack of superspices is **turmeric,** thanks to the unsurpassed antioxidant and anti-inflammatory activity of its very own bright yellow carotenoid called curcumin. It shines for relief of chronic pain and inflammation, overall liver support, improvement of digestion and fat absorption, reduction of cholesterol, and protection against heart disease, cancer, and even Alzheimer's. It may even improve fertility and reverse major depression. There are many reasons this golden powder has made its way to the top of the spice rack. Sprinkle ¼ to ½ teaspoon on your food daily or take it in capsule form, preferably with a smidge of black pepper to improve bioavailability. Learn more on page 188.

Other spices like **cinnamon**, **cumin**, **cloves**, **paprika**, and the **Italian herbs** (basil, parsley, thyme, oregano, marjoram) also all get high marks for their anti-inflammatory, antioxidant properties. A pinch of **cayenne** goes a long way and increases the activity of everything else as a circulation booster and synergist.

Mint-family tonics like **lemon balm**, **sage**, **rosemary**, and **spearmint** help keep your brain young, and each offers additional benefits. These mint-family herbs inhibit acetylcholinesterase; as a result, they boost levels of the important neurotransmitter acetylcholine in the brain. They're also all anti-inflammatory, antioxidant, and circulation enhancing. A handful of recent studies have found that healthy adults who took these herbs performed better on cognitive and memory tests. Typical food and tea doses work great. Learn more on page 172.

Green and white tea work their magic primarily thanks to potent antioxidant compounds called catechins, which are known to fight several types of cancer, human papillomavirus (HPV), heart disease, diabetes, obesity, and mental decline. Applied topically as a spritz, bath, compress, or herb-infused cream, tea helps fight wrinkles, sunburn, the effects of aging, and skin cancer. Enjoy several cups daily. Learn more on page 176.

Cacao is one of the most delicious heart tonics. Studies back its ability to improve overall heart health and endothelial lining, aid in weight management, and reduce cholesterol, blood pressure, plaque, and blood sugar. It's loaded with good-for-you polyphenols, and combining it with pure vanilla only improves its flavor and antioxidant capacity. Chocolate also boosts mood and picks up the pep. The higher the cocoa content (and the lower the sugar and milk), the better the effects. Enjoy a few squares of dark chocolate or a spoonful of cocoa powder, cacao, or nibs, but beware if you're supersensitive to caffeine. Learn more on page 155.

Longevity Elixirs *and* Adaptogens

The best-known longevity herbs are also noted adaptogens (plants that help your body resist and adapt to stress). These plants climbed the ranks of medicinal herbs across the world to become some of the most revered herbs in history. In general, they improve energy and vitality and help you resist disease. Interestingly, most also boost libido and reproductive health. Each superhero herb also has its own extra special powers, and some tend to be zippy while others promote a chill state of Zen. To figure out which herbs to try, first determine whether you want pep or calm energy, then consider the specific indications and side benefits for each. You can take adaptogens on an ongoing basis or pulse periodically (say, for a few weeks or months) as a pick-me-up. They blend fabulously with other tonic herbs, nutritives, medicinal mushrooms, and spices. For even more detail on adaptogens, see chapter 3.

Zippy Adaptogens

These stimulating adaptogens energize and revitalize the body while enhancing the function of a variety of body systems. Consider them when you're feeling old, tired, and depressed, when it's hard to get out of bed in the morning. Their stimulating nature can be too much for a sensitive heart or for people who suffer from anxiety, manic tendencies, or insomnia, though. Combining them with caffeine synergizes their energizing properties, not always for the better. You probably *don't* want to take them before bed.

▸ JIAOGULAN

Gynostemma pentaphyllum

Availability: G- C-

Key Properties: Jiaogulan's nickname, "immortality herb," underscores its longevity reputation. It's even reported to prevent hair loss. Jiaogulan is a fast-growing squash-family vine, widely cultivated in Korea and often used as a less expensive substitute for ginseng. It contains similar and identical constituents. Though it's reported to be a calming adaptogen, I find it quite zippy.

Additional Benefits: It supports immune health and is used in anticancer protocols. Jiaogulan also benefits overall heart health in many ways, specifically reducing blood pressure, cholesterol, triglycerides, and blood stickiness (platelet aggregation). It boosts your own production of antioxidants and is a classic antiaging adaptogen.

Preparation: This Asian herb is slowly becoming more available in American natural food stores and herb shops. It's very easy to grow and harvest in ample amounts in warm climates or as a houseplant — a distinct advantage over some of our more difficult-to-grow root adaptogens. However, you may have to search online to find seed starts. For medicinal purposes, use the aerial parts. Steep it for anywhere from just a few minutes to up to 40 minutes. Also consider tinctures or capsules. Standard herb doses apply (see page 298).

Cautions and Considerations: Jiaogulan may interact with blood thinners, sedatives, and other meds. Take it with food to avoid an upset stomach. High doses may cause a rash, fatigue, dizziness, or palpitations.

As you become accustomed to using herbs for health, you'll think nothing of taking a shot of elderberry syrup at the oncoming flu or mixing up a new blend to warm your bones or help you sleep. But many herbal newbies become paralyzed with uncertainty when dealing with children and animals. The use of herbs in children and pets is actually not so different from adults, though we'll want to lean toward gentle, safe options and keep a few guidelines in mind:

- Herbalism isn't an exact science. Because children and animals are (usually) smaller than adults, normally they are given smaller doses of herbs and remedies. With the safe and gentle herbs we tend to use for children and animals, higher doses are unlikely to pose problems but usually are not necessary.
- Start with a very low dose the first time you use an herb for a child or pet — just a drop or a sip — and slowly work your way up over hours or days (depending on how acute the need). Pay close attention to see how the individual responds. Does the remedy seem to be working? Are there any side effects or allergies? Slowly working in the herbs can also avoid negative reactions to a sudden new flavor.
- Use the gentlest herbs with the least risk of allergy or side effects first, before moving on to stronger herbs if needed. Gentle herbs include tonic and nutritive herbs. Gentle *forms* of herbs include homeopathic remedies and flower essences, tonic herbs as teas or in food, and low-dose liquid extracts. Avoid or limit incredibly potent remedies such as essential oils, which have a higher rate of side effects and toxicity for children and animals.
- Don't use honey for children under the age of 1. Glycerin and sugar syrups are safer for this age group.
- Be aware of contamination, especially for low-alcohol sweet remedies that easily grow germs, including glycerites, syrups, gripe water, and infused honey. These remedies should be refrigerated (especially for long-term storage), used up quickly, and tossed when they reach their expiration date. Don't put droppers directly into the mouth and then back into the bottle.
- Vinegar and alcohol are more shelf stable and less apt to harbor pathogens, but they may not be palatable for your patient. Even though we don't recommend significant doses of alcohol for children and pets, the small amount given (literally *drops*) as a tincture is usually fine. If you're not comfortable with alcohol, you have plenty of other options: vinegar, powder, tea, glycerite, et cetera.
- Stock your bookshelf with specific herbals geared for children or animals. Aviva Romm and Mary Bove offer modern, measured advice for herb use in pregnancy and for kids. For pets, consider *Herbs for Pets* by Wulff and Tilford, various herbals by Randy Kidd, and the textbook *Veterinary Herbal Medicine* by Wynn and Fougere. You'll often find varying viewpoints and tidbits, so it helps to read across a few sources to get a better sense of a particular health condition and the herbs themselves. This chapter is just a short introduction to these diverse areas of herbalism.
- Don't hesitate to ask a professional for advice, especially if you're new and unsure, or if a condition persists or becomes severe in spite of the care you give. Be aware of situations that can get dangerous quickly and may demand medical care, such as diarrhea, bleeding, difficulty breathing, severe allergic reaction, refusal of any food or water, and bad infections. Seek out a midwife or holistic pediatrician, naturopath, or herbalist for infant and children's care. For animals, find a holistic vet or an herbalist who specializes in animal care.

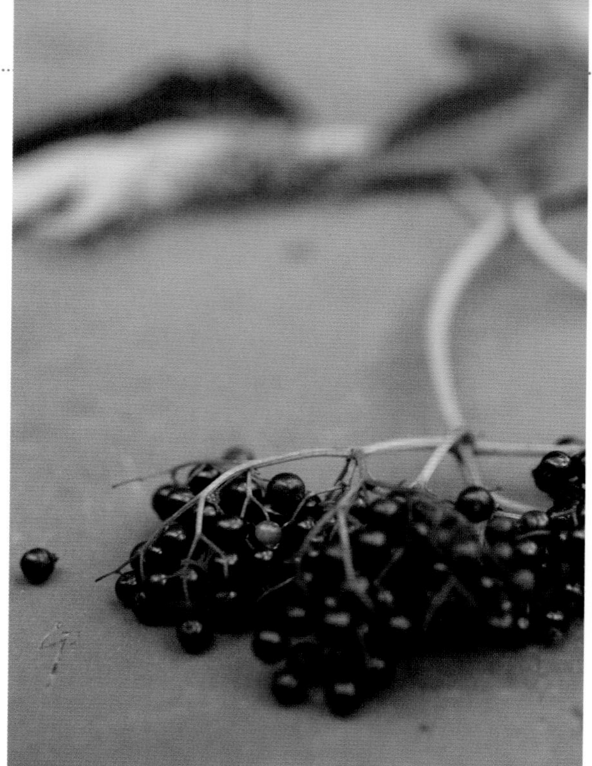

- If you're not comfortable making your own remedies, you can purchase premade products specially made for children or animals. Look to the children's lines of respected herb brands like Gaia Herbs and Oregon's Wild Harvest, or reputable companies like Herbs for Kids, Animals' Apawthecary, and Herbs for Life Pet Wellness Blends. Ask around, and you're likely to find a local herbalist who specializes in such products and may also offer consultations and teach classes.

While it may seem odd to discuss children and animals in the same section, their conditions and best herbs actually overlap quite a bit. In the few cases (elderberries, garlic) where safety varies, I've noted it in the cautions. Consider this chapter as a starting point, then turn to more specific books on children or animal care for further details, ideas, and herbs.

ADJUSTING THE DOSE

For most children and pets, you'll want to reduce the dose. Use age and/or body weight as your guide. Clark's rule can work for children and animals, dividing the dose down by body weight and assuming 150 pounds for the average adult:

Clark's rule: child/animal weight in pounds ÷ 150 × adult dose = child/animal dose

With safe tonic herbs, you have some wiggle room, and you may find that individuals may do better with higher or lower doses. Use the chart below as a guide.

Person's Age	Body Weight (Animal or Child)	Estimated Dose	Tincture Dose	Tea Dose
Adult	100–150+ lb	Full dose	60 drops	1 cup
Teen	around 100 lb	½ to full	30–60 drops	½–1 cup
Preteen	around 75 lb	½	30 drops	½ cup
Elementary	around 50 lb	¼	15 drops	¼ cup
Preschool	around 15–25 lb	⅛	8–10 drops	1–2 tablespoons
Toddler	around 10–15 lb	1/10	5–10 drops	2 teaspoons
Infant*	around 5–10 lb	1/16	2–5 drops	½–1 teaspoon

*Generally speaking, the less you give infants, the better. Lean toward the gentlest remedies, such as homeopathics and flower essences, as well as the herbs with a long history of use for infants, like chamomile. Don't hesitate to seek professional supervision.

Getting the Medicine Down

It's not always easy to reason with a child or animal when it comes time to "take their medicine," especially if it tastes nasty or you have a really finicky or anxious patient. You have two basic approaches: (1) force it down to get it over with quickly, or (2) hide it and improve palatability. If you can manage the second option, your patient will thank you!

Powder Possibilities

Having a powdered or finely cut/sifted herb offers many options for easy hiding, especially if it doesn't taste *really* disgusting. Depending on the flavor profile, mix it into oatmeal, applesauce, smoothies, eggs, honey, nut butter, honey-nut butter balls, et cetera. Many animals will eat whatever fresh or dry herbs you mix in their feed. A bit of powder holds more medicine than you'd think, too: 1 teaspoon equals approximately 10 capsules! Powder dose depends on the herb, and sometimes cut/sifted herb works just fine, too. Keep in mind that some herbs don't work as well once dried, such as echinacea, valerian, and lemon balm.

Teas and Liquid Extracts

With teas and liquid extracts, like tinctures, syrups, vinegars, and glycerites, sometimes adding or using a sweet base like syrup or honey is all you need, but other times you need to get more creative. You can hide these as you would powders, but often mixing them in sweet drinks works best. You might be able to add it straight to an animal's water or need to mix it in a favorite drink, such as milk or honey-sweetened water. With herbal formulas, consider trying better-tasting herbs first. Most kids lap elderberry syrup straight from the spoon but freak out if you give them straight-up echinacea or goldenseal tincture. If you *must* use a bad-tasting herb, try mixing it with better-tasting ones (e.g., licorice, peppermint) or a sweet base. For oily things like fish oil, try something fatty and thick, like a smoothie, eggnog, or stew (although grease-cutting orange juice works pretty well, too). If you plan to give a liquid remedy to your child or animal on a daily basis, start with a very small amount and slowly increase the dose each day so they get used to the taste.

Pills

We rarely use pills for young kids, but occasionally it makes sense for animals. You might be able to force it down the animal's throat, then hold the jaw shut until it swallows, though this can be stressful for both you and your pet. Try hiding it in cheese, a favorite food, or in a soft treat that you toss to your pet one by one (sneaking the medicine-infused treat in with regular treats). For older kids and teens who can't get over the pill-gag reflex (I was one of those!), practice with slippery, small softgels (e.g., cod liver oil) and warm water. Have them take a sip of water first to coat the throat and pill, which helps it go down more easily. Cats may be the most difficult of all, and a pill-pusher syringe with an extra flush of water may be needed to force it down (a treat afterward makes it slightly less horrific for your pet). With herbs, it's usually easier to simply stick to powders, tea, or liquid extracts and skip the pills. Some pills can be opened or crushed and added to food as a powder.

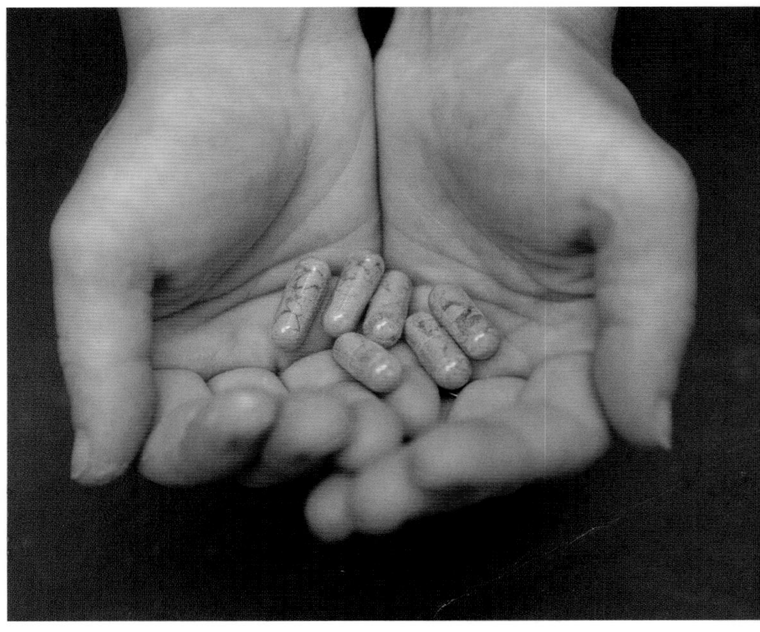

Basic Nutrition

Everyone needs vitamins and minerals, and nutritious herbs supply a nice variety in an easy-to-absorb form. Boosting nutrition with herbs can improve overall vitality and visibly enhance hair (or coat or feathers), skin, bones, and nails with regular use.

▸ Nettle

The supreme nutritive for humans and animals, nettle abounds with nutrients including calcium, magnesium, potassium, iron, and chlorophyll. It is the *super* dark leafy green. It improves overall vitality and nutrition and can be particularly helpful for growing pains and postexercise aches, which can be caused by an inadequate mineral supply. Add the dried herbs to recipes, feed, soup broth, tea, et cetera. It can be consumed in higher amounts than most herbs. It also decreases allergies and histamine, tightens and tones tissue (uterine, bladder, gut, respiratory system, kidneys), and acts as a diuretic (makes you pee, a lot!) to help flush toxins from the body.

Cautions: Though generally safe and well tolerated, the diuretic effect can be too much for some kids and animals. The fresh plant stings. Use spring greens before it flowers. For more on nettle, see page 33.

▸ Parsley

Parsley greens offer a nice addition to food, smoothies, and juices because of the mild yet perky flavor, nutrients (especially chlorophyll), and antioxidants. Stick to modest doses for small or young folks. It's a particularly nice addition to animal feed during the winter months, when forage opportunities are limited.

Cautions: Parsley is a potent diuretic, which might be too much for some. High doses may also lower blood pressure. The seeds can irritate kidneys, but the greens are usually okay.

▸ Violet

Violet leaves and flowers have a pleasant, mild flavor, even as a raw salad green, that almost anyone will enjoy, and they're rich in vitamin C and various minerals. Violet is a favorite forage plant for livestock and wild animals, too. Add it to food fresh or dry, tea, super infusions, and pesto. It's a gentle yet multipurpose herb. It also has a pleasant demulcent, cooling, moistening property, nice for dry folks and those for whom diuretic greens (ahem: nettle, parsley, dandelion) don't agree. Nice for respiratory irritation, coughs, and the skin, too. It moves the lymph, which aids detoxification and swollen lymph glands and is used for fatty tumors in older dogs.

Cautions: Pretty darn safe!

Similar herb: Chickweed offers similar nutrients, healing properties, and "yummy green" palatability. It's best fresh. True to its name, chickens particularly love nibbling on chickweed, as do kids. Chickweed also makes a great poultice for poison ivy and irritated skin.

▸ Rose Hips

Rose hips offer a different set of nutrients, mainly vitamin C, bioflavonoids, and blue-purple-red pigment antioxidants, all of which improve immune, respiratory, and skin/connective tissue health and decrease inflammation and oxidative stress. Rose hips taste pleasant: somewhat tart, sweet, and raisiny or tomatoey depending on the batch. The flavor improves and becomes fruitier with the addition of hibiscus flowers and honey. Use them for tea, for jam, in food, as a powder, in animal feed, and more.

Cautions: Generally very safe; however, the inner hairs can irritate the throat. If you buy crushed rose hips, the hairs have been removed already, but you'll have to scoop or strain them out (e.g., through fine cloth) if you process your own. For more on rose hips, see page 37.

▸ Dandelion

Dandelion roots and leaves have a mineral-rich nutrient profile similar to nettles. The bitter flavor will probably horrify most kids, but some animals (especially horses and chickens) *love* it. Use dandelion in food, tea, pesto, or vinegar extract. It also has digestion-enhancing, liver-detoxifying, and very potent diuretic effects, all of which make it useful as a kidney tonic and for poor digestion, allergies, skin woes (especially teen acne, used in combination with burdock), and high blood pressure. Tinctures capture most of dandelion's medicinal properties, but not the minerals. Also try tea, powder, and food forms.

Cautions: Generally safe, but the diuretic effect and bitter flavor don't work for everyone, and in rare cases the fresh plant causes contact dermatitis. Learn more about dandelion on page 37.

Nerves *and* Brain

Children and animals often present with overactivity, agitation, anxiety, insomnia, attention issues, and weak nervous-endocrine function. Nobody likes to feel this way! Try to identify and address the root cause. Certain nervines and calming adaptogens really shine in bringing things back into balance.

▸ Chamomile

Chamomile tea may be *the* most popular herb for infants and children worldwide. It has a gentle calming effect on the nerves that helps with agitation, anxiety, and insomnia. Only brew the tea for a minute or so to avoid unpleasant bitterness. Sweet liquid extracts and homeopathic preparations work well, too. Chamomile also famously improves digestion and helps dispel colic, gas, pain, and bloating. It has anti-inflammatory and pain-relieving properties, which partly explains its effectiveness for teething pain and topically for rashes.

Cautions: Chamomile is generally quite safe, but it aggravates allergies for some ragweed-sensitive people.

Similar herb: Catnip shares chamomile's calming and digestion/colic benefits and is less likely to cause allergy.

▸ Lemon Balm

Lemon balm shares chamomile's digestion-enhancing and calming properties but has a few extra tricks. Even though it's relaxing, the lemony essential oils gently lift mood and improve attention and cognition. Consider it for overactivity, attention deficit hyperactivity disorder, anxiety, memory, and insomnia. It tastes pretty good and is *loaded* with antioxidants. Use it as a tea, tincture/liquid extract, infused honey, and fresh or dry in food or added to animal bedding. It also has antiviral activity against the flu and herpes. For herpes, take it internally and also apply externally at the very first sign of outbreak. Lemon balm's essential oils block viruses from entering cells and replicating, and the herb also promotes healing.

Cautions: Generally very safe and well tolerated. Lemon balm loses potency quickly — dry leaves within a few months, and tinctures within a few years. You can still use older lemon balm, but it might not be as effective. Lemon balm may aggravate hypothyroid issues. See page 59 for more on lemon balm.

▸ Gotu Kola

Gotu kola, most famous as a calming adaptogen with brain-boosting effects, is fed to children in India when they go back to school. It energizes and helps the body adapt to stress while also improving cognition and memory and relieving anxiety. It can be eaten fresh or dry as a leafy green but is more commonly available as a tea, liquid extract, or powder. It has a mildly bitter and peppery flavor, akin to that of celery and watercress, but it is easy to mask with other ingredients. It also improves circulation and heart health, strengthens the vascular lining/capillaries and connective tissue, and promotes skin health and wound healing (both externally and internally). For this it can be applied topically and taken internally. It blends well with holy basil, lemon balm, and milky oat seed.

Cautions: Gotu kola is generally quite safe. See page 53 for more details on this herb.

Similar herb: Holy basil also offers broad benefits, including calm energy that is safe for children and animals (though it can lower blood sugar and may cause hypoglycemia if taken on an empty stomach in sensitive individuals). Learn more on page 53.

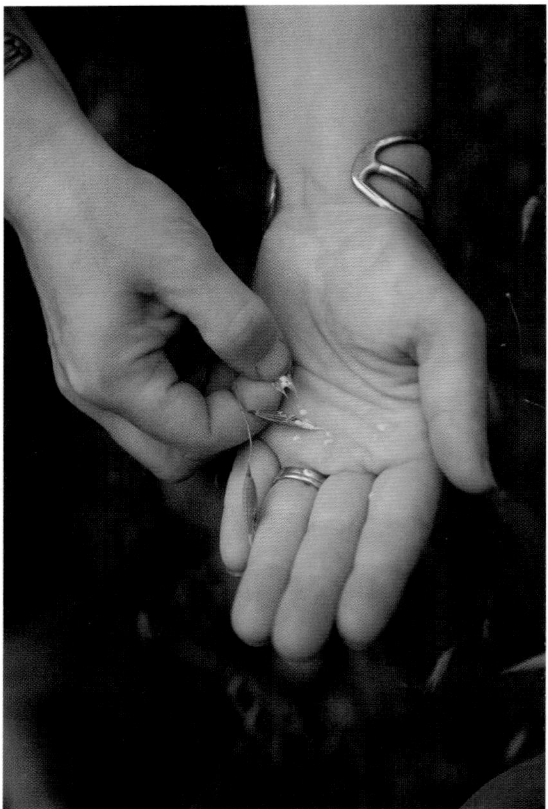

▸ Oats

Oats provide multiple remedies for children and animals. For the nerves, use milky oat seed, usually as a fresh liquid extract because the milky latex loses its benefit once dried. Milky oats nourish the nervous-adrenal system, improving its vitality while calming anxiety, hyperactivity, agitation, and overexhaustion. They work best when taken in steady doses over time and blend well with the other herbs in this section. They also act as a nutrient-rich food when taken as oat straw or oatmeal/grain, loaded with minerals (especially silica and calcium) and some B vitamins. Oatmeal/grain also has soothing slimy properties that benefit rashes, inflamed skin, and the digestive tract, and it's high in fiber.

Cautions: Generally safe, even at high doses, though gluten contamination is possible on the grains. Strain oat straw out of tea or broth before serving, unless it's for an animal that typically eats grass. See page 35 for more on oat straw.

Digestion

Digestive woes are common among children and animals, and herbs can help improve digestion, heal damaged and inflamed gut lining, and lessen diarrhea or constipation. If the digestive issues (especially diarrhea) are severe or don't improve, seek professional guidance immediately.

▸ Chamomile

Chamomile tea, as mentioned previously, remains the most popular remedy for indigestion, gas, pain, bloating, and colic, even for babies.

Similar herbs: Catnip and **lemon balm** offer similar benefits for digestion and also calm nerves. **Dandelion**, a digestive bitter, has stronger digestion-enhancing effects but may be less useful for nerves and colic.

▸ Apple Cider Vinegar

Apple cider vinegar, raw and unpasteurized, increases acidity in the gut, which can aid nutrient absorption and relieve indigestion and some cases of heartburn. You're unlikely to get children to take vinegar unless you add *lots* of honey; however, many animals do well with a splash in their drinking water. It also relieves sunburn and poison ivy itches when applied topically and makes a nice alternative to alcohol for liquid herbal extracts.

Cautions: Stop using vinegar if it seems to upset the stomach or cause heartburn. Be aware that vinegar corrodes most metals (and, over the long haul, rubber dropper tops) — use plastic, ceramic, or glass for serving instead.

▸ Mints

Peppermint and other mints improve digestion; ease gas, bloating, and colic; and can flavor formulas to make other herbs more palatable. It's most often used as a tea, but you can also eat it fresh or dried. Enteric-coated capsules target the lower GI tract and the pain of irritable bowel syndrome. Sweetened peppermint tea and candy ease nausea. It also helps open the lungs, perks up the spirits, and clears the sinuses. Of the mints, peppermint has the strongest pain-relieving and antispasmodic effects and is best for headaches, gut pain, and other complaints associated with muscle spasms. It acts as a mild diaphoretic to help break a sweat during fevers. Add fresh or dried mint (any type) to animal bedding to improve the scent and discourage rodents and bugs.

Cautions: Stop using peppermint if it upsets the stomach or causes heartburn. Learn more about peppermint on page 81.

Similar herb: Catnip shares peppermint's diaphoretic and digestive benefits.

▸ Slippery Elm

Slippery elm bark offers soothing, healing, slimy, mucilaginous, demulcent benefits. It temporarily coats the mucous lining of your digestive tract, which helps soothe irritation and promotes healing of inflammation and tissue damage (leaky gut, reflux, gastritis). Use it as a lozenge (look in the sore throat section of natural food stores) or tea, but it's most popular as a powder. Make a mucus-like gruel, which may be slightly less off-putting to finicky eaters in oatmeal, yogurt, or a smoothie. Slippery elm's flavor is mild and pleasant, akin to maple syrup. Add cinnamon, fennel, or licorice for better flavor. It also helps with sore throat, dry irritating cough and respiratory conditions, urinary tract inflammation, and topically for rashes.

Cautions: Slippery elm is pretty safe and well tolerated by most. The tea can be tricky to strain because it slimes the filter (cut/sifted herb works better).

Similar herbs: Marshmallow root is interchangeable and even more environmentally sustainable. **Plantain**, **violet leaf**, and **oatmeal** also have soothing, slimy, demulcent actions and blend well in formulas.

▸ Licorice

Licorice has the demulcent, mucilaginous, soothing, healing properties of fellow "slimers" like slippery elm and marshmallow — and similarly heals gut inflammation and damage, as well as sore throats, coughs, and respiratory issues; however, it's a complex plant offering a *lot* of extra properties. It has a greater variety of actions for gut inflammation, ulcers, and heartburn. It increases the production of mucous lining, offers extra anti-inflammatory properties, and fends off *H. pylori* infections. It also supports adrenal function and has some steroid-like properties that help with adrenal exhaustion (more often an issue in adults) and can also be used topically for eczema, rashes, and herpes outbreaks. It makes a nice flavoring agent for children's formulas.

Cautions: Best used in formulas and for occasional use, not in high doses as a solo herb, because licorice has some hormonal/estrogenic activity, can irritate the kidneys over time, and may interact with several meds. If you need high doses of licorice long term, consider the safer DGL form available in chewable tablets. See page 77 for more on licorice.

▸ Fennel Seed

Fennel seed may taste licorice-y and benefit gut health, but that's where the similarities to licorice end. It helps digestion in very different ways. Fennel and its relative anise have antispasmodic action that quickly relieves colic, gas, pain, bloating, and nausea, and they both have a delicious sweet flavor. Fennel is the key ingredient in many gripe water formulas, often combined with ginger and sodium bicarbonate. Nibble some seeds, use it in tea, food, liquid extract form, or infuse it into seltzer for "soda." It also provides antispasmodic action for coughs and respiratory complaints.

Cautions: Generally very safe in low-to-modest doses. The bulb and greens have similar but milder effects. See page 81 for more on fennel.

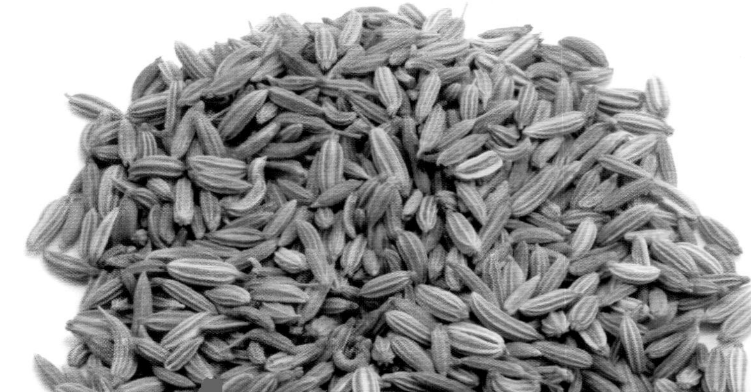

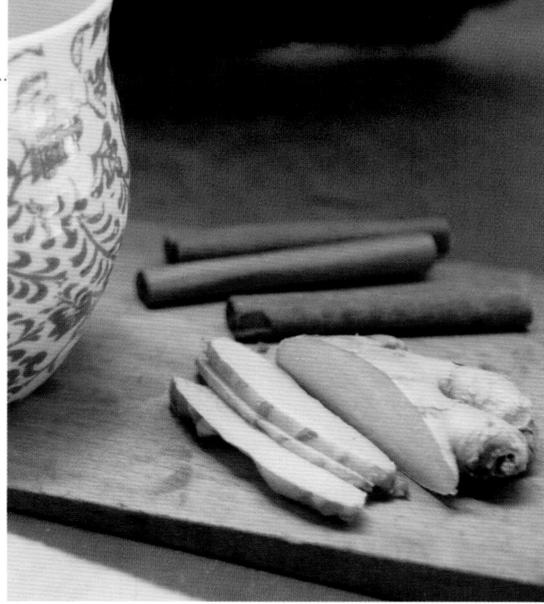

▸ Ginger

Ginger improves digestion, relieves lower gut pain and colic, warms the body, and prevents and treats nausea. Use it as a tea, liquid extract, honey infusion, soda, candy, in food, in the bath. It also is a potent anti-inflammatory for "cold" pain associated with tense muscles (arthritis, old injuries, headaches, and muscle cramps including menstrual cramps). Fresh ginger in tea or food fends off gut pathogens as well as colds and the flu. As a diaphoretic, it helps break a fever by causing you to sweat. Ginger makes an excellent synergist and flavor enhancer in a formula. Fresh ginger offers more antimicrobial benefits, while dried ginger may be better for nausea and pain.

Cautions: It's too spicy for some and thins the blood (contraindicated with blood thinners and bleeding disorders). It can also bring on or lengthen menstruation and isn't recommended in high doses during pregnancy. See page 83 for more on ginger.

▸ Probiotics

Probiotics help encourage good gut flora and level the playing field when pathogens proliferate: immune weakness, yeast infections, dysbiosis, stomach bugs, et cetera. They help normalize bowel function, easing chronic constipation *and* diarrhea issues as well as irritable bowel syndrome (IBS) and inflammatory bowel diseases (IBD). In dysbiosis, you may notice gas and loose stools at first, but this should pass as good bacteria take hold. Probiotics also improve your ability to digest fiber and certain foods, and make and assimilate various nutrients. Look for supplements that contain at least one billion live *Lactobacillus* and/or *Bifidobacterium* species. Fermented foods like yogurt, kefir, and fermented veggies (kraut, kimchi) also provide probiotics. Probiotics help with the overall health of the skin and immune system, too, and they decrease inflammation.

Cautions: Generally quite safe, though quality and dose vary brand from brand, and some need to be kept refrigerated. Homeostatic soil organism (HSO) probiotics including *Saccharomyces* have caused microbe overgrowth in rare cases; stick to *Lactobacillus* and *Bifidobacterium.* Avoid excessive dairy probiotics for chickens; it gives them the runs. In fact, anyone with a dairy allergy or intolerance will be better off with nondairy sources of probiotics.

▸ Cinnamon

Cinnamon has astringent, anti-inflammatory, and antimicrobial properties, which help tighten, tone, and heal gut damage, ease diarrhea, and discourage pathogens. Mix the powder in applesauce, oatmeal, yogurt, smoothies, or other food (it gets slimy), or make tea with the sticks or chips. Cinnamon makes a superb flavoring agent for children's remedies. It also lowers blood sugar and cholesterol and improves heart health.

Cautions: Generally safe, but keep the doses modest, and take it with food (due to hypoglycemic effects). Some concerns have been raised about the coumarin content in most species of cinnamon — including the *Cinnamomum cassia* that is most often sold as "cinnamon" in the United States. Looking at historical use, cinnamon-coumarin concerns appear unfounded, but if you wish to err on the side of caution, seek out "true" or "sweet" cinnamon (*C. verum*, syn. *C. zeylanicum*), also called Ceylon and Sri Lanka cinnamon. It contains fewer coumarins but also loses potency more quickly during storage. See page 148 for more on cinnamon.

Skin

Skin woes are incredibly common among adults, children, and animals, and many of our most effective herbs are appropriate for all. The following herbs specifically address rashes, wounds, stings, bites, and irritations. You'll be amazed by how effective yet safe they are!

▸ Calendula

Calendula flower, usually infused in oil or made into a salve, is the go-to herb for almost any kind of rash. It often works quickly to sooth irritation and promote healing. It's fabulous for infants and children with diaper rash, cradle cap, or eczema or as an ingredient in everyday skin care. (The Weleda company's baby line centers around calendula.) For animals, use it on hot spots, surface wounds, or rashes. It's food-safe, just in case anyone licks it off, but you may want to put it under a bandage so the herb has a chance to stay put and do its work. Though calendula offers mild antiseptic action, other herbs (yarrow, oregano, berberine-rich plants) are more specific for infections and infected wounds. You can make calendula-infused oil via any process; I find that using the dry herb and combining the alcohol intermediary *and* heat methods makes the strongest and longest-lasting oil. (Learn how to make oils on pages 313 to 315.) You can also use calendula in the bath; as a compress, salve, or cream; or infused in alcohol or vinegar.

Cautions: Calendula is generally very safe and well tolerated as a topical herb. Allergies are possible but rare; test it on a small, sensitive patch of skin first. Herbal oils get moldy and rancid over time, so you may need to change your oil every 6 to 12 months. Oils made via the alcohol intermediary method tend to have a better shelf life than other methods. Learn more about calendula on page 41.

Similar herb: St. John's wort oil blends nicely with calendula and works exceptionally well for healing skin wounds, burns, rashes, and nerve pain and damage. Learn more about St. John's wort on page 57.

▸ Plantain

Fresh plantain leaf, mashed up or chewed and applied as a poultice, brings relief within seconds for bee stings, insect and spider bites, and poison ivy. It works better than calendula in these specific instances, and you can also use plantain in all-purpose anti-itch blends. The sooner you apply plantain, the better it works. Dry plantain and plantain- infused oils work in a pinch but aren't quite as effective as the fresh poultice. Plantain draws out venom and irritants, quells the itch, reduces inflammation, and promotes wound healing with light astringent and demulcent actions. If by chance it ends up in someone's mouth, it's fortunately food-safe. Also consider it in a topical tincture or vinegar spritz, salve, bath, or cream.

Cautions: Plantain is generally extremely safe; just make sure you've correctly identified it. See page 220 for more about plantain.

Similar herbs: For poison ivy rashes, my colleague and animal herbalist Mimi Alberu also loves a combination of **witch hazel**, **sweet fern**, **jewelweed**, and **St. John's wort** in a convenient low-alcohol tincture spray. Learn more about healing rashes and other skin issues in chapter 14.

▸ Yarrow

Yarrow leaves have many, many uses. Topically, yarrow is one of the most effective fresh poultices you can apply to stop bleeding, discourage infection, and promote fast healing for wounds with minimal scarring. Dried herb, infused oil/salve/cream, and liquid extracts can be used, but the fresh mashed/chewed leaves work best on wounds. Yarrow also can be applied as a wash, bath, or compress to promote healing, tighten and tone tissue (including varicosities), improve circulation to the area, reduce inflammation, and act as an antiseptic.

Cautions: Generally very safe. See page 222 for more about yarrow, including internal use.

Similar herb: Chaparral has similar benefits for wound healing and is a stellar antimicrobial herb.

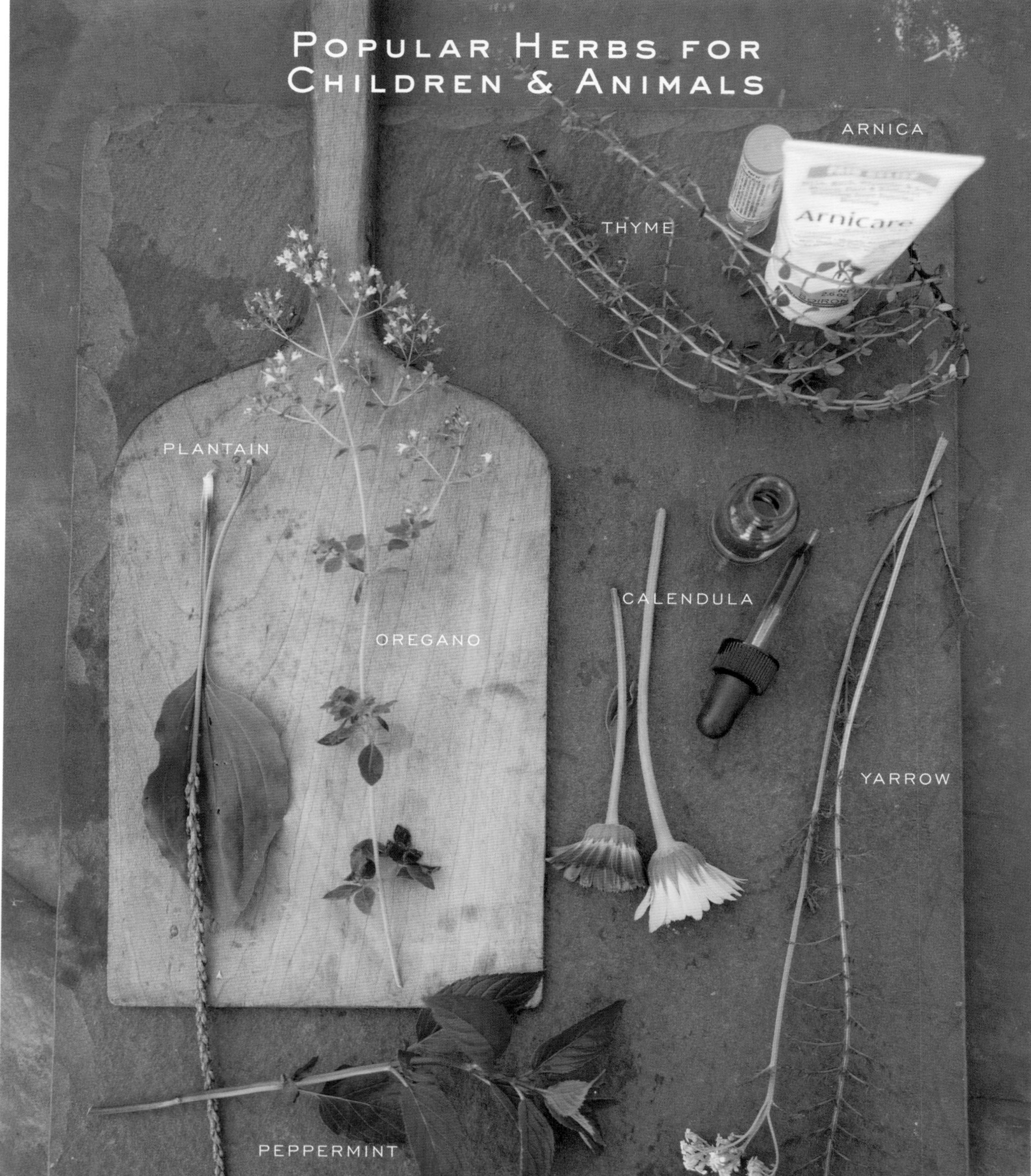
Popular Herbs for Children & Animals
ARNICA
ArniCare
THYME
PLANTAIN
OREGANO
CALENDULA
YARROW
PEPPERMINT

▸ Arnica

Arnica homeopathic topical formulas can be applied as soon as possible to reduce bumps, bruises, and aches from trauma or injury. Arnica also can be used internally in a homeopathic preparation (for example, 30C pills) for the same use.

Cautions: Arnica shouldn't be applied to broken skin (including rashes) and is toxic in standard herb doses, but the homeopathic preparations (which are incredibly dilute) and topical applications are fine for all ages and species.

Similar herbs: To help prevent and heal bruises, consider **gotu kola** internally and externally as well as regular consumption of **blueberries** and **dark purple grape juice. Elder leaf** or **comfrey** topical remedies can be substituted for arnica, but they should not be taken internally due to potential toxicity.

Immune Support, Infections, *and* Infestations

For infants, seek professional supervision when dealing with immune issues. In the first year of life, their immune systems are young, tender, and still forming. Many herbal immune remedies may not be appropriate. However, toddlers, older children, and animals take well to herbal therapies that can strengthen their immune systems and help them overcome illness and issues more quickly.

Remember that it's normal for children to get sick frequently while they're young — studies show that this strengthens their immune systems so that they're healthier as adults. Also remember that most fevers do not need to be artificially reduced with medications; the fever response helps kill pathogens, and dulling it can drag infections on longer than necessary. Support the fever, and work to keep your patient as comfortable and hydrated as possible. When in doubt about a high fever, check with your practitioner.

One good online resource is HealthyChildren.org, the website of the American Academy of Pediatrics. You can find a lot of information about common childhood ailments there and, in particular, good guidelines on when to call the pediatrician regarding your child's fever and other conditions.

▸ Elder

Elderberry and elderflower offer complementary immune remedies for children. Elderberries prevent viruses from entering cells and replicating, which helps avert or shorten a cold or flu if taken at the first sign of infection. They strengthen the overall immune response as well. Elderflowers act as a diaphoretic to help break a fever and also reduce the histamine response to ease both infection and allergy symptoms. Both the berry and the flower are generally well tolerated and taste good, especially when sweetened. Use them together or separately in a syrup, tea (tea works best as a diaphoretic), or tincture.

Cautions: Though totally safe for kids when properly prepared, fresh elderberries and flowers have mild cyanide-related compounds. Use them dried or cooked only, and strain out elderberries rather than eating them whole — the seeds can be quite nauseating for sensitive folks. Don't use the leaves or twigs internally. All parts of the elder plant can be toxic for most pets and livestock and, as such, elder is rarely used for animals. For more on elder, see page 116.

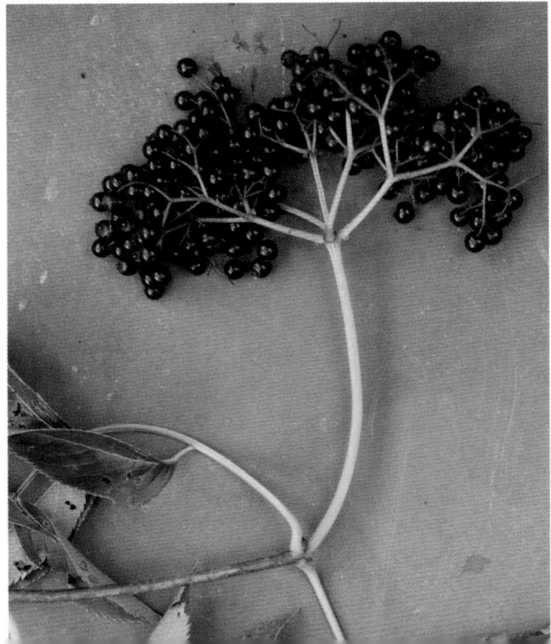

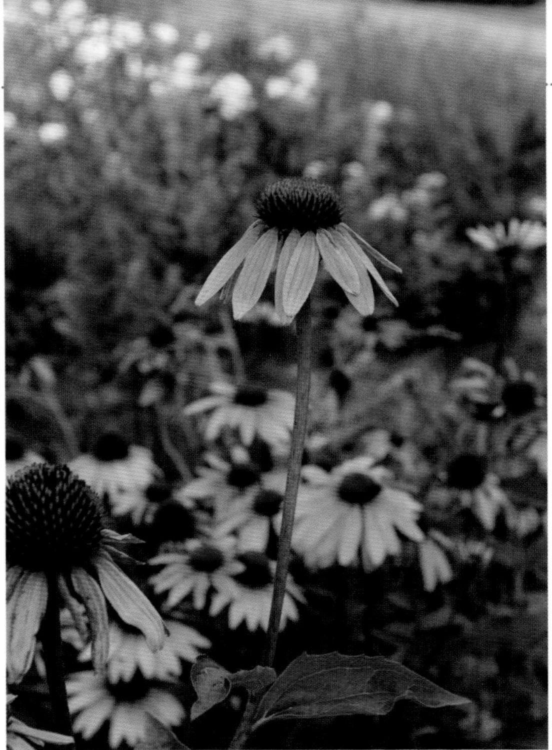

▸ Echinacea

Echinacea stimulates immune function to prevent and treat the cold and flu when taken in high, regular doses at the first signs of infection. It helps the body fight both bacterial and viral infections. As a spray, it numbs and heals sore throats and topical wounds on contact (note that a vinegar or alcohol base might sting). Taking it internally and applying it topically may limit the spread and irritation of non-life-threatening bites of various sorts; it numbs, cleans, and has antivenin properties. The fresh root tincture is strongest, though all parts of the plant provide benefit. Consider it for children as well as animals. It does *not* taste great and has a numbing, saliva-increasing effect on the tongue. Blending it with ginger and lemonade improves the taste, and ginger improves the action. For animals, add the tincture to food or drinking water. Echinacea also acts as an alterative to aid detoxification, move the lymph, and "clean" the blood and interstitial fluid.

Cautions: Echinacea sometimes aggravates autoimmune conditions and should be approached with caution. Allergy is rare but possible for this daisy-family flower. For more on echinacea, see page 118.

▸ Mullein

Mullein leaves help with respiratory and lung issues (including asthma, bronchitis, and coughs) by opening the airways and soothing irritation. The soft, fuzzy leaves can be used fresh or dry as a tea or liquid extract and blend well with other respiratory herbs. Infuse the flowers in oil that can be dripped in the ear for earache pain, used solo or in combination with garlic, calendula, and St. John's wort oils. Mullein also can be used topically for other issues. Make a poultice with the leaf to draw out splinters and boils and ease aches, including backache and foot aches. Mullein root works well internally and externally for tendon/ligament issues, sprains, and pain.

Cautions: Generally safe, but the little hairs on the leaf can irritate the throat and should be well strained from teas and liquid extracts through a coffee filter or tightly woven cloth. Some people are also sensitive to the hairs topically; test by rubbing the leaf on a small sensitive patch of skin before using it as a poultice. For more on mullein, see page 125.

▸ Oregano and Thyme

Oregano and thyme are common culinary/garden herbs with a range of benefits for children and animals. They have potent antimicrobial and antiseptic properties that aid respiratory, oral, topical, and gastrointestinal infections of various sorts — bacterial, viral, fungal/yeast, even worms. They aid respiratory issues, including nonacute asthma and chest congestion; open the lungs; and ease coughs and sneezes. Oregano targets the gut and thyme the lungs, but both are relatively interchangeable. They make excellent liquid extracts, including palatable cough syrups, tea, broth, et cetera. You can add the dried herb to animal bedding, add the tea to a child's bath, make a steam or compress, and so on. Oregano and thyme also improve and support digestion, much like peppermint, by increasing digestive juices and easing gas, bloating, and pain. For animals, add these herbs and peppermint to bedding to ward off insects, lice, mites, and rodents, though they may not be sufficient in a full-on infestation.

Cautions: Generally safe in low to modest doses, but don't use high doses and avoid the unnecessarily potent and potentially toxic essential oil. Therapeutic doses are contraindicated for pregnant animals due to an emmenagogue effect.

Similar herbs: Similarly scented **mint-family herbs**, including bee balm and savory, are relatively interchangeable with oregano and thyme. **Elecampane** shares the respiratory, digestive, antimicrobial, and deworming properties but should be kept to low to modest doses due to high-dose toxicity. **Catnip** and **lemon balm** also have some similar yet gentler actions.

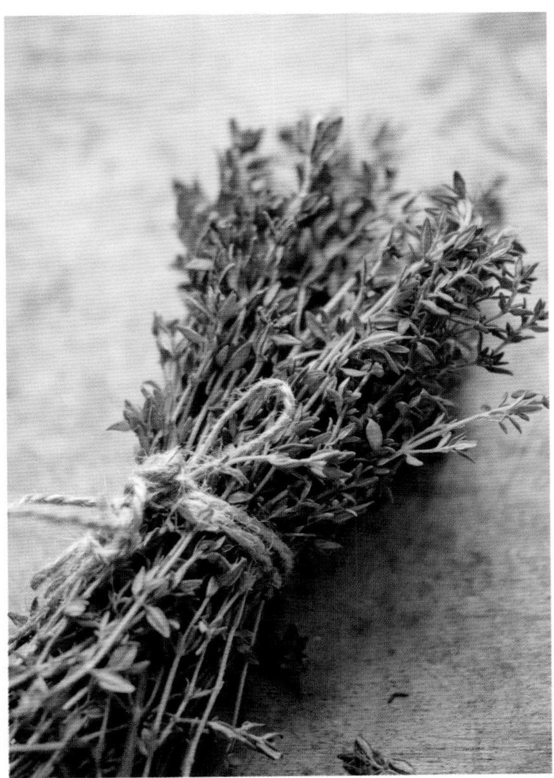

▸ Garlic

Garlic provides well-known potent antimicrobial properties. Historically used to ward off evils, raw garlic improves the immune system's ability to fight viral and bacterial invaders, cancer, and yeast/fungus. Regular use reportedly makes you less appealing to biting insects, including mosquitoes, ticks, and fleas. Garlic infused in honey or milk is an old-time remedy for chest congestion and cough for children, as is garlic mashed with vinegar and honey for almost any ailment in livestock. Tincture or infused vinegar made with raw garlic works in a pinch, and powdered garlic granules in food offer weaker benefits. Use the infused oil topically for earaches, and apply crushed garlic to warts. Garlic also supports heart health and digestive function in humans but not for all animals.

Cautions: Though generally safe for humans, garlic oil may irritate the skin and mucous membranes of sensitive folks, so test a little bit before using ear oil or applying it raw to the skin. Garlic's use in animals is controversial because many animals can't digest disulfide compounds in the allium family, which can lead to gastrointestinal upset, anemia, and poisoning. The risk-benefit ratio varies by dose and animal breed. Low doses may be fine for most dog breeds and horses, but high doses are not recommended. Chickens generally tolerate garlic granules and occasional raw garlic (but not onions). Cats and Japanese dog breeds should not be given *any* amount of garlic. If you're unsure, consult a holistic vet. For more on garlic, see page 263.

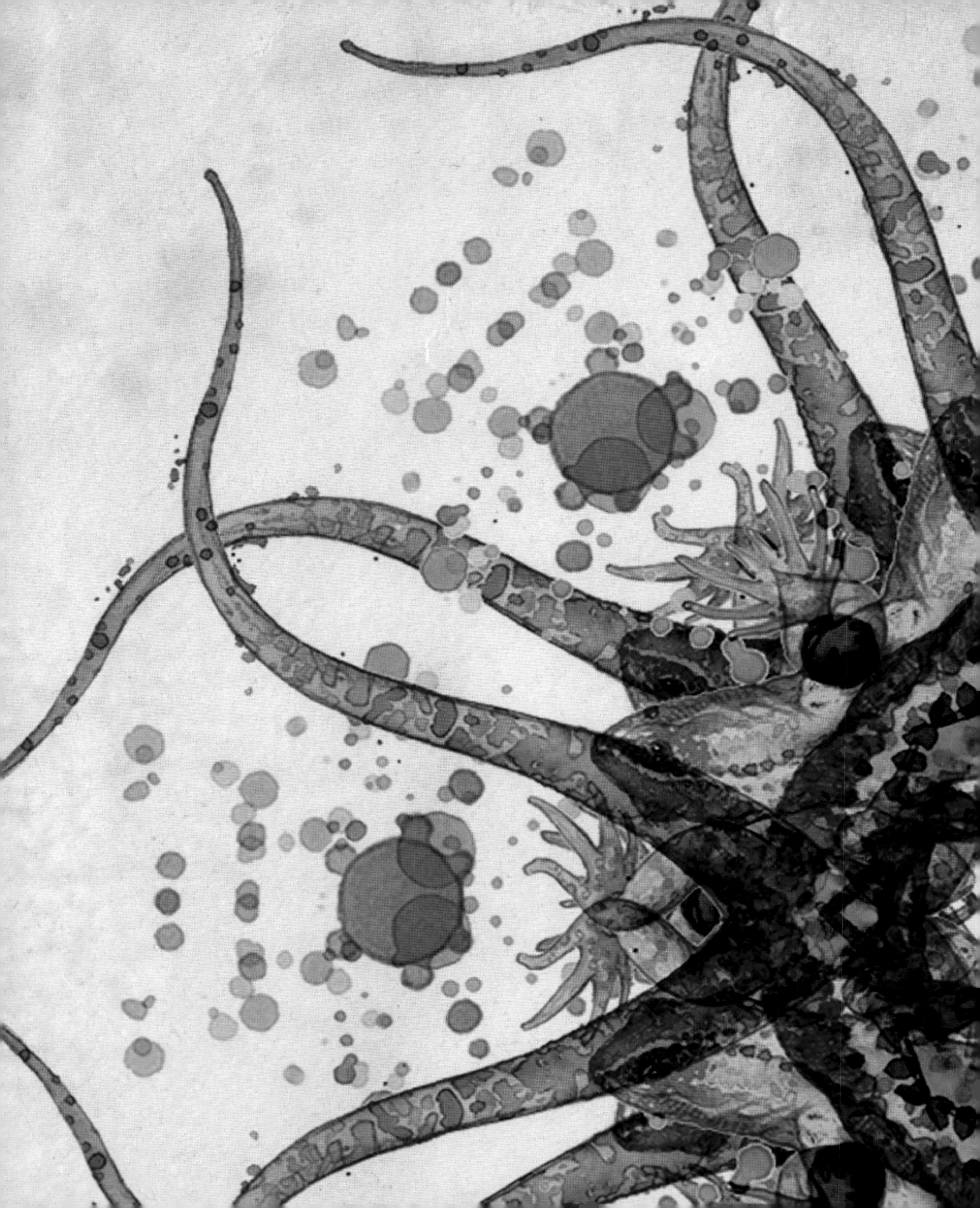

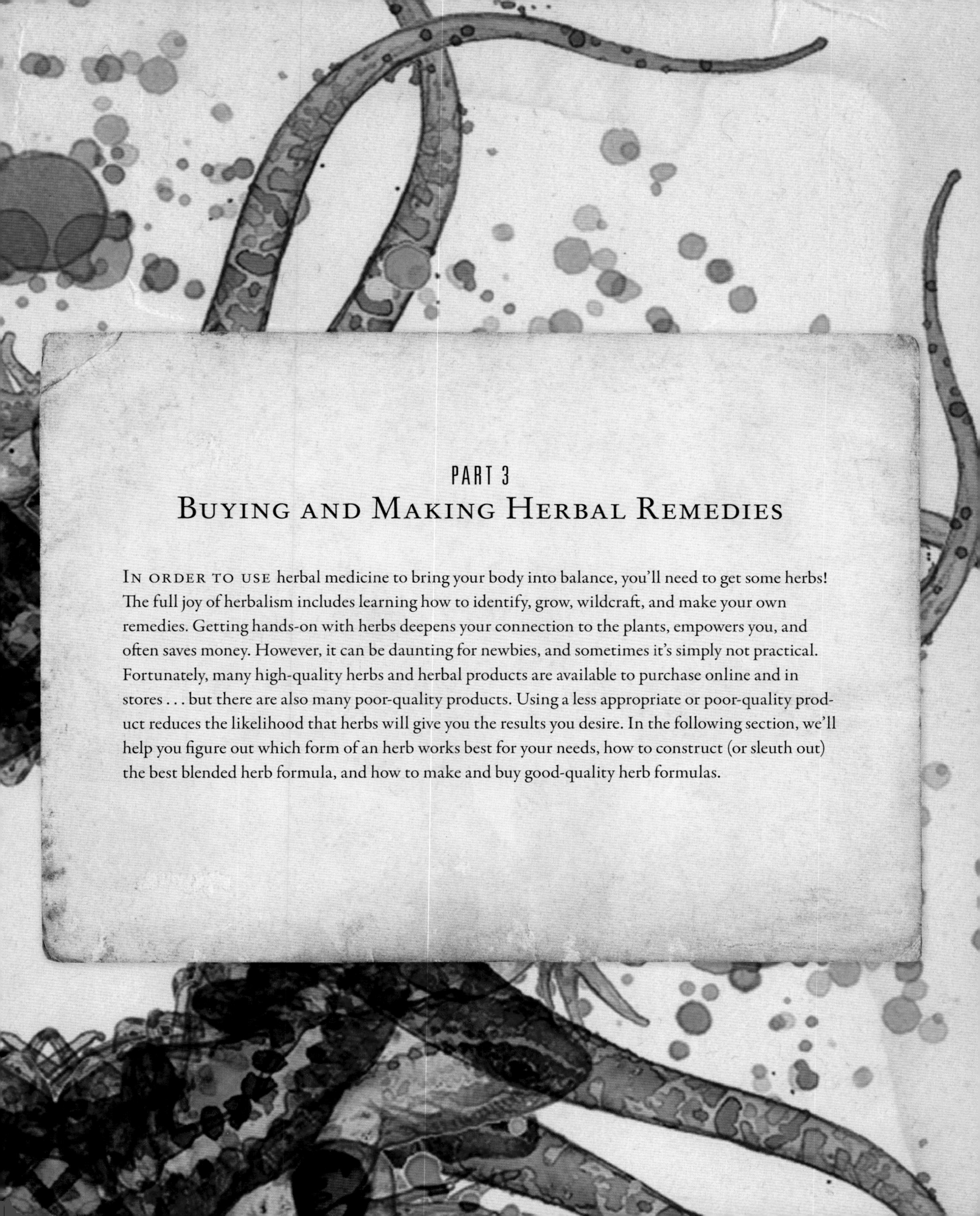

PART 3
Buying and Making Herbal Remedies

In order to use herbal medicine to bring your body into balance, you'll need to get some herbs! The full joy of herbalism includes learning how to identify, grow, wildcraft, and make your own remedies. Getting hands-on with herbs deepens your connection to the plants, empowers you, and often saves money. However, it can be daunting for newbies, and sometimes it's simply not practical. Fortunately, many high-quality herbs and herbal products are available to purchase online and in stores . . . but there are also many poor-quality products. Using a less appropriate or poor-quality product reduces the likelihood that herbs will give you the results you desire. In the following section, we'll help you figure out which form of an herb works best for your needs, how to construct (or sleuth out) the best blended herb formula, and how to make and buy good-quality herb formulas.

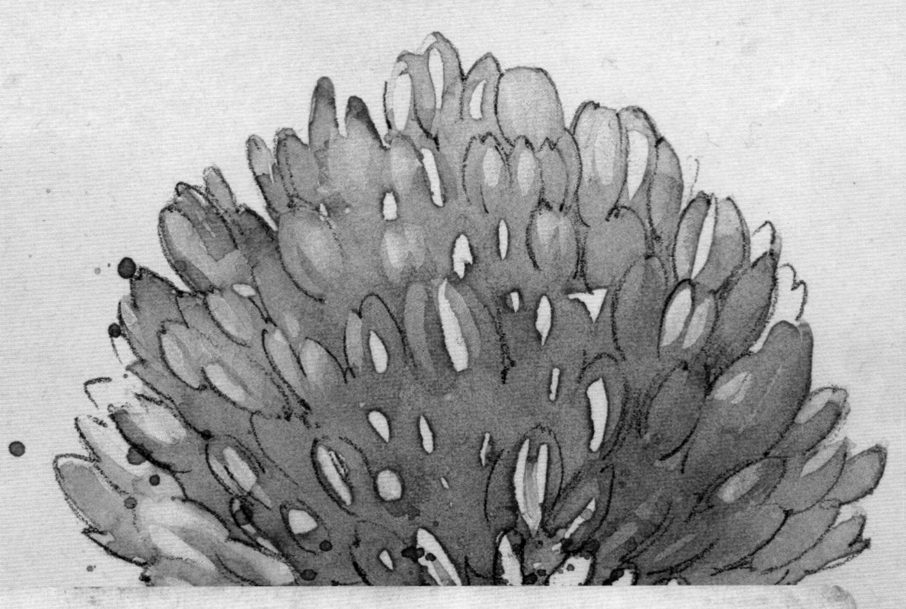

Chapter 18

Harvesting, Buying, Storing, and Using Herbs

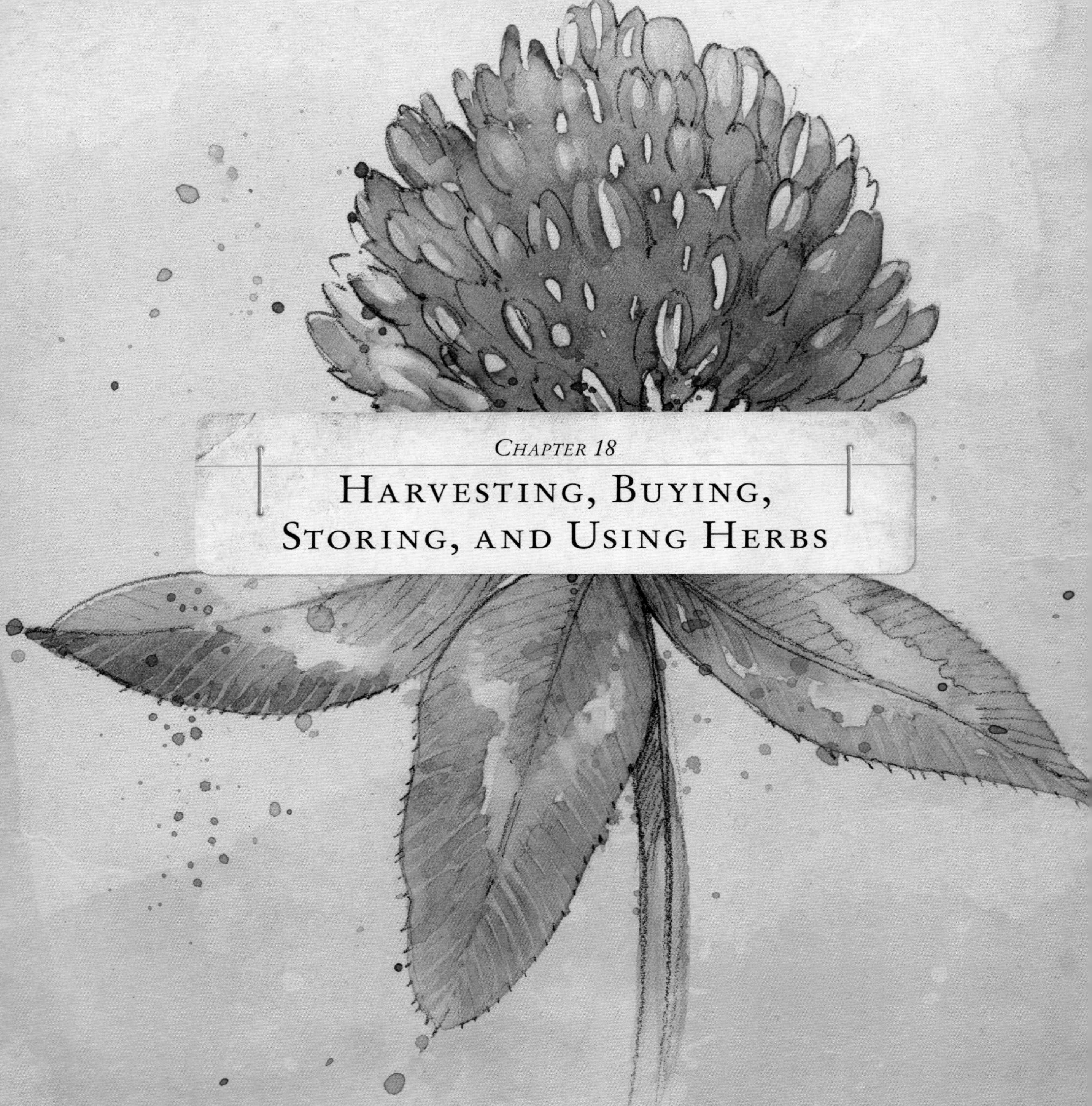

Crafting herbal medicine by hand offers one of the greatest joys of plant medicine; however, sometimes it's simply more convenient to buy them. Truth be told, most herbal newbies start out with store-bought herbs and remedies. Maybe you don't have herbs growing at easy access or you're still learning how to properly identify them. Maybe you're just short on time or feel daunted by the process. Fortunately, many truly wonderful herbs and remedies are available for purchase in stores, at farms and farmers' markets, and online.

Whether you grow your own, wildcraft, or buy herbs, you'll want to store them properly to best maintain their active principles, and you'll need to know how to dose them properly for best effect. We'll cover all these details in this chapter.

Harvesting Herbs

Always seek out happy, healthy plants to harvest.

- **Leaves and aerial parts:** Harvest the top one-quarter to three-fourths of the plant when the plant looks vibrant and happy, usually in spring or summer. Be sure to leave at least a few sets of leaves so it can continue to grow. Also consider leaving some flowers to set seed for future plants and help support pollinators.
- **Flowers:** Pinch off the top flower head. For most flowers, you can include the green bract (e.g., calendula, chamomile) and any leaves that are adjacent to the head (e.g., St. John's wort, red clover). Harvest as it begins to bloom and still looks vibrant, usually in summer.
- **Roots:** Gently dig up the plant with a fork, shovel, or digging stick. Rinse your harvested roots clean with cold water, use a potato scrubber if needed. Harvest roots in spring before the plant sends up flowers or in fall once it has died back. If possible (depending on the plant), leave some root matter behind to support future growth.
- **Bark:** Prune off branches up to 1 inch in diameter. Use a knife or peeler to strip the bark away from the woody pith (the inner tissue of a stem or branch) collecting both the outer bark as well as the inner bark (often green, juicy, fragrant — where the most medicine is at). You can simply chop up twigs. On larger (i.e., fallen) trees, you will need to remove the outer bark with a special saw, but this is not necessary for younger, smaller branches. Harvest bark in fall (for some plants spring is also okay), preferably when there are no leaves on the trees or they are in the process of falling off.
- **Berries:** Harvest berries at their peak color and flavor, often in summer or fall. If you're drying them, be sure to use a higher drying temp to avoid spoiling.

WILDCRAFTING TIPS

IF YOU'RE HARVESTING HERBS from the wild — as opposed to using plants cultivated for the sole purpose of being harvested — only pick from large stands and be sure not to take any more than 10 percent of the population. Make sure you have permission from the landowner. Be aware of local laws that may prohibit picking any plants or specific plants, such as those that are endangered or invasive. Go back regularly to both observe the impacts of your harvesting and also to be a good steward of the land. Harvest in a way that ensures your presence is barely perceptible and that the plants and ecosystem thrive. Visit www.unitedplantsavers.org to learn how you can help preserve medicinal plants at risk of being overharvested.

Drying Processes

Use dried herbs for tea, seasoning, and making remedies. Most dried herbs will keep for 1 to 2 years stored in an airtight glass container in a cool, dark, dry spot. (If you use plastic bags, store them all in a big, sealed plastic tub.) Delicate herbs like calendula, skullcap, and lemon balm begin to lose potency within 3 to 6 months. Roots and mineral-rich herbs may last longer than 2 years. In spite of its popularity, the method of hanging herbs to dry is generally not the best.

- **My favorite method (the car dehydrator):** Loosely place recently harvested herbs — stems and all — in a brown paper bag. (It's not necessary to wash, but do discard any dirty or damaged leaves and bugs first.) Fold shut and let sit in the windshield of your car, in the sun, until fully dry, approximately 1 to 3 days.
- **Dehydrator method:** Place herbs loosely in the dehydrator set to 95° (in a dry climate) to 115°F (in a humid climate) for leaves and flowers. Herbs at risk of molding or fermenting, including wintergreen leaves and red clover blossoms, do best in the dehydrator. Fruits generally require higher temps, 125° to 135°F.

Flowers should be dried in a single layer; be sure the middles are totally dry before storing. I prefer to use a dehydrator for them.

Check daily for dryness. An herb's leaves will crumble easily between your fingertips when ready. Immediately remove the leaves from the stems or "garble" the herb with your hands until the mixture is cut/sifted (broken up into small pieces). Compost the stems, and store the dried herb in a sealed glass container in a cool, dark, dry place.

Freezing Process

Some herbs lose their flavor or potency once dried, and for them, freezing is an excellent storage option. Frozen herbs keep well for 2 months to 1 year, depending on the plant and air exposure.

- **Whole herbs:** Some herbs can simply be placed in a freezer bag and tucked into the freezer with good results: lemongrass stalks, chives. Try to remove as much air as you can. Herbs that bruise and blacken easily (basil, lemon balm, tarragon) will do better if you vacuum-seal them in individual serving-size bags. Consider a Seal-a-Meal or FoodSaver machine (best) or the ThriftyVac (affordable). If you want to avoid plastic, get accessories to allow you to vacuum-seal herbs in glass mason jars.
- **Herb ice cubes:** For individual use, you can add chopped herbs to ice cube trays and then cover with water or oil. Baby food storage trays work well.
- **Frozen herbal paste:** Some herbs, like parsley, cilantro, and chives, lose too much flavor once dried. In these cases, you can purée the herbs fresh with olive oil. Sweeter herbs like mint and lemon balm can be puréed with canola oil for future baking ventures. Put the mix in ziplock bags, flatten and remove the air, then freeze. To use, break off chunks as needed.

Buying Herbs *and* Remedies

When it comes to purchased herbal products, not all are created equal. Well-made products will be more potent, effective, and sustainable, and less apt to be adulterated.

Buying Fresh-Cut Herbs and Potted Plants

Fresh plants often taste and work best, especially if you plan to make remedies with them. Look to well-stocked produce departments, local farms, and online herb farms.

- Choose local, organic (or chemical-free) suppliers who have intimate knowledge of plant medicine and can help you pick out the right plant for your needs.

- Purchase plants that look happy, not wilted, mushy, or moldy.
- Double-check the identity of plants with reliable field guides. Mistakes often happen, especially if two plants have the same common name or there has been a species or variety mix-up.
- If you plan to plant the herb in your garden, ask or research what growing conditions it prefers and if the seedling needs to be "hardened off" before being planted outdoors.
- Use fresh-cut herbs as quickly as possible. If you must wait a few days, ask the supplier or research how best to keep it fresh in the meantime.

Buying Dry "Bulk" Herbs

Use bulk herbs for tea and spice blends and to make your own remedies. They're invaluable, inexpensive, and often more potent than prepackaged tea, but quality varies widely on the market. Look to local herb growers, herb shops, natural food stores, and quality online suppliers.

- Choose organic (or ethically wildcrafted) brands that specialize in medicinal plants.
- Use your senses to gauge quality: even when dried, herbs should have bold colors, flavors, and scents; they should not be brown, "dusty," and bland. Herbs are best stored out of direct light. Good "marker" herbs for quality include calendula (bright yellow or orange), red clover (purple blossoms), nettle (verdant green), spearmint (strong Doublemint gum scent), cayenne (bold red-orange), and hawthorn whole berries (more burgundy than brown, minimal white cast). It's easy to observe quality before purchasing in a store. For online purchasing, try placing a small order first or asking for a "tester" sample to see if the supplier passes muster.
- Though powders are handy, they lose quality quickly and are easy to adulterate. Choose the most whole form that is still convenient for your use.
- If you can, find out where the plants were grown and when they were harvested. Herbs grown in China (or bought/sold through China) are often adulterated and may not adhere to quality standards even if labeled as organic. Ask if/how the supplier tests for identity, quality, and contaminants.

FRESH VS. DRIED?

THE MAJORITY OF HERBS can be used fresh or dry. In most cases, fresh plants make better medicine (especially for tinctures) if you have the choice. Most of us use dried herb only when the method requires it (tea, powder, capsules) or when the fresh plant isn't available.

Best Fresh

- Echinacea, milky oat seed, valerian, pulsatilla, and lemon balm: these herbs lose significant potency once dried.

Always Use Dried

- Elderberries, elderflowers, and cherry bark: to eliminate cyanide-related compounds, nausea, and possible toxicity; elder can also be cooked.
- Alder bark and twigs: to eliminate the nausea-inducing emetic effects.
- Ginseng, codonopsis, ashwagandha: the dried form is traditional for maximizing potency.

Buying Prepared Remedies

The average consumer walking down an aisle stocked with herbal pills has no way of knowing all the production details that take place behind the scene. Short of doing a lot of research and calling individual companies with a list of questions, the simplest approach will be to purchase from companies that are truly dedicated to quality and have an excellent reputation in the herbal/supplement community.

- For big brands, look for "GMP" on the label or ask if and how the company abides by Good Manufacturing Practice regulations. Legally, *any* company that makes and sells herbal dietary supplements (including tinctures and capsules, though not always teas and food-like remedies) must comply with stringent GMP regulations set by the FDA. These regulations include identity testing, quality testing, contaminant testing, and cleanliness. That said, the regulations are relatively new, and companies still slide under the radar.

- Purchase from companies that specialize in herbal products and are run by herbalists. These will generally be of higher quality than mass-market herbal products. Some of my personal favorites include Herb Pharm, Gaia Herbs, Oregon's Wild Harvest, and MegaFood. Nature's Way is a good-quality multinational company with phytopharmaceutical connections in Germany.

- Seek certified organic herbs and ingredients when possible. They're usually better quality and have a solid paper trail to reduce the likelihood of identity, adulteration, and unethical wildcrafting issues.

- Read the ingredients list (including any fine-print "inactive ingredients") to see what herbs or other ingredients are included. Beware of synthetic ingredients, artificial colors, artificial flavors, and preservatives.

Buying Local: Special Considerations

Herbalism *thrives* in small-scale, grassroots circles, and many of the best herbal remedies are produced by hand in small batches. Unfortunately, small-scale, local product makers often struggle to comply with the FDA's regulations (which are geared toward large manufacturers but don't offer exemptions based on company size or sales). Even though the FDA believes *everyone* should be GMP-compliant, personally I recommend supporting small-scale suppliers regardless. Here are some questions to ask to ensure good-quality products:

- Where are the herbs grown, and how quickly are they processed after being harvested? Does the product maker grow them him/herself or buy them elsewhere? If purchased, from where?

- How does the herbalist ensure plant identity? Avoid adulteration? Are *all* ingredients listed on the product label? They should be!

- Where are the finished remedies made? If they're made in a home kitchen, how does the herbalist ensure cleanliness? Can you visit the production space? (For personal privacy, they may not allow you to see the space, but it's nice if they do.)

- How long do they store their products? Is there a batch or lot number on the product that allows the producer to know when each product was made?

- How do they ensure prepared remedies are shelf stable? How long are the products expected to last after you buy them? This is of particular concern for low-alcohol extracts, body cream, herbal honey/syrup, oils, and so on. Some herbalists think their products have longer shelf lives than they really do.

Storing Your Herbs *and* Remedies

All herbs do best in a cool, dark, dry spot. Heat, light, oxygen, and moisture spoil or reduce the potency of almost any remedy. Shelf-stable remedies and dried herbs do best in a pantry or cabinet. If you store them out in the open for an extended period of time, use dark glass or opaque containers.

- **Long-term shelf-stable:** Dry herbs, tinctures, vinegars, thick infused honeys, salves, cordials, capsules
- **Short-term shelf-stable (a few months to 1 year):** Creams and topical oils; hydrosols, oxymels, glycerites, and syrups preserved with alcohol may last for a few months on the shelf but keep longer and maintain freshness better in the fridge
- **Best refrigerated:** Hydrosols, oxymels, glycerites, syrups, watery infused honey, culinary oils (1 week), herbal soda (1 day)
- **Consider freezing:** Fresh herbs (preferably vacuum-sealed), pastes, and any extra batches of cream, oil, salves, or syrups for later use

Using Herbs: General Doses *and* Tips

The exact dose that you need of an herb will vary depending on the person, the herb, the preparation, and even the practitioner. Sometimes just a few drops of a well-chosen herb will elicit a favorable response, and many herbalists prefer these almost-homeopathic doses. On the other side of the spectrum, traditional Chinese medicine herbalists often prefer to hit things heavy with large doses of herbs. Don't let this get overwhelming; herbs work well in a wide range of doses.

Following are very basic guidelines to using herbs as medicine. When in doubt, please don't hesitate to seek professional guidance.

- Most herbs do best taken with food, especially if you have a sensitive stomach. This is particularly true for bitter, strong-tasting, astringent, and hypoglycemic herbs.
- Take a tiny dose the first time, just a few drops of tincture or sips of tea, to see if the remedy agrees with you, especially if you tend to be sensitive and reactive to foods and medicines. Gradually work up to the recommended dose. Pay attention to how you *feel* when you take the remedy. At first you might just get a vague sense that it resonates with you — or doesn't. As time goes on, are you getting the desired effects? Any other changes?
- If you notice a negative side effect, stop taking the remedy. Do your research: is this reaction common or known? Depending on the reaction, consider trying the remedy again once or twice more to confirm whether it was caused by the remedy. If you do have a negative side effect from the herb, stop taking it or seek professional guidance. Take note and be cautious with herbs that have similar actions or are related.
- If you're not seeing results from the recommended dose within a reasonable amount of time (this varies by herb and condition, but some improvements will generally be seen within 1 to 2 weeks), consider increasing the dose. If you're not seeing results within a month or two, consider different herbs or therapies.
- If your condition is serious or worsens, get professional guidance.
- If you notice that you're not sleeping well while taking a remedy, consider taking it earlier in the day or find a less stimulating formula.
- Depending on your level of sensitivity, you may not want to drink large cups of tea or take diuretic herbs before bedtime to avoid having to get up in the night to pee.

STANDARD HERB DOSES

The following dose recommendations work well for most people and most herbs. Please note that the measurement equivalents are approximate. If you purchase a product with a recommended dose, start with that. Otherwise, start with a low dose and work your way up as needed.

Remedy	Standard Dose
Tea	Dried herb: 1 teaspoon–1 tablespoon dried herb per 8 ounces water, 1–3 times per day Fresh herb: 1 large handful fresh herb per 8 ounces water, 1–3 times per day Medicinal/super infusion: 1 ounce dried herb per 32 ounces water, sipped throughout the day (or over 2 days)
Tincture	1–2 squirts, 1–3 times per day or as needed, preferably diluted in some water or other drink; up to a 4-squirt dose is often fine if needed (1 squirt = 1 mL = 30 drops = 1/5 teaspoon)
Vinegar	Tincture doses or up to 1 teaspoon, 1–3 times per day, straight or diluted in some water or other drink
Syrup, elixir, oxymel, or honey	½ teaspoon–1 tablespoon, 1–3 times per day
Cordial	1 ounce daily, usually as a treat!
Capsule	Crude or ground herb: 1–4 capsules, 1–2 times per day, usually before/with food and a full glass of water (1 capsule = 500 mg) Standardized, soft gels, or liquid capsules: Follow the dosage instructions on the product label
Powder	1/8–1 teaspoon daily, all at once or divided throughout the day, usually mixed in some water or other drink, honey, milk, ghee (for fat-soluble constituents), smoothies, or other food (1 teaspoon = 10 capsules)
Flower essence	1–5 drops, 1–3 times daily or as needed, on the tongue, in water, as an air mist, or rubbed into the skin

Choosing *the* Best Remedy *for* You

As you come to research and better understand herbs, your ability to make or buy the best formula for your particular needs will improve dramatically. This means that the herbs you take will be more apt to work, and you'll feel more engaged and empowered in the healing process.

While single herbs can be very therapeutic, many herbalists prefer to make (or purchase) blends. Sometimes herbal newbies approach the creation of blends with trepidation, afraid they'll screw up or combine herbs that don't belong together. The truth is that you have a *lot* of leeway for herbal combinations, and herbs are more apt to improve the efficacy of one another rather than produce negative results.

Herbal Simples

"Simples" are herbal remedies that rely on just one herb. If you're just getting started with plant medicine, using the herbs individually will help you get to know and understand the taste and action. This may mean that you just make one small cup of tea or a few drops of tincture and then try the standard dose. Or you may decide to really explore one herb for an extended period of time, taking it daily in a variety of forms and noting how your body responds.

Many herbs work very well as simples, and you may do just fine with turmeric capsules for your pain, valerian tincture to sleep, or chamomile tea for nervous indigestion. If you have a lot of sensitivities or allergies, you might take comfort in working with simple herbs that you know agree with you. Many wise women and community herbalists rely heavily on just a few tried-and-true herbal simples with fabulous results. A well-matched simple can often work wonders, particularly if it is chosen with its homepathic or flower essence indications in mind.

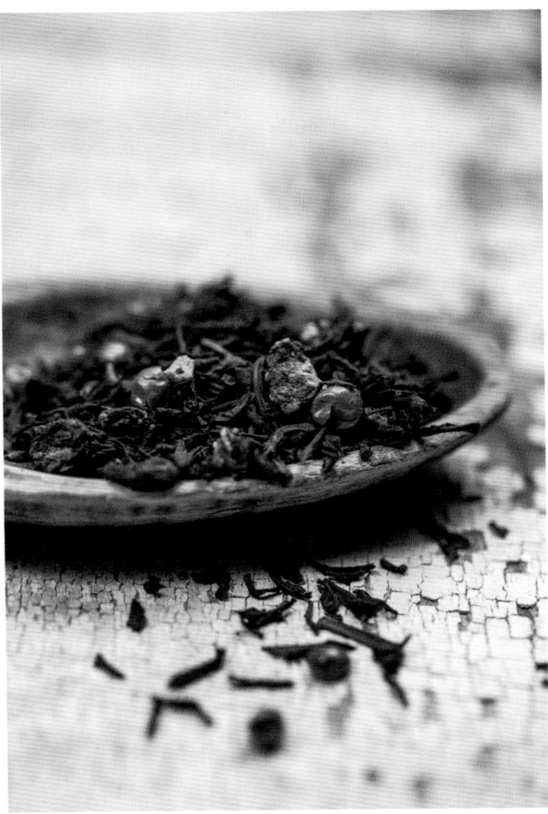

Multi-herb Formulas

In spite of the efficiency and ease of herbal simples, formulas sometimes open more doors. Traditional Chinese medicine and Ayurveda almost exclusively rely on complex formulas. Why? Because you can address more facets of healing, support various issues in one blend, buffer strong herbs to avoid side effects, improve the flavor, and synergize the whole blend so that it works better.

Formulation techniques range from very simple to exceedingly complex; however, I love the easy-to-understand concepts put forth by herbalist Rosemary Gladstar. She breaks formulas down into three parts: primary herbs, supportive herbs, and synergists. (I also like to add some "good vibrations" when inspired.) Your first formulas might consist of just two or three herbs, but the possibilities are endless. You can use these basic concepts for making tasty teas, medicinal blends, tinctures — really anything!

CHOOSING THE BEST REMEDY FOR THE JOB

You have a range of options at your disposal. The three most common forms of herbs are tea (water extract), tincture (alcohol extract), and capsule (usually powdered herb), but you can also use powders mixed in food (milk, smoothies, nut butter, honey) or make syrups, honeys, cordials, vinegar . . . Each method has pros and cons. Some herbs extract better in certain solvents. Some remedies are more easily absorbed or have longer shelf lives. Consider the following options, keeping in mind the individual herbs you hope to work with as well as your personal preferences.

Extract Method	Pros	Cons
Tea (water extract)	Inexpensive, gentle, hydrating, easily absorbed. The tea ritual — making and drinking it — alone is therapy.	Generally limited to dry plants (and some herbs lose potency once dry). Less palatable for certain herbs. Inconvenient for some. Difficult to mix herbs with different steeping times/styles (e.g., roots vs. leaves). Not a good solvent for resins.
Tincture (alcohol extract)	Extracts most herbs (fresh or dry) well and is easily absorbed. Easy to take, portable, shelf stable for many years.	Not everyone tolerates alcohol. Can take 1 month to make (unless using percolation method). Doesn't extract minerals, mucilage, or polysaccharides (like those in mushrooms) well (unless using low-alcohol decoction tincture method). High-proof alcohol is best for resins and fat-soluble constituents.
Vinegar (usually apple cider vinegar) or oxymel (vinegar and honey)	Similar to tincture but alcohol-free. Different solvency, particularly good for minerals and alkaloids. Vinegar itself benefits digestion and other issues. Plain vinegars have a decent shelf life (1 or 2 years).	Not as long-lasting or as good a solvent as alcohol for most herbs. Some may not like the taste. Vinegar corrodes metal lids and, eventually, dropper tops. Oxymels have a short life span and may aggravate sugar issues. Vinegar may aggravate heartburn and some digestive issues.
Syrups (sugar or honey, sometimes also water and alcohol), cordials and elixirs (alcohol and sweetener), honey, and glycerites (glycerin)	Very tasty and palatable. Can be made with fresh or dried herbs. Relatively gentle. Can be made alcohol-free (except cordials). Honey and syrups soothe sore throat and cough.	May not be potent enough. May aggravate sugar and alcohol issues. Shorter shelf life compared to vinegar and tinctures. Without alcohol, they grow microbes easily and should generally be kept refrigerated.
Powders (loose or in capsules)	Convenient to take. Homemade powders and capsules are affordable. Capsules have minimal flavor. Powders can be mixed in honey, nut butter, food, and drinks and offer better absorption than capsules. Some store-bought herb pills are filled with concentrated liquid extracts or carbon dioxide extracts, and these tend to be much more potent (but you can't make them at home due to the specialized equipment needed).	Homemade capsules are time consuming to make. You rely on your digestive strength to absorb them, which is a particular issue for capsules. Powdered herbs degrade quickly, are often of poor quality, and are easy to adulterate. Limited to dry herbs (except store-bought liquid caps and soft gels). Standardized extracts do not use the whole herb as nature intended and may involve unlabeled solvents. Vegetarians will want to seek out veggie capsules.

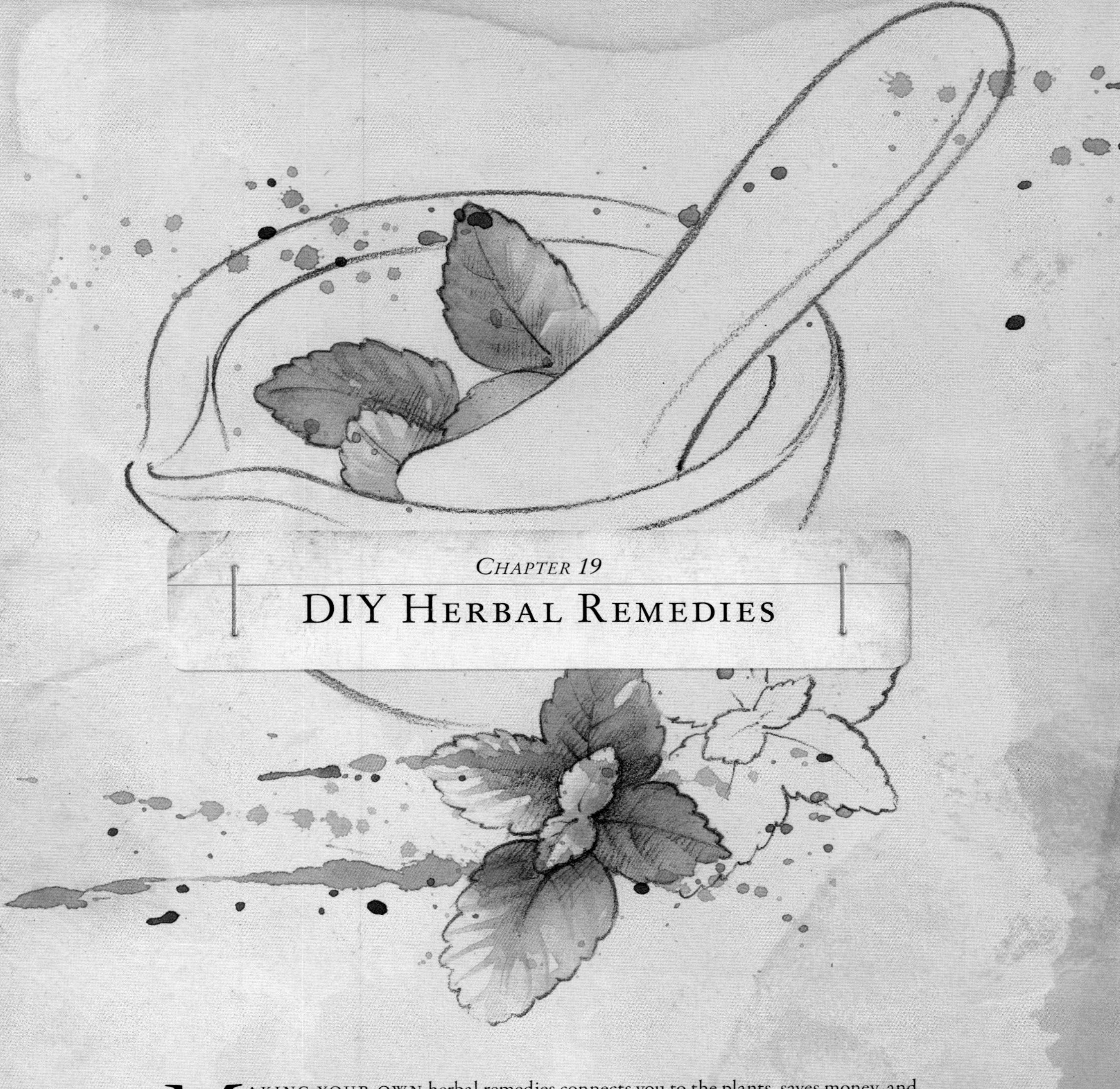

Chapter 19

DIY Herbal Remedies

Making your own herbal remedies connects you to the plants, saves money, and gives you access to the freshest, best-quality medicine! As my teacher Michael Moore would say, "This isn't lab science, it's herbology." In other words, you can make the same basic remedy via a variety of methods, and they usually all come out well. (It's more like cooking — how many recipes for chicken soup are there?) I once interviewed six herbalists and asked them how to dry herbs; each one said a different technique worked *best*. So, use these recipes (*my* personal favorites) as a guide, not a rule. Even if you "make a mistake," it will usually still work.

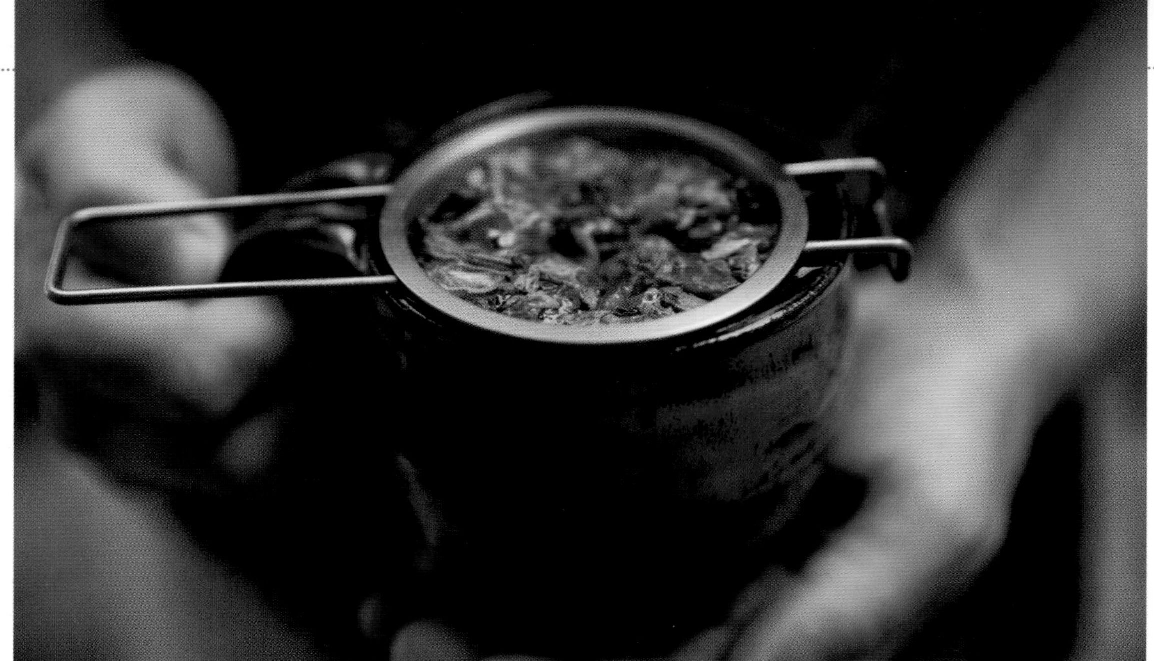

Herbal Teas: Infusion (Steep)

This method is best for delicate parts of a plant, like leaves and flowers. When you make tea from a teabag, you're making an infusion. Larger amounts of herb and longer steeping times make stronger-tasting teas; less herb and time make a lighter tea.

1. Add 1 teaspoon to 1 tablespoon of dried herb per cup of water to a mug (with or without a strainer, as you prefer) or French press.
2. Pour boiling or near-boiling water over the herbs.
3. Cover the mug and let steep for 5 to 20 minutes. Putting a lid on helps retain more of the herbs' volatile oils.
4. Strain and drink.

Variation: Super Infusion. Add 1 ounce of herb (by weight) to a 32-ounce jar or French press. Fill the container to the top with boiling water. Put on the lid and let steep for at least 4 hours and up to overnight. Use the press or wring out the herbs in a cloth to get as much tea as possible.

Variation: Fresh Herb Infusion. Fresh herbs are not generally as medicinally potent in tea as dried. However, fresh aromatic herbs and sliced fresh fruit often taste much better than their dried counterparts — especially lemon balm, mints, citrus fruits, thyme, sliced or grated ginger, and evergreen needles. The solution? More time and more herbs. To make a fresh tea, bring water to a boil. Add a handful of herbs (or 1 tablespoon ginger) per 2 cups of water, cover, and let sit for 1 to 2 hours.

Note: Some herbs — cinnamon, roses, cherry bark — extract or taste better if steeped in tepid water for a longer period of time because it minimizes bitter astringent tannins and won't destory less stable compounds.

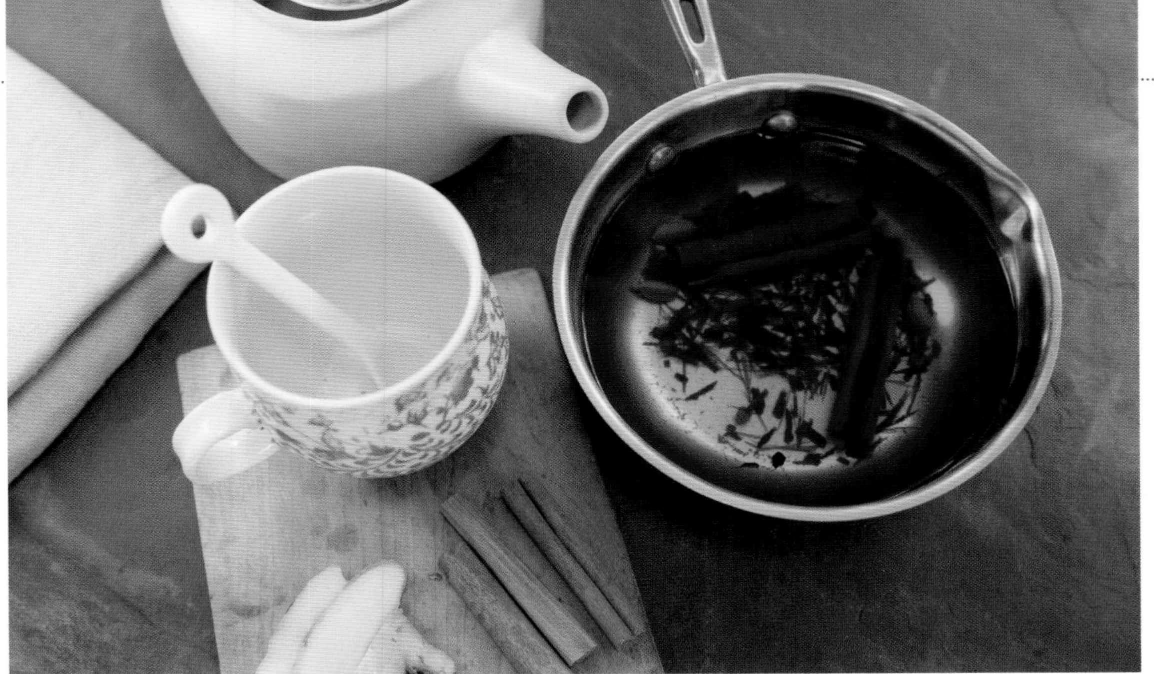

Herbal Teas: Decoction (Simmer)

The decoction method is best for harder parts of herbs: roots, bark, and seeds. These parts of the plant often make a weak tea if only allowed to infuse; simmering/decocting extracts their active ingredients and flavor faster. Larger amounts of herb and longer simmering times make stronger-tasting teas; less herb and time make a lighter tea.

1. Add 1 teaspoon to 1 tablespoon of dried herb per cup of water to your pot on the stove.
2. Simmer for approximately 20 minutes.
3. Strain and drink.

Variation: Thinking beyond the Teapot. You can infuse or decoct herbs in something other than tea! Remember: soup is a tea! Consider tonic and nutritive herbs, mushrooms, and seaweed for long-simmered broths.

HOW TO STRAIN HERBAL REMEDIES

PLACE A FINE-MESH STRAINER over a bowl and line it with cheesecloth or a clean, nonabsorbent cloth/jelly bag. Pour the herb mixture through. Wring the liquid (oil/tincture/honey/vinegar) out of the cloth and discard the herbal dregs. (For quick teas and chunky herbs like roots that don't hold a lot of liquid, it's fine to skip the cloth.) If you want to improve the clarity of the remedy, let the strained liquid sit for a while, giving any little bits time to settle, and then decant it or strain it through a coffee filter.

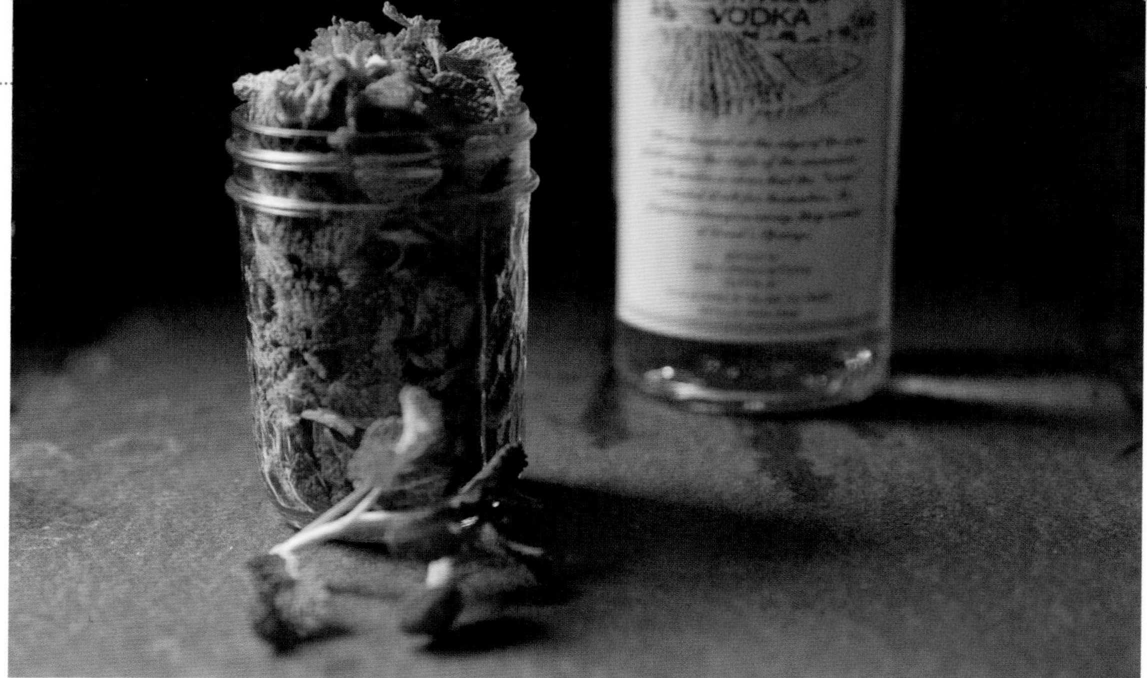

Fresh Herb Tincture

Without measuring anything, this technique makes an approximately 1:2 extract. That is, for every 1 ounce (by weight) of herb, you'll add 2 ounces (by volume) of alcohol.

1. Chop up your fresh herb material, and *really stuff* it in a jar until you can't fit any more.
2. Fill the jar to the brim with whole-grain alcohol, high-proof vodka, or brandy. A day later, the liquid level will have dropped a bit; top off the jar with more alcohol.
3. Let the jar sit in a dark spot for at least 1 month (or as long as you like). If the ingredients (e.g., roots) settle, shake the mixture periodically.
4. Strain the tincture, using a fine-mesh strainer and muslin or cheesecloth to squeeze out the last bit.

TINCTURE STORAGE

ALONGSIDE TEAS, tinctures may be the most popular form of herbal medicine, particularly for at-home remedies. Store your finished tincture in an airtight (preferably dark glass) container in a cool, dark, dry spot. Most tinctures will keep for up to 10 years, though some may lose potency earlier or get unpleasantly gloppy.

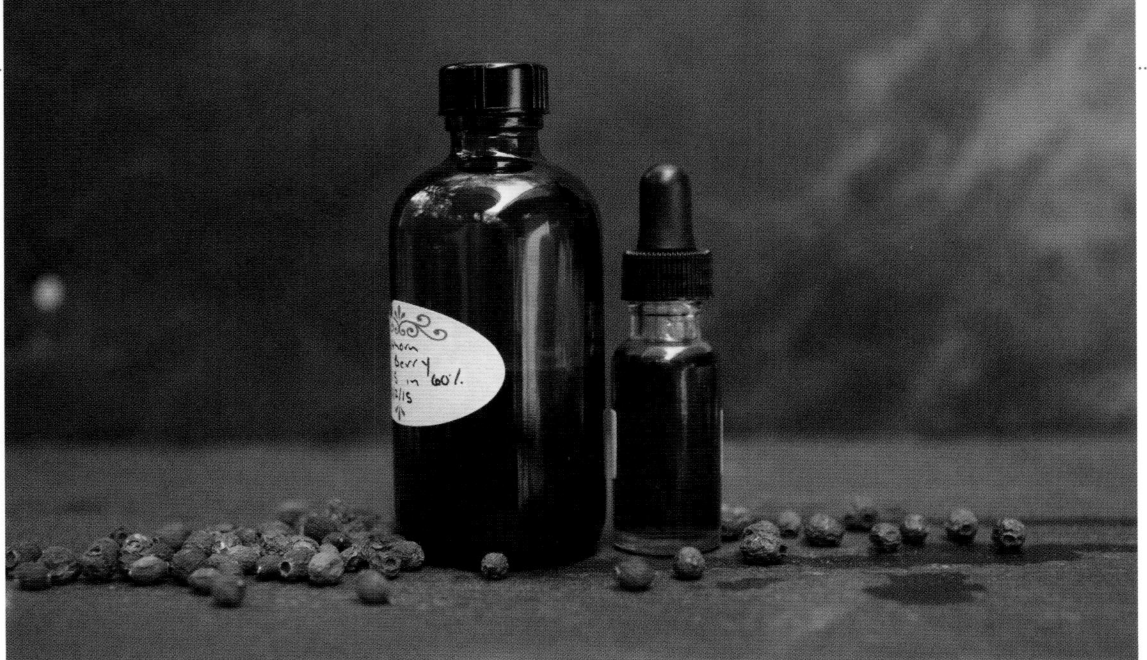

Dry Herb Tincture

The density of dried herbs varies widely, which means it's very difficult to eyeball their weight. Therefore, this technique comes out much better if you use a scale or purchase a known weight of herb.

1. If possible, grind your herb with a mortar and pestle or grinder. Grinding isn't absolutely necessary, but it makes a better extract (and fluffy herbs might not fit in the jar unless they're ground). Put the herbs in a glass jar.

2. For every 1 ounce (by weight) of herb, add 5 ounces of alcohol to the jar. Most dried plants extract best in 40 to 60 percent alcohol. A 100-proof or 80-proof vodka or brandy works well. Do not use ethanol unless it's diluted with distilled water.

3. Let the jar sit in a dark spot for at least 1 month (or as long as you like). Shake your jar every day or so.

4. Strain the tincture, using a fine-mesh strainer and muslin or cheesecloth to squeeze out the last bit. If there's still a lot of sediment, strain it again through a coffee filter.

Variation: Percolation Tincture Method. This variation on a dry herb tincture is complete within 24 hours and requires perfectly powdered herb and a special percolator cone. It borrows from old pharmacy methods and is a bit complicated. See my website (www.wintergreenbotanicals.com) for a free video and instructions.

Decoction Tincture

A decoction tincture (a.k.a. double-extraction tincture) is made using a combination of tincture and decocted tea techniques. It works well for those herbs — especially those that are mucilaginous (marshmallow), mineral-rich (nettle), or polysaccharide-rich (astragalus, echinacea), as well as mushrooms — that extract best when simmered for hours in hot water.

You'll need to know the weight of the herb(s) you're using before you begin. The technique is easier with dried herb because you can more accurately calculate how much alcohol to use, but you can use fresh herb as long as you take the fresh material's estimated water content into consideration; I generally double the herb weight in the ratios in step 3.

1. Decoct: Simmer the herb in water for 1 to 3 hours. Mushrooms can go all day.
2. Concentrate: Strain out and set aside the dregs (don't throw them away!). Simmer the tea, uncovered, to your desired volume to concentrate it. (This step is optional but preferred to increase potency.)
3. Tincture: Combine your concentrated tea, dregs, and alcohol in a glass jar. You'll want at least 25 percent alcohol to prevent your formula from growing mold and bacteria. As an example, if you have 190-proof alcohol, you'll want approximately 3 ounces (by volume) of tea and 2 ounces (by volume) of alcohol for every 1 ounce (by weight) of dried herb. For 100-proof alcohol, you'd use 2½ ounces of tea and 2½ ounces of alcohol for every ounce of dried herb.
4. Let the jar sit in a dark spot for at least 1 month. Shake your jar every day or so.
5. Strain the tincture, using a fine-mesh strainer and muslin or cheesecloth to squeeze out the last bit. If there's still a lot of sediment, strain it again through a coffee filter.

Note: Some herbalists tincture the plant first and then strain the dregs (a.k.a. the marc) to simmer and add to the finished tincture. Or they make two totally separate extracts — using fresh material for each — and then combine them. It all works. The math can get confusing, but the technique itself is quite easy!

PROOF AND PERCENTAGE: CHOOSING YOUR ALCOHOL

TINCTURES WORK SO WELL because they extract both water- and alcohol-soluble constituents from plants, which covers almost everything except fiber and minerals. Most of what we consider "alcohol" is actually only a percentage alcohol; the rest is water.

190-proof ethanol (95 percent alcohol), often called "whole grain" (it can also be made from sugarcane or grapes), makes a potent extract. I prefer it for almost all fresh plant tinctures (it desiccates the fresh plant, which adds water and water-soluble constituents to your final product) as well as dry resins (which repel water). You can dilute ethanol with distilled water to achieve any desired alcohol percentage, and old pharmacy techniques relied on it.

151-proof spirits (75 percent alcohol) is increasingly available as whole grain, rum, and vodka and works well as an ethanol substitute.

100-proof vodka (50 percent alcohol) works well for almost any tincture, including those made with dried plants (which generally require some water in the solvent since there is none in the plant). Although different dried plants have different solvency ranges, 50 percent alcohol covers almost all bases quite nicely. Resins and turmeric do better at 70 percent alcohol or higher.

80-proof vodka or brandy (40 percent alcohol) works in a pinch for almost any tincture and is preferred in many wise-woman herbal techniques because it's what is commonly available to the everyday person. The lower alcohol percentage also makes your tincture less harsh tasting and more appropriate for cordials; it's also more appropriate for topical remedies.

20 to 30 percent alcohol is the minimum amount of alcohol needed to preserve your tincture or other recipe (cordials, syrups) for shelf stability. You make it by cutting alcohol with water, honey, or simple syrup (being sure to calculate for the percent of water already in some spirits). Water-soluble mucilaginous herbs (comfrey, marshmallow), which repel alcohol, and mushrooms do better at a lower alcohol percentage, preferably via the decoction tincture method.

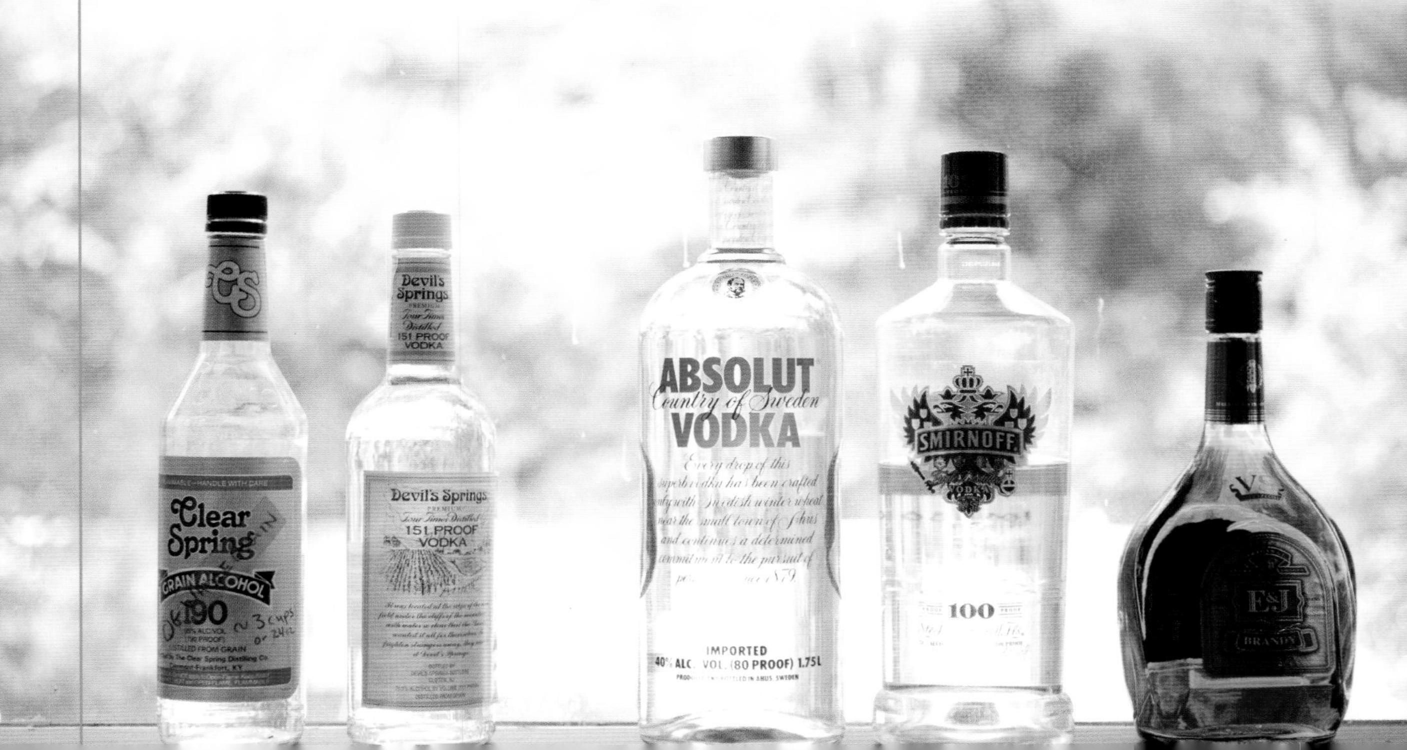

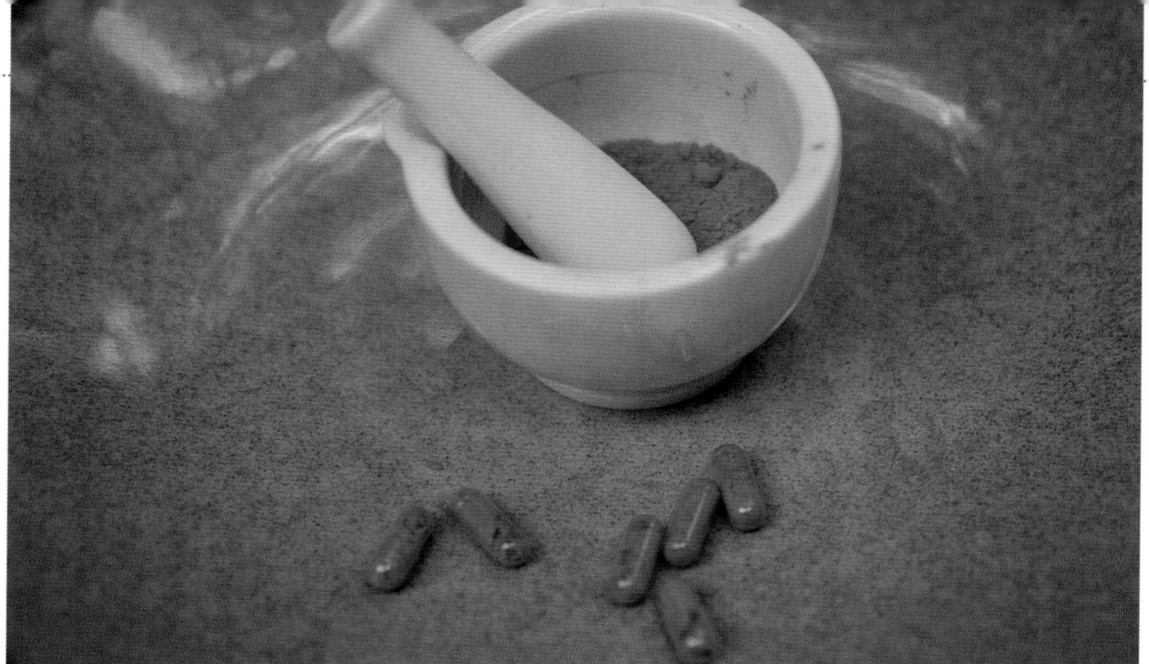

Capsules

Capsules and capsule machines come in sizes. One full "00" capsule holds about 500 mg. Size "0" is smaller, "000" is larger. Be sure your machine and capsules are the same size. Veggie caps are less apt to get stuck in the machine (and are preferred by vegetarians), but gelatin caps cost less. Making capsules is tediously time consuming — it's a good job to do while watching a movie — but it saves money and allows complete control over ingredients.

1. Start with dried, powdered herb. If you have cut/sifted herb, grind it, using a coffee grinder, bullet-style grinder, or mortar and pestle. Sift through a fine-mesh strainer to get a finer powder, if desired.
2. Using a capsule machine or your hands, fill the large end of the empty capsules.
3. Snap on the top cap.
4. Store your finished capsules in an airtight (preferably dark glass) container in a cool, dark, dry spot for up to 1 year.

Herbal Honey

"Cooking" herbs in honey works well for tasty and aromatic herbs, such as lemon balm, anise hyssop, or mint, as well as those used as expectorants or cough/cold remedies, such as bee balm, thyme, ginger, and fresh spring pine branches. Save the dregs and use them to make sweet tea.

1. Chop up your fresh or dried herb, as needed.
2. For every ½ cup of chopped fresh herb or ¼ cup of dried herb, add 2 cups of honey.
3. Bring to nearly a boil, then turn off the heat and let cool.
4. Repeat at least once and up to three times daily for 3 days. (Fresh, juicy herbs need at least a few heatings. Aromatic herbs may need less, while subtle herbs like rose petals and root medicines do well with repeated heatings over a few days.)
5. After the last heating, pour the warm mixture through a strainer and into glass jars. Let cool with the lid off.
6. Once the honey has cooled, check the viscosity. If it's as thick as or thicker than plain honey, it should be shelf stable for at least a year. If it's more watery, the moisture from the plant will shorten the shelf life significantly, and you should refrigerate it; it will keep for up to 3 months. It's okay if herbal honey crystallizes, but throw it away if you notice any signs of mold or fermentation.

Variation: Raw Herbal Honey. This alternative method is very easy but takes more time. It also takes advantage of the benefits of raw honey that would be lost if you cooked it. Just chop up your herb and loosely pack it in a jar. Cover with honey to the top. Seal and let sit for a few weeks or so. Every day or two, flip the jar. When the honey tastes good, plunk the jar in warm water to get the honey runny. Strain it through a fine-mesh strainer, pressing on the herbs with a spoon to push out as much honey as you can.

Note: The moisture in fresh plants increases the likelihood of spoilage and fermentation, especially with the raw method. Evaporating the moisture through cooking, drying the herbs, or wilting the fresh plants in advance, or refrigerating the honey and using it up quickly, will lessen the risk.

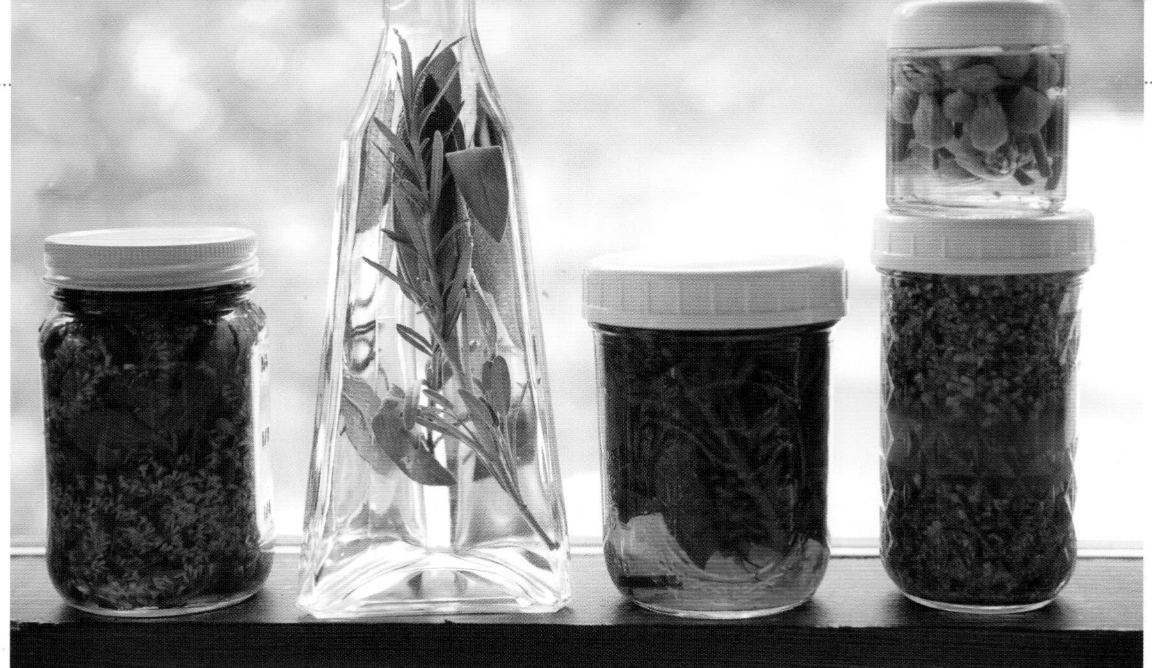

Herbal Vinegar

Minimally processed raw apple cider vinegar has its own healing properties and is preferred for nutritive and medicinal vinegars as well as fire cider. White wine and rice vinegars have more neutral flavor and color to really show off culinary herbs. Distilled white vinegar is more heavily processed and often tastes and smells bad, though organic white vinegar is better. Tarragon vinegar is classic. Chive blossoms make a lovely and delicious pink vinegar. Bronze fennel, purple basil, and raspberries make red-magenta vinegars. Garlic occasionally turns vinegar teal blue.

1. If you're using fresh herbs, chop them.
2. Pack the fresh herbs into a jar. If you're making a nutritive vinegar, pack the herbs loosely; if you're making a medicinal vinegar, pack them tightly. If you're using fresh herbs, fill the jar to almost the top; if you're using dried herbs, fill it only about halfway. Add enough vinegar to completely fill the jar. Seal with a *plastic* cap; vinegar eats metal lids.
3. Let the vinegar steep on your kitchen counter or in your pantry. Taste it every day or two. It's ready when it tastes good. (For medicinal vinegars, wait a whole month.)
4. Strain out the herbs. Store the vinegar in a glass bottle with a plastic lid in a cool, dark, dry spot. It should keep for 1 to 2 years. You may opt to put a whole sprig of herb into a finished vinegar for visual appeal.

Variation: Oxymel. Use a mix of honey (30 to 50 percent of the total) and vinegar. An oxymel may only keep for a few months and is best refrigerated for a longer shelf life.

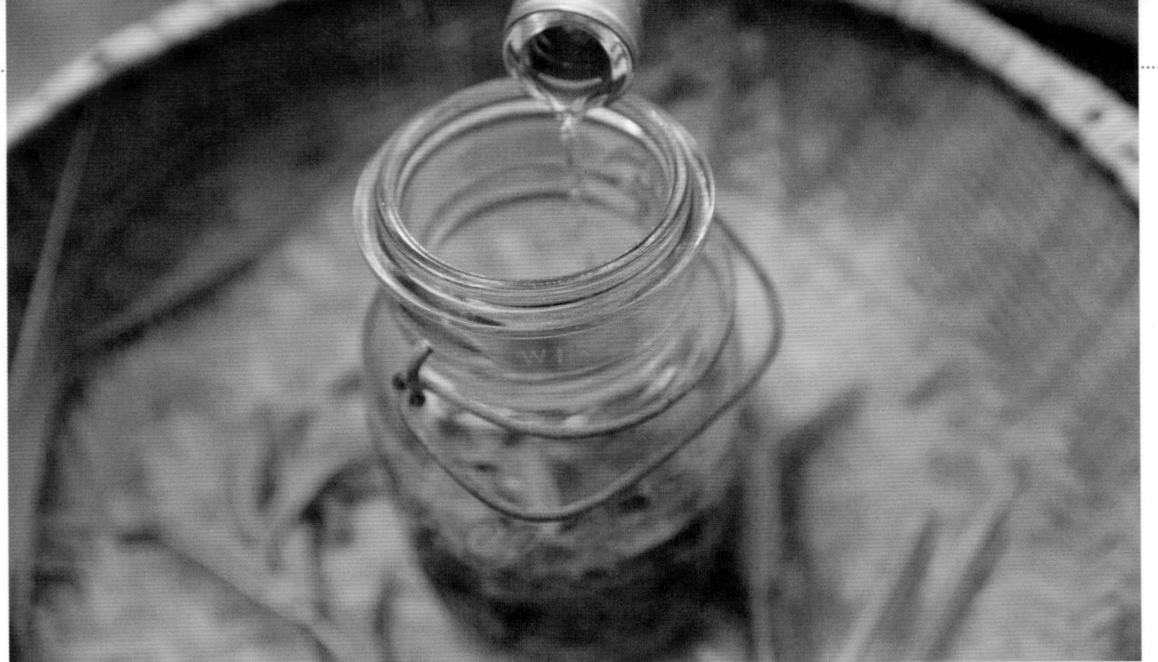

Herbal Cordial

Perfect for special events and a delicious dessert! Consider vanilla (one bean for every 4 to 8 ounces of cordial), licorice-y plants (anise hyssop, anise, fennel, star anise), lemony plants (balm, grass, thyme, verbena), and fruits of all kinds, as well as herbal bitters and fruity antioxidants blends.

1. First, make simple syrup by simmering 2 cups of sugar with 1 cup of water until clear. (Alternatively, you can use plain honey or maple syrup in place of simple syrup.)
2. Loosely fill a jar with fresh herbs or fruit or both (or a lesser amount of dried herb).
3. Fill to the top with a mix of 30 to 40 percent simple syrup and the rest good-tasting spirits like brandy or quality vodka. Aim for at least 20 percent true alcohol in your finished product for shelf stability.
4. Cover, shake, and taste every few days. Strain when it tastes good (sometimes just a day or two) or after 1 month. Store in an airtight glass container in a cool, dark spot. It will keep for 1 to 2 years.

FRESH HERBAL SODAS AND WATERS

A DELICIOUS WAY TO ENJOY HERBS. I particularly enjoy lemongrass, mints, fennel, Korean licorice mint or anise with vanilla extract, a whole rose blossom (most flavorful after several hours), or a few whole, dry hibiscus blossoms. Clear glass bottles really show off the herbs and start conversations at parties. Simply stuff a few sprigs of herbs into a bottle, cover with plain seltzer, and refrigerate for at least 30 minutes before serving. Drink it the same day. If desired, sweeten with maple syrup or simple syrup to taste. If you don't like bubbles, use plain water.

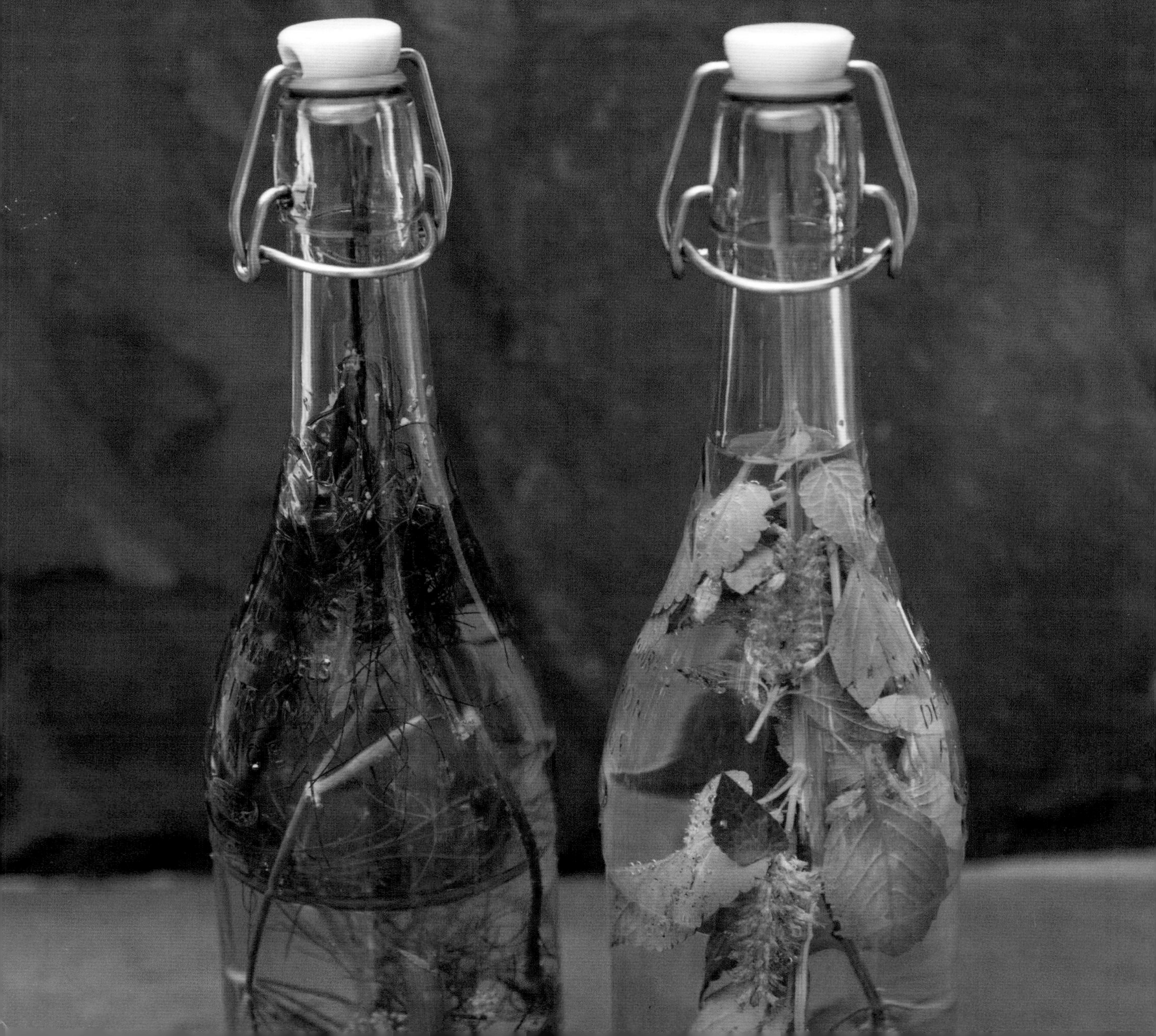

Herb-*Infused* Oils

Herb-infused oils form the base of many topical preparations because of their moisturizing, soothing activity. They can be used as is, rubbed into the skin, or as an ingredient in skin remedies. However, oil easily harbors and promotes the growth of bacteria and mold. Some create visible "clouds" and mold, but you can't see, taste, or smell botulism (a rare but real risk). For this reason, culinary infused oils should be stored in the fridge and used within 1 week, maximum, unless they've been pasteurized or have had preservatives added. Spoilage is less of a concern for topical infused oils, but it can still occur. Using dried herbs and the alcohol-intermediary technique reduces the risk, but some herbs (St. John's wort, chickweed) are more potent when infused fresh.

Topical infused oils usually keep for 6 months to 1 year, sometimes longer. Make small batches to ensure freshness.

You can use any kind of oil or fat as your base, but extra-virgin olive oil is preferred due to its affordability, long shelf life, healing properties, and low risk of allergy. Grapeseed (less shelf stable but also odorless and lighter colored) and coconut (lightly heated to make it liquid) oils also work well. Jojoba has the longest shelf life and is fantastic for skin but is also quite expensive and not always good at extracting herbal properties. Indigenous cultures used rendered animal fat to make ointment-consistency extracts, and some locavore herbalists have moved back to that.

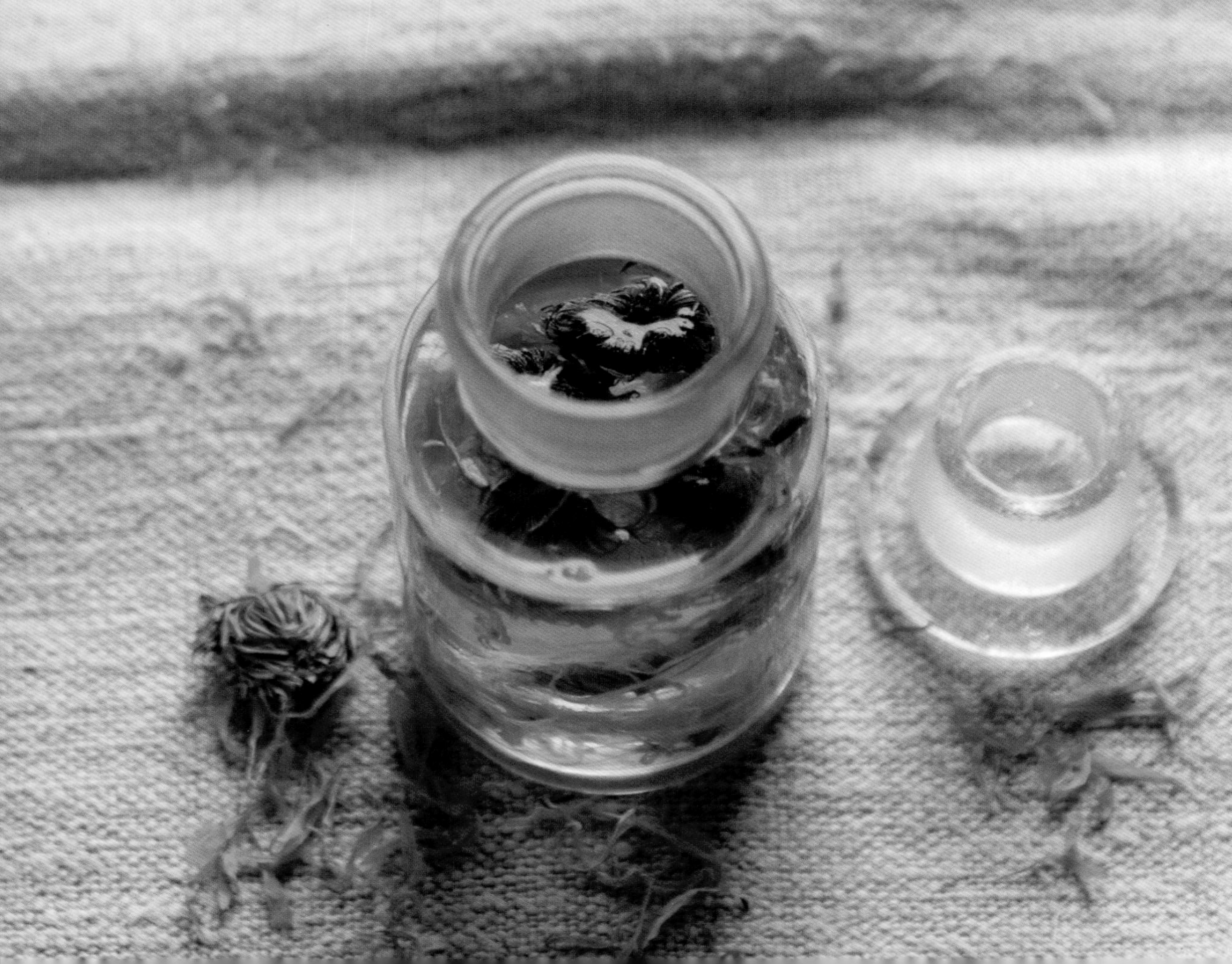

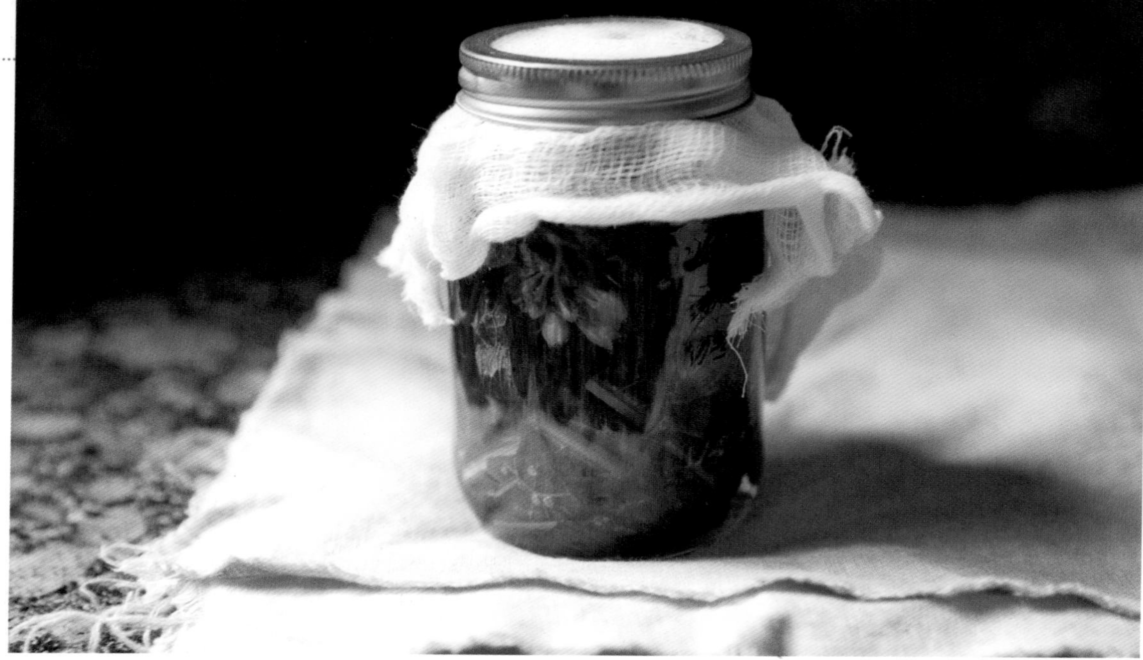

Herbal Oil: Basic Maceration

This is the classic method, which will work for any herb in any form. The technique is akin to that for tinctures and vinegars except that you should press out the oil within 2 weeks. It tends to spoil quickly when made with fresh herbs.

1. Loosely fill a glass jar with fresh or fresh-wilted herb. Or for dried herb, use 1 ounce of coarsely ground or cut/sifted herb per 4 to 8 ounces of oil.
2. Add enough oil to fill the jar completely and cover the herbs. Cover tightly. If you're using fresh herbs, you may prefer to cover the jar with cheesecloth to allow moisture to escape, which makes a more stable oil.
3. Let the jar sit in a warm, sunny spot — like a windowsill — for 2 weeks. Stir or shake it *daily*, which is especially important for fresh herbs (and even more so if you're using cheesecloth for a lid), which get funky quickly when they rise to the top. A glass fermentation weight helps everything stay submerged.
4. Strain the herbs from the oil. Store the oil in an airtight glass container in a cool, dark, dry spot for up to 1 year, watching for signs of microbial growth or rancidity. Oil will eventually break down rubber droppers and jar liners, but plastic and metal lids should be fine.

Variation: Heated Herbal Oil. Using the same proportions given above for dried or fresh herbs, heat the herbs in the oil for a few hours to a few days. The ideal temperature is 90°F to 110°F. If you use a slow cooker or double boiler (which won't stay as low as 110°F), you may need to shut it off periodically so that it doesn't get so hot as to fry the herbs and oxidize the oil. You may also use a greenhouse, dehydrator, yogurt maker, or stove with a pilot light; in fact, these locations tend to provide a more desirable heat range. When the oil is infused to your liking, strain and store as usual.

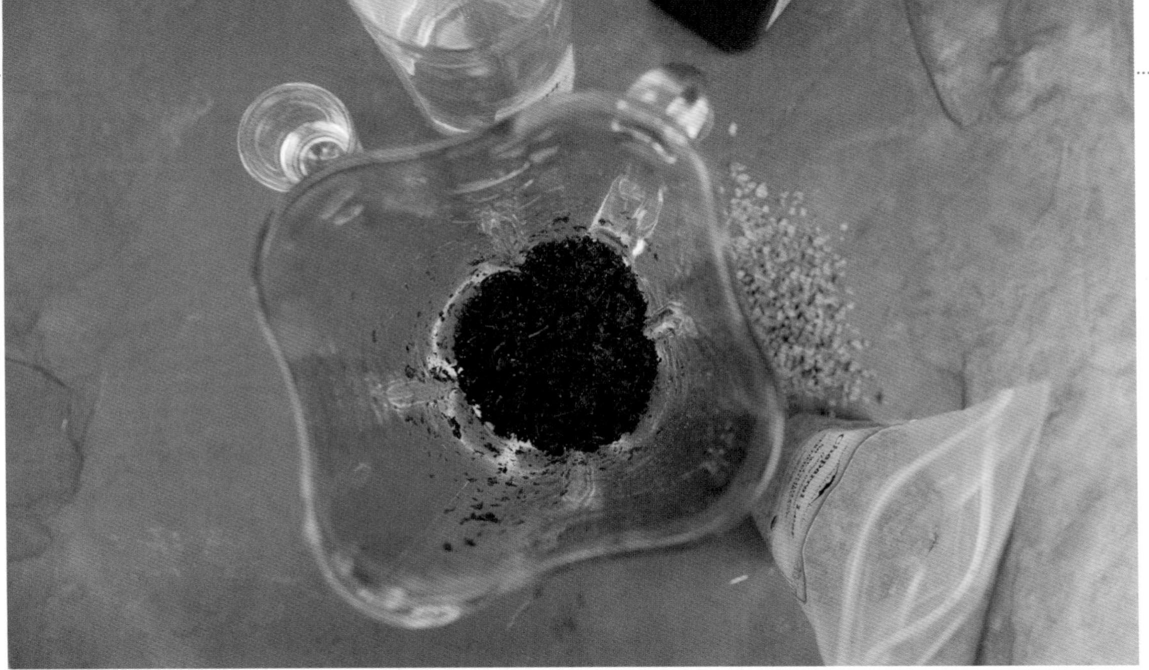

Herbal Oil: Alcohol Intermediary

My favorite method! This technique makes surprisingly potent, colorful, long-lasting oils thanks to the use of alcohol. It only works for dried plants, so you can't use this method for herbs that are best infused fresh (St. John's wort, chickweed, cleavers). For all other herbs, I highly recommend this technique.

1. Grind up the herb in a blender to a coarse powder.
2. For every ounce of herb (by weight), you'll need ½ ounce of grain alcohol or high-proof vodka. Combine the herb and alcohol in a jar and mix thoroughly. The mixture will be damp, like beach sand or potting soil.
3. Cover and let sit overnight (or for several days or weeks, as long as the lid is airtight).
4. Scrape the herb-alcohol mix into a blender. For every ounce of dried herb that you started with, add 7 ounces of oil. Process until the blender gets warm, 5 to 10 minutes.
5. Strain the oil. If there is a lot of sediment, strain again through a coffee filter. Store in an airtight glass container in a cool, dark, dry spot, where it will keep for up to a year.

Variation: Alcohol Intermediary and Low Heat. This method follows the alcohol intermediary technique; however, instead of straining the oil after blending it with the alcohol-herb mixture, pour all the "slop" into a jar and let it sit someplace warm (like the car) for a few days. Shake daily, then strain. This technique works well for fat- and alcohol-soluble plants. I primarily use it for calendula; after testing all the techniques I feel this makes the most potent calendula oil.

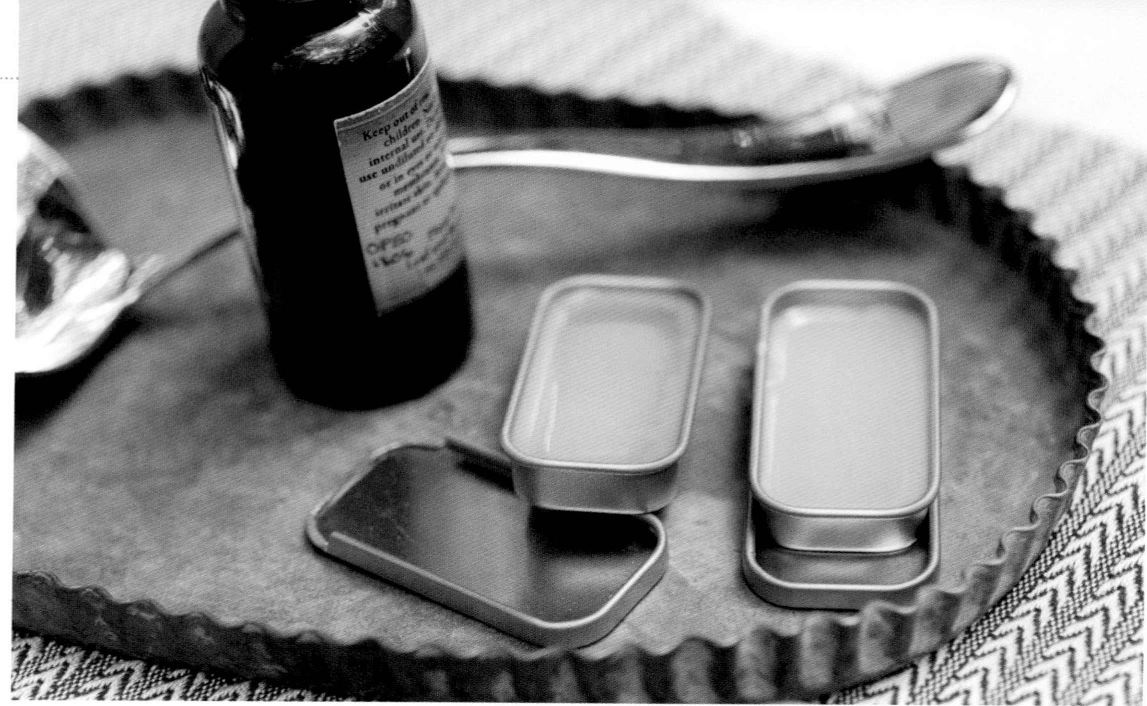

Salves & Lip Balms

Salves and lip balms are basically the same, differing only in the types of oils and herbs you use.

1. Melt 1 ounce of beeswax in a double boiler.
2. Add 4 ounces of oil, plain or herb infused. I prefer to wait until the beeswax has melted to add the oil to reduce the heat exposure, but you can add them all at once if you wish. Stir to combine.
3. Once the beeswax has melted and you've mixed in the oil, remove the mixture from the heat. If you want to add essential oils (10 to 20 drops per batch) or other ingredients, mix them in now.
4. Quickly pour or ladle the mixture into heat-safe containers while it's still liquid. I prefer a small gravy spoon with an edge for pouring, but most people use a glass liquid measuring cup. If the wax begins to harden prematurely, scoop it back into the double boiler to warm it back up.
5. Let the salve fully cool and harden, then cap the container. Store in a cool, dark, dry spot. It should keep for at least 1 year. You can extend its shelf life by freezing it.

ABOUT BEESWAX

MOST HERBALISTS USE BEESWAX to thicken and harden topical formulas including salves, lip balm, and cream. It's long-lasting, minimally processed, locally available, safe, and relatively affordable. When purchasing beeswax, quality varies widely. Chunks and blocks are better than pelletized or granulated beeswax (which is often rancid and oddly white). Good beeswax should be yellowish brown and smell honeylike, not rancid. Local beekeepers often sell small quantities of beeswax, and you can also buy it from most natural food stores, herb shops, and bulk herb suppliers. Wrap the chunk in a clean, sturdy cloth and whack with a hammer on a solid surface (e.g., rock, concrete floor) to break it into smaller bits that are easier to measure and melt. You can also use a grater, but it's very tough to grate and almost impossible to clean off the grater.

Some vegans prefer not to use beeswax because animals produce it and instead opt for cocoa butter (not quite as hard) or vegetable waxes (which may be more expensive and heavily processed) instead. You'll need to tinker with the ratio of oil to wax or butter to get the thickness you like. Keep a handful of spoons in the freezer and dip them into your hot mix to test the consistency. For something softer, add more oil; if you want it harder, add more wax.

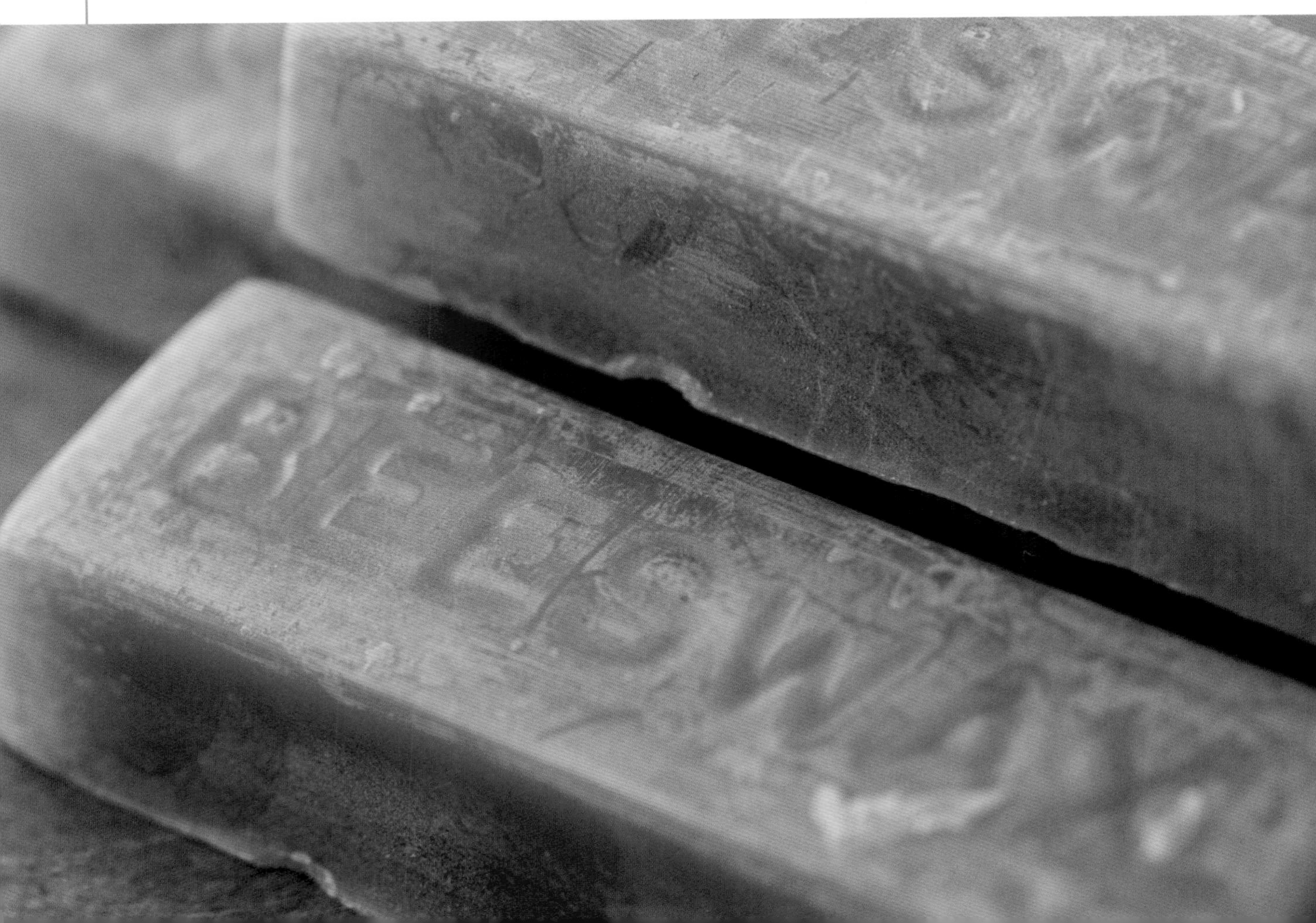

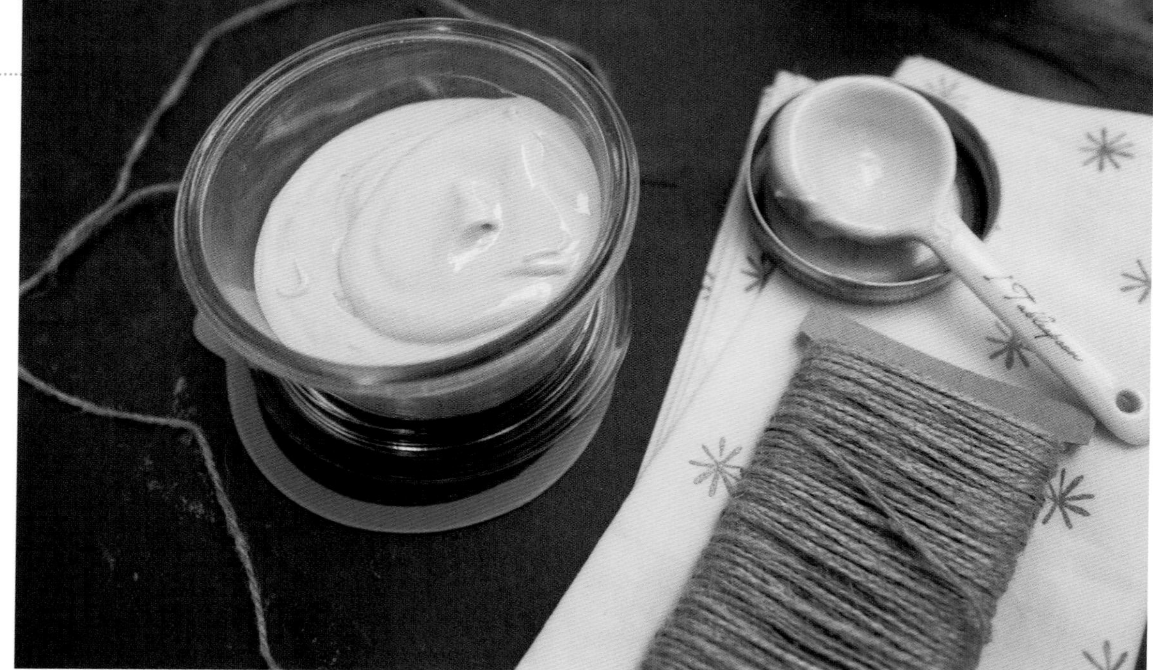

Creams

Creams make unique and lovely topical remedies because they combine oil- and water-based ingredients, which sink into the skin as the cream moisturizes. Unfortunately, water and oil don't always blend well, especially without chemical preservatives and stabilizers. Hats off to herbalist Rosemary Gladstar for her ever-popular "perfect cream" recipe. Here, I've made a few alterations and deconstructed it a little so that you can easily adapt the ingredients. You can use almost any ingredient in this recipe; however, every ingredient must be shelf stable or it will mold. The freshness and stability of your ingredients will determine your cream's shelf life. This should be shelf stable for 6 months to 1 year in a cool, dark, dry spot. If it separates, stir it with a spoon.

OILS

- ½–1 ounce beeswax (depending on desired thickness)
- ¾ cup (6 ounces) "liquid oils" (grapeseed, olive, herb-infused oil . . .)
- ⅓ cup (2½ ounces) "solid fats" (coconut oil, cocoa or shea butter . . .)

WATERS

- ⅔ cup (5½ ounces) "waters" (distilled water, vanilla extract, hydrosol, tincture . . .)
- Few drops of essential oil (optional)

1. In a double boiler over low heat, melt the beeswax. Then add the liquid oils and solid fats and heat just enough that everything melts together. Heating (and cooling) your oils *slowly* makes it less likely for cocoa and shea butter to form granules in your cream over time. (They won't spoil the cream, but you might not like the consistency.) If you want to get really technical, look online for how to "temper" various butters.

2. Pour the oils mixture into a quart glass jar (for use with an immersion blender, which I find works best), a blender, or a bowl for a mixer. Let cool until it is just warm or at room temperature. The mixture should become thick, semisolid (ointmentlike), and opaque.

3. While the oils are cooling, pour the "waters" and essential oil, if using, into an easy-pour container. Let sit until they reach room temperature. The cream will form much more easily if the oils and waters are approximately the same temperature when blended and none of your equipment is overly cold.

4. When both mixtures have reached room temperature (1 to 2 hours), use an immersion blender, regular blender, or hand/standing mixer to mix the oils at high speed. With the blender or mixer going, slowly drizzle the waters into the whirling oils. If necessary, stop blending occasionally to mix with a spoon or spatula until everything has combined.

5. Pour or scoop the cream into clean jars with clean caps, preferably sterilized to discourage mold and bacteria growth. Store in a cool, dry place. The cream will thicken as it sets. Neat trick: if you put your fresh-made cream in the freezer for a few days, your cocoa and shea butter will be less apt to crystallize and make the cream grainy over time. Thaw on the counter before using. The cream will keep for 6 to 9 months at room temperature; you can freeze extra batches as needed for a longer shelf life.

Note: Rosemary Gladstar also uses ⅓ cup (2½ ounces) aloe gel or juice in her recipe, but I prefer the thicker consistency and extended shelf life without it. If you choose to use it, opt for shelf-stable aloe with preservatives or your cream will eventually get moldy. Definitely do not use fresh-from-the-plant aloe. If you'd prefer a thinner cream that works in a pump dispenser, use aloe, add a couple of more ounces of "waters," or use less beeswax.

MY FAVORITE CREAM

THE QUALITY AND STABILITY of my creams improved dramatically when I started using about 1 ounce of cocoa butter for the solid fats (coconut for the rest) and 2 ounces of vanilla or other alcohol-based extract for the waters, and I began using an immersion blender. The oils and waters rarely separate. My creams never mold and take nearly a year before they begin to turn rancid. Also, cocoa and vanilla give my creams a heavenly scent! For my other ingredients, I use grapeseed oil (or infused olive oil), coconut oil, distilled water, and ¾ ounce of beeswax.

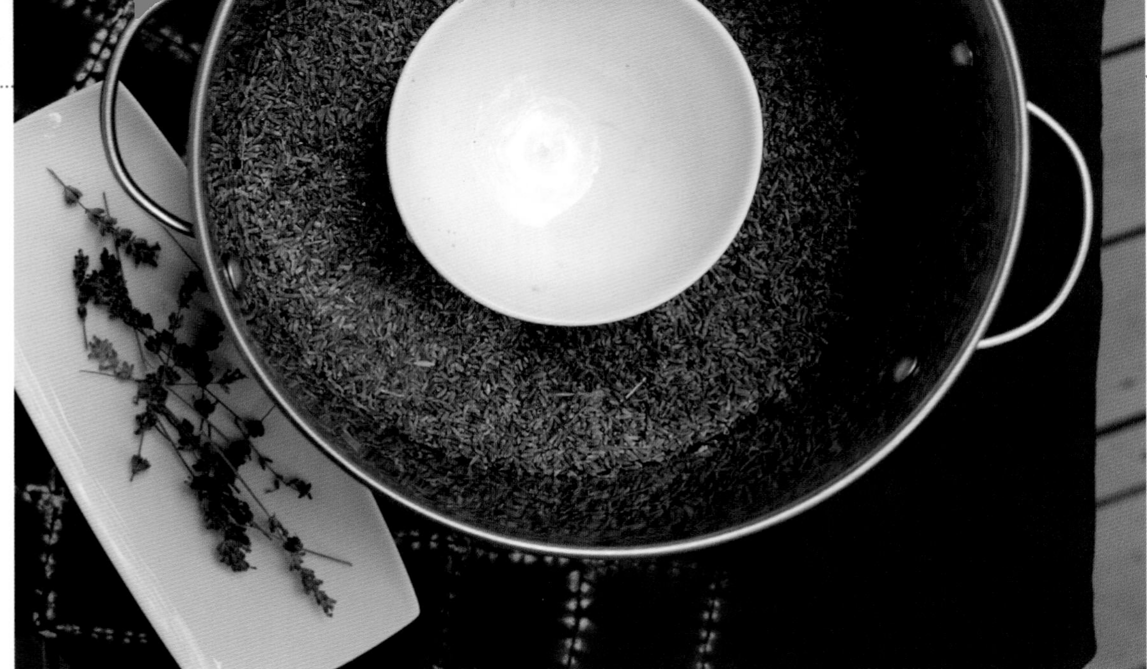

Hydrosols/Flower Waters

Fragrant essential oils are nearly impossible to make at home because you need special equipment and lots of plant material (many pounds, sometimes tons!) to make just 1 ounce of oil. Hydrosols, on the other hand, extract a small amount of the plant's essential oils in distilled water. They're gentler and safer, yet they still offer a nice scent and are very easy to make at home with any aromatic plant that holds up to heat. Try this with rose petals, mint-family aromatic herbs, lavender, et cetera.

1. Pour a few inches of water into a large stainless steel pot. Put a clean brick in the middle and a bowl on top (or use a bowl that will stay put and not float around in the water). Place several fistfuls of herb material in the water around (not in) the bowl.

2. Put the pot lid on *upside down* and fill with ice to promote condensation (I freeze water in a metal mixing bowl and put this on top of the lid — much less messy!).

3. Bring the water to a light boil, then simmer gently until you have about 4 ounces of flower water in the bowl.

4. Scoop the liquid into a clean container. Hydrosols have finicky shelf lives. Using sanitized equipment helps. Although your hydrosol might stay shelf stable for a year, it's best kept refrigerated (or frozen) and used quickly. Toss it if you see any funky floaters (mold, bacteria).

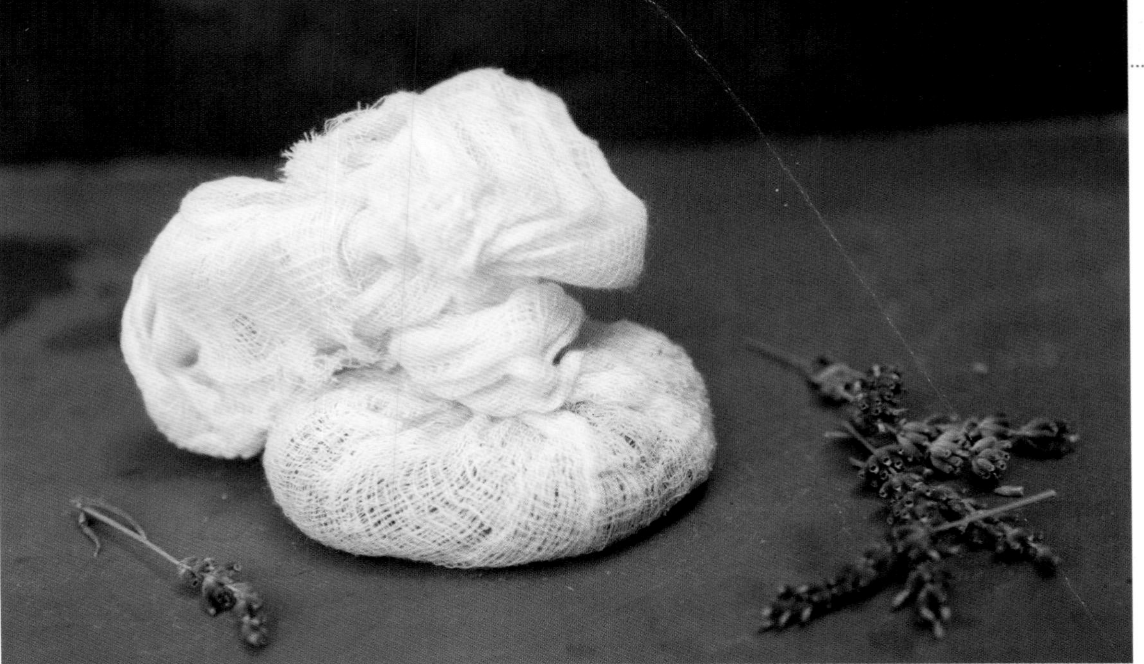

Poultices, Compresses & Baths

Poultice: Chew or mash up fresh plant material (for dry, grind it to a powder and add water or other liquid). Apply where needed on the skin. Cover with a bandage if needed to keep it in place. Remove and apply a new poultice every few hours or as needed.

Compress: Make a strong tea. Dip a cloth into it. Apply the dampened cloth to the affected area of your skin. (Or you may prefer to wrap your loose herb in a cloth, tie it in a bundle, dip it in hot water to saturate, and apply the bundle to the affected area.)

Bath: Make a large batch of strong tea. Pour it into the tub and soak for 15 to 30 minutes. Or fill a clean sock or nylon with dried herbs and tie it under the faucet as the bath fills. You could also shake the herbs into the water directly, which works great but can be quite a mess to clean. Don't just think of baths as a skin remedy. Your skin will absorb some of the herbs' properties into your bloodstream; baths can be an effective way to deliver medicine to babies, children, and adults. If you want to add a few drops of essential oil to your bath (for adults only), be sure to mix the oil with milk, vegetable oil, or bath salts first. Also try footbaths.

APPENDIX I

The Latin Names of Herbs

acerola (*Malpighia emarginata*)
aconite (*Aconitum* spp.)
agastache (*Agastache* spp.)
agrimony (*Agrimonia* spp.)
alaria (*Alaria* spp.)
alder (*Alnus* spp.)
alfalfa (*Medicago sativa*)
aloe (*Aloe vera*)
amanita (*Amanita* spp.)
American ginseng (*Panax quinquefolius*)
amla (*Phyllanthus emblica*)
andrographis (*Andrographis paniculata*)
angelica root (*Angelica* spp.)
anise (*Pimpinella anisum*)
anise hyssop (*Agastache foeniculum*)
aralia (*Aralia* spp.)
arnica (*Arnica montana*)
artichoke leaf (*Cynara scolymus*)
ashwagandha (*Withania somnifera*)
Asian ginseng (*Panax ginseng*)
Asian pennywort (*Centella asiatica*)
aspen (*Populus* spp.)
astragalus (*Astragalus propinquus*, syn. *A. membranaceus*)
atractylodes (*Atractylodes macrocephala*)
autumn olive (*Elaeagnus umbellata*)
avens (*Geum* spp.)
bacopa (*Bacopa monnieri*)
balsam root (*Balsamorhiza sagittata*)
barberry (*Berberis* spp.)
bay leaf (*Laurus nobilis*)
bee balm (*Monarda* spp.)
beggar's-ticks (*Bidens frondosa*)
bilberry (*Vaccinium myrtillus*)
birch (*Betula lenta, B. alleghaniensis*)
bitter melon (*Momordica charantia*)
blackberry (*Rubus* spp.)
black cohosh (*Actaea racemosa*, syn. *Cimicifuga racemosa*)
black-eyed Susan (*Rudbeckia laciniata, R. hirta*)
black haw (*Viburnum prunifolium*)
black pepper (*Piper nigrum*)
black tea (*see* tea)
black walnut (*Juglans nigra*)
bladderwrack (*Fucus vesiculosus*)
blessed thistle (*Cnicus benedictus*)
blueberry (*Vaccinium* spp.)
blue cohosh (*Caulophyllum thalictroides*)
blue vervain (*Verbena hastata*)
boneset (*Eupatorium perfoliatum*)
boswellia (*Boswellia carteri, B. serrata*)
brahmi (*see* gotu kola *or* bacopa)
broad dock (*Rumex obtusifolius*)
buckthorn (*Rhamnus cathartica*)
bugleweed (*Lycopus virginicus*)
burdock (*Arctium* spp.)
butterbur (*Petasites hybridus*)
cacao (*Theobroma cacao*)
calendula (*Calendula officinalis*)
California poppy (*Eschscholzia californica*)
Canadian fleabane (*Conyza canadensis*)
caraway (*Carum carvi*)
cardamom (*Elettaria cardamomum*)
carob (*Ceratonia siliqua*)
cascara sagrada (*Rhamnus purshiana*)
catnip (*Nepeta cataria*)
cayenne (*Capsicum annuum*)
celandine (*Chelidonium majus*)
celery (*Apium graveolens*)
chaga (*Inonotus obliquus*)
chamomile (*Matricaria recutita*)
chaparral (*Larrea tridentata*)
chaste tree berry (*see* vitex)
cherry, tart (*Prunus cerasus*)
chia (*Salvia hispanica*)
chickweed (*Stellaria media* and related species)
chicory (*Cichorium intybus*)
Chinese ephedra (*Ephedra sinica*)
chives (*Allium schoenoprasum*)
cinnamon (*Cinnamomum* spp.)
cinquefoil (*Potentilla* spp.)
cleavers (*Galium aparine*)
cloves (*Syzygium aromaticum*)
codonopsis (*Codonopsis pilosula* and related species)
comfrey (*Symphytum officinale, S.* x *uplandicum*)
coptis (*Coptis* spp.)
cordyceps (*Ophiocordyceps sinensis*, syn. *Cordyceps sinensis*)
coriander (*Coriandrum sativum*)
corn (*Zea mays*)
cosmos flower (*Cosmos* spp.)
cotton root bark (*Gossypium* spp.)
cramp bark (*Viburnum opulus*)
cranberry (*Vaccinium macrocarpon*)
cumin (*Cuminum cyminum*)
damiana (*Turnera diffusa*)
dandelion (*Taraxacum officinale*)
datura (*Datura* spp.)
digitata kelp (*Laminaria digitata*)
dill (*Anethum graveolens*)
dong quai (*Angelica sinensis*)
dulse (*Palmaria palmate*)
echinacea (*Echinacea* spp.)
elder (*Sambucus nigra*)
elecampane (*Inula helenium*)
eleuthero (*Eleutherococcus senticosus*)
enoki (*Flammulina velutipes*)
ephedra (*Ephedra* spp.)
eyebright (*Euphrasia* spp.)

fennel (*Foeniculum vulgare*)
fenugreek (*Trigonella foenum-graecum*)
feverfew (*Tanacetum parthenium*)
fir (*Abies* spp.)
fireweed (*Chamerion angustifolium*)
flax (*Linum usitatissimum*)
foxglove (*Digitalis* spp.)
garden sage (*Salvia officinalis*)
garlic (*Allium sativum*)
gentian (*Gentiana lutea*)
germander (*Teucrium chamaedrys*)
ginger (*Zingiber officinale*)
ginkgo (*Ginkgo biloba*)
ginseng (*Panax* spp.)
goji (*see* lycii)
goldenrod (*Solidago* spp.)
goldenseal (*Hydrastis canadensis*)
goldthread (*Coptis trifolia*)
gotu kola (*Centella asiatica*)
green tea (*see* tea)
grindelia (*Grindelia* spp.)
guarana (*Paullinia cupana*)
guggul (*Commiphora wightii*)
gymnema (*Gymnea sylvestre*)
hawthorn (*Crataegus* spp.)
hemlock (*Tsuga* spp.)
hibiscus (*Hibiscus sabdariffa*)
hijiki (*Sargassum fusiforme*, syn. *Hizikia fusiformis*)
holy basil (*Ocimum sanctum*, syn. *O. tenuiflorum*)
hops (*Humulus lupulus*)
horehound (*Marrubium vulgare*)
horny goat weed (*Epimedium* spp.)
horse chestnut (*Aesculus hippocastanum*)
horseradish (*Armoracia rusticana*, syn. *Cochlearia armoracia*)
horsetail (*Equisetum arvense*)
hyssop (*Hyssopus officinalis*)
Irish moss (*Chondrus crispus*)
Jamaican dogwood (*Piscidia piscipula*)
jewelweed (*Impatiens capensis*)
jiaogulan (*Gynostemma pentaphyllum*)
jujube dates (*Ziziphus jujuba* var. *spinosa*)
juniper (*Juniperus* spp.)
kava (*Piper methysticum*)
kelp (*Laminaria* and *Nereocystis* species)
kombu (*Laminaria japonica* and others)
Korean licorice mint (*Agastache rugosa*)
kudzu (*Pueraria* spp.)
lady's mantle (*Alchemilla vulgaris*)
lamb's-quarter (*Chenopodium album* and related species)
lavender (*Lavandula angustifolia*)
laver (*Porphyra umbilicalis*)
lemon balm (*Melissa officinalis*)
lemongrass (*Cymbopogon* spp.)
lemon verbena (*Aloysia citrodora*)
licorice (*Glycyrrhiza glabra*)
linden (*Tilia* spp.)
lion's mane (*Hericium erinaceus*)
lithospermum (*Lithospermum officinale*)
lobelia (*Lobelia inflata*)
lycii (*Lycium barbarum*, *L. chinense*)
maca (*Lepidium meyenii*)
magnolia (*Magnolia* spp.)
maitake (*Grifola frondosa*)
mallow (*Malva* spp.)
marshmallow (*Althaea officinalis*)
mastic gum (*Pistacia lentiscus*)
meadowsweet (*Filipendula ulmaria*)
milk thistle (*Silybum marianum*)
milky oats (*Avena sativa*)
mimosa (*Albizia julibrissin*)
mint (*Mentha* spp.)
motherwort (*Leonurus cardiaca*)
muira puama (*Ptychopetalum* spp.)
mulberry (*Morus* spp.)
mullein (*Verbascum thapsus*)
myrrh (*Commiphora* spp.)
nettle (*Urtica dioica*, *U.* spp.)
nori (*Porphyra* spp.)
oak (*Quercus* spp.)
oats (*Avena sativa*)
ocotillo (*Fouquieria splendens*)
onion (*Allium cepa*)
Oregon grape (*Mahonia* spp.)
oregano (*Origanum vulgare*)
osha (*Ligusticum porteri*)
oyster mushroom (*Pleurotus ostreatus*)
parsley (*Petroselinum crispum*)
partridgeberry (*Mitchella repens*)
passionflower (*Passiflora incarnata*)
pau d'arco (*Handroanthus impetiginosus*, syn. *Tabebuia impetiginosa*)
pedicularis (*Pedicularis* spp.)
peony (*Peonia* spp.)
peppermint (*Mentha* x *piperita*)
pigweed (*Amaranthus* spp.)
pine (*Pinus* spp.)
pineapple (*Ananas comosus*)
plantain (*Plantago major*, *P. lanceolatam*, *P. rugelii*)
pleurisy root (*Asclepias tuberosa*)
poke root (*Phytolacca decandra*)
polar (*Populus balsamifera*, *P.* spp.)
pulsatilla (*Anemone patens*)
pumpkin (*Cucurbita* spp.)
purple loosestrife (*Lythrum salicaria*)
purslane (*Portulaca* spp.)
pygeum (*Prunus africana*)
ramps (*Allium tricoccum*)
raspberry (*Rubus idaeus*, *R.* spp.)
red clover (*Trifolium pratense*)

red root (*Ceanothus americanus*)

reishi (*Ganoderma lucidum, G. tsugae*)

rhodiola (*Rhodiola rosea*)

rooibos (*Aspalathus linearis*)

rose (*Rosa* spp.)

rosemary (*Rosmarinus officinalis*)

sage (*Salvia officinalis, S.* spp.)

sarsaparilla, Jamaican (*Smilax regelii*)

savory (*Satureja* spp.)

saw palmetto (*Serenoa repens*)

schizandra (*Schisandra chinensis*)

self-heal (*Prunella vulgaris*)

senna (*Senna alexandrina*)

shatavari (*Asparagus racemosus*)

sheep sorrel (*Rumex acetosella*)

shiitake (*Lentinula edodes*)

skullcap (*Scutellaria lateriflora*)

slippery elm (*Ulmus fulva, U. rubra*)

Solomon's seal (*Polygonatum biflorum*)

sorrel (*Rumex acetosa*)

Spanish sage (*Salvia lavandulifolia*)

spearmint (*Mentha spicata*)

spikenard (*Aralia racemosa*)

spilanthes (*Acmella oleracea*, syn. *Spilanthes acmella*)

spruce (*Picea* spp.)

star anise (*Illicium verum*)

stevia (*Stevia rebaudiana*)

St. John's wort (*Hypericum perforatum*)

strawberry (*Fragaria* spp.)

suma (*Pfaffia paniculata*)

sunchoke root (*Helianthus tuberosus*)

sweet fern (*Comptonia peregrina*)

tamarind (*Tamarindus indica*)

tart cherry (*Prunus cerasus*)

tea (*Camellia sinensis*)

tea tree (*Melaleuca alternifolia*)

thuja (*Thuja occidentalis, T. plicata*)

thyme (*Thymus* spp.)

tribulus (*Tribulus terrestris*)

turkey rhubarb (*Rheum palmatum*)

turkey tails (*Trametes versicolor*)

turmeric (*Curcuma longa*)

umcka (*Pelargonium sidoides*)

usnea (*Usnea* spp.)

uva ursi (*Arctostaphylos uva-ursi*)

valerian (*Valeriana officinalis*)

vanilla (*Vanilla planifolia*)

violet (*Viola* spp.)

vitex (*Vitex agnus-castus*)

wakame (*Undaria pinnatifida*)

white oak (*Quercus alba*)

white tea (*see* tea)

wild cherry (*Prunus serotina*)

wild lettuce (*Lactuca* spp.)

wild strawberry (*Fragaria vesca*)

wild yam (*Dioscorea villosa*)

willow (*Salix* spp.)

wintergreen (*Gaultheria procumbens*)

witch hazel (*Hamamelis virginiana*)

wood betony (*Stachys officinalis*)

wormwood (*Artemisia vulgaris*)

yarrow (*Achillea millefolium*)

yellow dock (*Rumex crispus*)

yerba mansa (*Anemopsis californica*)

yerba maté (*Ilex paraguariensis*)

yerba santa (*Eriodictyon* spp.)

yohimbe (*Pausinystalia yohimbe*)

APPENDIX II

Learn More

For an expanded and up-to-date list of recommended reading, links to online resources, and other good information, visit my website: www.wintergreenbotanicals.com.

Great Starter Herbals

Although many herbals deserve a spot on your shelf, these four are the ones I recommend to my students to start with because of the quality of information, quantity of herbs covered, and photographs. Of the four, Tilgner's offers the most up-to-date scientific herbal information as well as safety data.

Bruton-Seal, Julie, and Matthew Seal. *Backyard Medicine.* Castle Books, 2012.

Chevallier, Andrew. *Encyclopedia of Herbal Medicine*, 2nd ed. DK Publishing, 2000.

Gladstar, Rosemary. *Rosemary Gladstar's Medicinal Herbs: A Beginner's Guide.* Storey Publishing, 2012.

Tilgner, Sharol. *Herbal Medicine: From the Heart of the Earth*, 2nd ed. Wise Acres, 2009.

More Excellent Herbal Resources

These books will also guide you to a great mix of quality information about herbs. Some are scientific, while others are traditional or historical, and yet others provide more detailed information on foraging and wild medicines, traditional Chinese medicine, Ayurveda, or general holistic health and dietary supplements. Another great resource is the American Botanical Council (www.herbalgram.org).

Grieve, Margaret. *A Modern Herbal.* 2 vols. Dover, 1971. First published 1931 by Harcourt, Brace & Co. *Available online at www.botanical.com.*

Haines, Arthur. *Ancestral Plants.* Anaskimin, 2010.

Hoffmann, David. *The Holistic Herbal*, 3rd ed. Thorsons, 2002.

Kress, Henriette. *Practical Herbs.* Printed by author, 2011.

Masé, Guido. *The Wild Medicine Solution.* Healing Arts Press, 2013.

Moore, Michael. *Medicinal Plants of the Pacific West.* Museum of New Mexico Press, 1993.

Murray, Michael T., and Joseph Pizzorno. *The Encyclopedia of Natural Medicine*, 3rd ed. Atria, 2012.

Tierra, Lesley. *Healing with the Herbs of Life.* Crossing Press, 2003.

Tierra, Michael. *Planetary Herbology.* Lotus Press, 1992.

———. *The Way of Herbs.* Pocket Books, 1998.

Tillotson, Alan Keith. *The One Earth Herbal Sourcebook.* Kensington Publishing, 2001.

Winston, David, and Steven Maimes. *Adaptogens.* Healing Arts Press, 2007.

Safety Resources

Some herbals, especially Tilgner's book, provide thorough safety data; however, you may also want to look to these safety- and interaction-specific guides (which tend to give you a wider range of less likely safety concerns). Don't forget that you can also ask your pharmacist about herb-drug interactions or find a skilled herbalist or naturopathic doctor when a case is complicated.

Gardner, Zoë, and Michael McGuffin. *American Herbal Products Association's Botanical Safety Handbook*, 2nd ed. CRC Press, 2013.

National Center for Complementary and Integrative Health. "Herbs at a Glance."
Visit online at https://nccih.nih.gov/health/herbsataglance.htm.

Skidmore-Roth, Linda. *Mosby's 2016 Nursing Drug Reference*, 29th ed. National Center for Complementary and Integrative Health. Elsevier, 2016.
This is my favorite for information on herb-drug interactions.

University of Maryland Medical Center. "Complementary and Alternative Medicine Guide." 2013.
Visit online at https://umm.edu/health/medical/altmed.

INDEX

Page numbers in *italic* indicate photographs; numbers in **bold** indicate main entries or charts.